Borderline Personality Disorder

The Guilford Personality Disorders Series
John F. Clarkin, Elsa Marziali, and Heather Munroe-Blum
Series Editors

BORDERLINE PERSONALITY DISORDER:
CLINICAL AND EMPIRICAL PERSPECTIVES
John F. Clarkin, Elsa Marziali, and Heather Munroe-Blum, *Editors*

BORDERLINE PERSONALITY DISORDER

Clinical and Empirical Perspectives

Edited by
JOHN F. CLARKIN
ELSA MARZIALI
HEATHER MUNROE-BLUM

THE GUILFORD PRESS
New York   London

© 1992 The Guilford Press
A Division of Guilford Publications, Inc.
72 Spring Street, New York, NY 10012

Printed in the United States of America

This book is printed on acid-free paper.

Last digit is print number: 9 8 7 6 5 4 3 2

Library of Congress Cataloging-in-Publication Data

Borderline personality disorder: clinical and empirical perspectives
  / edited by John F. Clarkin, Elsa Marziali, Heather Munroe-Blum.
      p.   cm. — (The Guilford personality disorders series)
  Includes bibliographical references and index.
  ISBN 0-89862-262-X
  1. Borderline personality disorder. I. Clarkin, John F.
II. Marziali, Elsa. III. Munroe-Blum, Heather, 1950–   IV. Series.
  [DNLM: 1. Borderline Personality Disorder. WM 190 B72893]
RC569.5.B67B688   1992
616.85'852—dc20
DNLM/DLC
for Library of Congress   91-28304
                                                         CIP

Contributors

Lorna Smith Benjamin, PhD   Department of Psychology, University of Utah, Salt Lake City, Utah

John F. Clarkin, PhD   Department of Psychiatry, Cornell University Medical College, New York Hospital–Cornell Medical Center, Westchester Division, White Plains, New York

John P. Docherty, MD   Nashua Brookside Hospital, Nashua, New Hampshire; Department of Clinical Psychiatry, Tufts University, Boston, Massachusetts

Arlene F. Frank, PhD   Nashua Brookside Hospital, Nashua, New Hampshire; Department of Psychiatry, Harvard Medical School, Boston, Massachusetts

Heidi L. Heard, BA   Department of Psychology, University of Washington, Seattle, Washington

Stephen W. Hurt, PhD   Department of Psychiatry, Cornell University Medical College, New York Hospital–Cornell Medical Center, Westchester Division, White Plains, New York

Jeffrey M. Jonas, MD   Clinical Development III, Upjohn Laboratories, Kalamazoo, Michigan

Otto F. Kernberg, MD   Department of Psychiatry, Cornell University Medical College, New York Hospital–Cornell Medical Center, Westchester Division, White Plains, New York

Paulina Kernberg, MD   Department of Psychiatry, Cornell University Medical College, New York Hospital–Cornell Medical Center, Westchester Division, White Plains, New York

Harold Koenigsberg, MD   Department of Psychiatry, Cornell University Medical College, New York Hospital–Cornell Medical Center, Westchester Division, White Plains, New York

Marsha M. Linehan, PhD   Department of Psychology, University of Washington, Seattle, Washington

Paul S. Links, MD, FRCP(C)   Department of Psychiatry, Faculty of Health Sciences, McMaster University, Hamilton, Ontario, Canada

Elsa Marziali, PhD   Faculty of Social Work, University of Toronto, Toronto, Ontario, Canada

Gloria M. Miele, MA   Department of Psychology, New School for Social Work, New York, New York

Theodore Millon, PhD   Department of Psychology, University of Miami,
Coral Gables, Florida; Department of Psychiatry, Harvard Medical School,
Boston, Massachusetts

Heather Munroe-Blum, PhD   Faculty of Social Work, University of
Toronto, Toronto, Ontario, Canada; Departments of Psychiatry and of Clinical
Epidemiology and Biostatistics, McMaster University, Hamilton, Ontario,
Canada

Harrison G. Pope, MD   Biological Psychiatry Laboratory, McLean Hospital, Belmont, Massachusetts; Department of Psychiatry, Harvard Medical
School, Boston, Massachusetts

James Reich, MD, MPH, MRCP   Department of Psychiatry, Harvard
Medical School, Boston, Massachusetts

Michael Selzer, MD   Department of Psychiatry, Cornell University Medical
College, New York Hospital–Cornell Medical Center, Westchester Division,
White Plains, New York

M. Tracie Shea, PhD   Department of Psychiatry and Human Behavior,
Brown University, Providence, Rhode Island; Veterans Administration Medical
Center, Providence, Rhode Island

Michael H. Stone, MD   Department of Clinical Psychiatry, Columbia
University College of Physicians and Surgeons, New York, New York; De-
partment of Psychiatry, New York State Psychiatric Institute, New York,
New York; Department of Clinical Psychiatry, Albert Einstein College of
Medicine, Bronx, New York (visiting); Middletown Psychiatric Center, Mid-
dletown, New York

Sarah M. Tilly, BA   Department of Psychology, New School for Social
Research, New York, New York

Robert J. Waldinger, MD   Department of Psychiatry, Harvard Medical
School, Boston, Massachusetts; Massachusetts Mental Health Center, Boston,
Massachusetts

Thomas A. Widiger, PhD   Department of Psychology, University of
Kentucky, Lexington, Kentucky

Frank Yeomans, MD   Department of Psychiatry, Cornell University
Medical College, New York Hospital–Cornell Medical Center, Westchester
Division, White Plains, New York

Preface

With this volume on borderline personality disorder (BPD) we introduce a series of books to be published by The Guilford Press, each focused on one of the personality disorders as defined in the revised third edition of the *Diagnostic and Statistical Manual of Mental Disorders* (DSM-III-R), Axis II. The specific focus of both this volume and the entire series is on the growing knowledge from empirical investigation of the personality disorders.

It is no accident that BPD was chosen to introduce a series emphasizing empirical work concerning the personality disorders. Since their introduction in DSM-III in 1980, the personality disorders have been empirically investigated at a phenomenal rate. However, there has not been an equal distribution of attention to all 11 of the Axis II disorders, and a casual glance of articles in print suggests that BPD is by far the most heavily researched personality disorder.

From both a research and a clinical point of view, the significance of the personality disorders is only beginning to emerge. One need only contrast Axis I disorders with Axis II disorders for a moment in order to consider this statement. Axis I describes symptoms and symptom clusters that exist at one point in time (state). In contrast, Axis II describes characteristic (trait), longstanding behaviors and attitudes that typify the individual. The utility and power of the multiaxial diagnostic system is that it emphasizes the importance of the combinations of the various axes. While the nature of the relationship between the Axis I and Axis II disorders is complex and needs further research explication, the enduring Axis II conditions are the bedrock for understanding the life course of the individual, and must play a central role in treatment planning.

In organizing this volume, we have obtained the cooperation of the leading researchers and theoreticians on the assessment and treatment of BPD. Each chapter contains a review of the latest empirical work in a specific topic area. There are, of course, many earlier books on BPD (Volkan, 1987; Kernberg, 1975; Kroll, 1988; Masterson, 1981; Stone, 1980) that provide theoretical and treatment directions. The present volume is unique in its focus on empirical work. While theoretical discussions are valuable and necessary for understanding and developing hypotheses, it is in the research results that the firm ground of our understanding of this most serious and destructive disorder will develop.

Given its content and organization, we are hopeful that this book will be of interest to a range of individuals concerned with the personality disorders. Our students—medical students, residents in psychiatry, graduate students in psychology and social work—have heard versions of some of these chapters, and we anticipate that the book will be useful for advanced courses on the personality disorders and psychopathology in general. The practicing clinician needs summaries of the data on BPD patients, and we intend for the chapters to provide an integration of up-to-date knowledge useful to clinical practice. Finally, it is hoped that personality researchers themselves will find this volume a complete overview of the status of the field at the present time.

We wish to thank our chapter authors for their acceptance of the task of summarizing the research in their areas of expertise. Their generous and collegial cooperation made the book possible. We also wish to thank our editor at The Guilford Press, Seymour Weingarten, whose wise view of the field and its literature indicated the timeliness and importance of this project.

JOHN F. CLARKIN
ELSA MARZIALI
HEATHER MUNROE-BLUM

REFERENCES

Kernberg, O. F. (1975). *Borderline conditions and pathological narcissism*. New York: Jason Aronson.

Kroll, J. L. (1988). *The challenge of the borderline patient*. New York: Norton.

Masterson, J. (1981). *Borderline and narcissistic disorders*. New York: Brunner/Mazel.

Stone, M. H. (1980). *The borderline syndromes*. New York: McGraw-Hill.

Volkan, V. D. (1987). *Six steps in the treatment of borderline personality organization*. Northvale, NJ: Jason Aronson.

Contents

PART IV. TREATMENT

PART V. CONCLUSIONS

Borderline Personality Disorder

PART ONE

INTRODUCTION

The Borderline Construct: Introductory Notes on Its History, Theory, and Empirical Grounding

THEODORE MILLON

This introductory review of the borderline construct is more narrowly focused than it would otherwise have been—that is, if it encompassed notions such as "borderline schizophrenia," "pseudoneurotic schizophrenia," and "latent psychoses," each of which is considered by some as part of a broad borderline spectrum (Dahl, 1990). These latter clinical entities are bypassed in the present rendering of the *Diagnostic and Statistical Manual of Mental Disorders* (DSM) borderline concept. Complicating this review further, the particular traits that comprise the DSM borderline syndrome have historical and theoretical precursors that antedate the current designation; hence, this discussion cannot be limited to propositions that employ the recent diagnostic label "borderline." There is a substantial body of literature on syndromes *not* termed "borderline," but possessing clinical features that clearly represent the pattern of affective and interpersonal instability characteristic of the DSM personality type. This introduction, therefore, does not begin with the borderline concept, but with formulations that differ in designation but are closely akin to it clinically.

Further sources of difficulty in furnishing a comprehensive yet relevant survey of the borderline construct are the plethora of terms used in the literature and the not inconsiderable disagreement that exists among theorists concerning the prime attributes of the syndrome. Popular among psychoanalytic thinkers is the position that borderline personality is best conceived of as a structural configuration or character organization that exists at a level of personality cohesion midway between neurotic and psychotic levels. By contrast, biologically oriented researchers hold the view that it is best conceived of as a set of personality variants within the affective disorders spectrum. More recently, theorists have turned their attention to the possible impact of recent cultural changes in fostering the deficient psychic cohesion that typifies the

DSM syndrome. Those who consider the term to represent an incipient precursor or inchoate substrate for schizophrenia may best review the literature on the new DSM "schizotypal personality" designation. Still others have formulated the construct as a stable and moderately severe level of functioning that encompasses a variety of different personality subtypes. Before a few of these diverse viewpoints are elaborated upon, attention should be directed toward the central features of the disorder, although they are still controversial.

CLINICAL FEATURES

Overdiagnosed and elusive as the borderline syndrome has been—approached from innumerable and diverse perspectives (e.g., Eriksonian, Kernbergian, Gundersonian, and Mastersonian, to name only those of an analytic persuasion), as well as clothed in an assortment of novel conceptual terms ("identity diffusion," "self-object representations," "projective identification")—there remain, nevertheless, certain shared observations that demonstrate the astuteness and heuristic fertility of the clinical mindset. Whatever doubts one may have with respect to either the logical or methodological merit of conjectures posed by our modern cadre of clinical thinkers, they deserve more than passing commendation for their perspicacity in discerning and portraying the key features of a new and major clinical entity. Overlooking for the present the seemingly intractable conflicts among and within analytic, biological, and social learning schools of thought, let us note the key borderline features that contemporary clinicians appear to judge salient and valid.

There is reasonable consensus that pervasive instability and ambivalence intrude constantly into the stream of borderlines' everyday lives, resulting in fluctuating attitudes, erratic or uncontrolled emotions, and a general capriciousness and undependability. These individuals are impulsive, unpredictable, and often explosive; it is difficult for others to be comfortable in their presence. Both relatives and acquaintances feel "on edge," waiting for these patients to display a sullen and hurt look or become obstinate and nasty. In being unpredictably contrary, manipulative, and volatile, borderlines often elicit rejection rather than the support they seek. Displaying marked shifts in mood, they may exhibit extended periods of dejection and apathy, interspersed with spells of anger, anxiety, or excitement.

Dejection, depression, and self-destructive acts are common. The anguish and despair of borderlines are genuine, but they also constitute a means of expressing hostility, a covert instrumentality to frustrate and retaliate. Angered by the failure of others to be nurturant, borderlines employ moods and threats as vehicles to "get back" or "teach them a lesson," so to speak. By exaggerating their plight and by moping about, borderlines avoid responsibilities and place added burdens on others, causing their families not only to care for them, but to suffer and feel guilt while doing so. In the same way, cold and stubborn silence may function as an instrument of punitive blackmail, a way of threatening others that further trouble is in the offing. Easily nettled and offended by trifles, borderlines are readily provoked into being sullen and contrary. They are impatient and irritable unless things go their way.

Cognitively capricious, borderlines may exhibit rapidly changing and often antithetical thoughts concerning themselves and others, as well as the odds and ends of passing events. They voice dismay about the sorry state of their lives, their sadness, their resentments, their "nervousness." Many feel discontent, cheated, and unappreciated; their efforts have been for naught; they have been misunderstood and are disillusioned. The obstructiveness, pessimism, and immaturity that others attribute to them are only reflections, they feel, of their "sensitivity" and the inconsiderateness that others have shown. But here again, ambivalence intrudes: Perhaps, they say, their own unworthiness, their own failures, and their own "bad temper" are the true causes of their misery and the pain they bring to others.

The affective and interpersonal instability of borderlines may be traced in great measure to their defective psychic structures—their failure to develop internal cohesion and hierarchical priorities. Both a source and a consequence of this lack of inner harmony is the borderlines' uncertain sense of self; they experience either an immature, nebulous, or wavering sense of identity. Hence, the deeper structural undergirding for intrapsychic regulation and interpersonal processing provides an inadequate scaffolding for both psychic continuity and self-integration. Segmented and fragmented, subjected to the influx of their own contradictory attitudes and enigmatic actions, they feel that their very sense of being is precarious. Their erratic and conflicting inclinations continue as both cause and effect, generating new experiences that feed back into and reinforce an already diminished sense of wholeness.

Two additional features distinguish borderline personalities from individuals with personality disorders at less severe levels. One may be termed deficient social competence; this is evident in the erratic personal history of many borderline patients, and their failure to attain a level of social achievement commensurate with their natural aptitudes and talents. Faulty starts and repeated disruptions characterize their educational, vocational, and marital lives. In contrast to those with less severe disorders, who progress and achieve a modicum of social and vocational effectiveness, borderlines tend to create endless complications for themselves and experience the same setbacks time and again. Despite these failures, many are able to "pull themselves together" and "make a go of it again." This recovery process contrasts with the fate of those at more severe levels of personality decompensation, who exhibit a more persistent downhill regression that eventuates in prolonged and often total social invalidism.

As evident from the foregoing, periodic but reversible psychotic episodes constitute another feature of borderlines. These severe transient disorders are characterized by the loss of reality contact and by both cognitive and emotional dyscontrol. Psychotic thought processes occur with some frequency, but their reversibility differentiates them from those of a schizophrenic character. Reality breaks tend to be brief and transitory, whereas in more severely decompensated personalities such breaks are often prolonged, prominent, and permanent. Caught in tendencies to foster new difficulties and self-defeating circles, borderline personalities experience constant upsets in their equilibrium and are subject to emotional eruptions and uncontrollable behaviors and thoughts. However, once these feelings are discharged, they regain a modicum of psychic balance—until such time as their tensions again mount beyond manageable proportions.

HISTORICAL FORERUNNERS

The following sections provide some examples of how theoretically dissimilar perspectives have conceptualized the same clinical picture in highly divergent ways. First, however, it is illuminating to record the observations of astute clinicians of the past who reported cases highly similar to those we designate today as "borderline personalities."

From the earliest literary and medical history, writers have recognized the coexistence within single persons of intense and divergent moods such as euphoria, irritability, and depression. Homer, Hippocrates, and Aretaeus described with great vividness the related character of impulsive anger, mania, and melancholia, noting both the erratic vacillation among these "spells" and the personalities likely to be subject to them. However, like most other medical and scientific knowledge, these early descriptions were suppressed in medieval times. With the advent of the Renaissance, many of the observations of early Greek and Roman physicians were brought again to light, and studies of these patients were begun anew.

The first theorist to revive the notion of the covariation between impulsive and erratic moods in a single syndrome was Bonet, who applied the term *folie maniaco-mélancolique* in 1684. In the 18th century, Schacht and Herschel reinforced the view suggested in Bonet's terminology that these erratic and unstable moods followed a rhythmic or periodic regularity of highs and lows. Fixed in the minds of all subsequent clinicians was the belief in an inevitable periodicity of the manic–depressive covariation. In fact, the case histories described by Bonet, Schacht, and Herschel rarely followed so regular a pattern. Rather, they were episodic, erratic, and desultory in sequence, shifting almost randomly from depression, to anger, to guilt, to elation, to boredom, to normality, and so on in an unpredictable and inconsistent course. In 1854, Baillarger and Jean-Pierre Falret summarized the results of 30 years' work with depressed and suicidal persons. They reported that a large portion of these patients showed a course of extended depression, broken intermittently by periods of irritability, anger, elation, and normality. The terms *la folie circulaire* (Falret, 1854) and *folie à double forme* (Baillarger, 1854) were applied to signify the syndrome's contrasting and variable character.

It was Kahlbaum who, in 1882, clearly imprinted the current belief in the fixed covariation of mania and melancholia. Although he saw them as facets of a single disease that manifested itself in different ways at different times—occasionally euphoria, occasionally melancholy, and occasionally excitability or anger—it was the primacy of the former two that rigidified further conceptions of the syndrome and redirected thinking away from its more typical and fundamental affective instability and unpredictability. Kahlbaum termed the milder variant of the illness, notable for its frequent periods of normality, "cyclothymia." A more severe and chronic form of the same pattern was designated *vesania typica circularis*.

By the turn of the century, a number of French and German clinicians elucidated other characteristics of these "circular" or emotionally inconsistent patients—those who today would be referred to as exhibiting a borderline disorder. Jules Falret (1890), the gifted son of Jean-Pierre Falret, elaborated the features of what he termed *folie hystérique*—notably emotional volatility, impulsivity, contradictoriness, and proneness to controversy. For them, "love transforms into hatred, sympathy into disdain, desire into repulsion" (1890, p. 502; my translation), each in rapid order. Similar characterizations of the emotionally unstable pattern of those patients we term borderlines today were depicted in the incisive clinical portrayals of Pierre Janet (1901).

→ Emil Kraepelin, the great 19th-century nosologist, borrowed heavily from his German predecessor, Kahlbaum, but sought to separate the "personality" and "temperament" variants of what Kahlbaum termed "cyclothymia" from the manifest or clinical state of the disease. Nevertheless, he proposed that the name "maniacal–depressive insanity" be employed for "the whole domain of periodic and circular insanity," including such diverse disturbances as "the morbid states termed melancholia . . . [and] certain slight colorings of mood, some of them periodic, some of them continuously morbid" (1896, p. 161; my translation). Convinced of the unitary character of this disease, Kraepelin wrote:

> I have become convinced all these states only represent manifestations of a single morbid process. It is certainly possible that later a series of subordinate groups may be . . . entirely separated off. But if this happens, then according to my view those symptoms will certainly not be authoritative which hitherto have usually been placed in the foreground. (1896, p. 164; my translation)

As evident, Kraepelin viewed "circular insanity" as a unitary illness. Every disorder that gave evidence of mood disturbances—however regular or irregular; whatever the predominant affect, be it irritability, depression, or mania—was believed to be a variant or "rudiment" of the same basic impairment. To him, the common denominator for these disturbances was an endogenous metabolic dysfunction that was "to an astonishing degree independent of external influences" (1896, p. 173; my translation).

In the eighth edition of his monumental *Lehrbuch* (1909–1915), Kraepelin began to formulate a number of subaffective personality conditions that are quite comparable to current borderline criteria. Still later, he wrote:

> There are certain temperaments which may be regarded as *rudiments of manic–depressive* insanity. They may throughout the whole of life exist as peculiar forms of psychic personality, without further development; but they may also become the point of departure for a morbid process which develops under peculiar conditions and runs its course in isolated attacks. Not at all infrequently, moreover, the permanent divergencies are already in themselves so considerable that they also extend into the domain of the morbid without the appearance of more severe, delimited attacks. . . . (1921, p. 118; italics in original)

Kraepelin identified four temperament variants disposed to clinical manic–depressive disease. The irritable temperament, elsewhere described by Kraepelin as the "excitable personality," was conceived of as a "mixture of the fundamental states." It parallels the borderline features closely, as illustrated in the following excerpts:

> The patients display from youth up extraordinarily great fluctuations in emotional equilibrium and are greatly moved by all experiences, frequently in an unpleasant way. . . .
> They flare up, and on the most trivial occasions fall into outbursts of boundless fury.
> The coloring of mood is subject to frequent change . . . periods are interpolated in which they are irritable and ill-humored, also perhaps sad, spiritless, anxious; they shed tears without cause, give expression to thoughts of suicide, bring forward hypochondriacal complaints, go to bed. . . .
> They are mostly very distractible and unsteady in their endeavors.
> In consequence of their irritability and their changing moods their conduct of life is subject to the most multifarious incidents, they make sudden resolves, and carry them out on the spot, run off abruptly, go traveling, enter a cloister. (1921, pp. 130–131)

Of special note is the extent to which Kraepelin's description encompasses the central criteria of the DSM borderline diagnosis, especially the impulsivity, unstable relationships, inappropriate and intense anger, affective instability, and physically self-damaging acts.

Kretschmer (1921/1925) provided another precursor of the borderline in portraying patients who exhibited what he considered a "mixed cycloid–schizoid" temperament. Not quite as apt or congruent as is Kraepelin's text,

Kretschmer's description nevertheless captures a number of important elements of the borderline syndrome:

> Cases of agitated melancholia with violent motility symptoms, alien influences in the constitution . . . may be distinguished [by] . . . an admixture of humourless dryness, of a hypochondriacal, hostile attitude towards the world . . . of sharpness, nervousness, and jerky restless moodiness (not rhythmic cyclic modifications), of insufficient affective response, of a grumbling dissatisfaction, and of a display of sulky pessimism. (1921/1925, p. 140)

Schneider, Kretschmer's prime European contemporary, came even closer to the mark of the borderline in his 1923 portrait of the "labile" personality. In his characterization of this type, Schneider wrote:

> The labile . . . has no chronic moodiness but is specifically characterized by the abrupt and rapid changes of mood which he undergoes.
>
> Sometimes the smallest stimulus is sufficient to arouse a violent reaction. . . . It appears that there is some constitutional tendency toward sporadic reactions of a morose and irritable character. . . .
>
> We are only interested here in behavior which clearly arises from periodic lability of mood. Such behavior has sometimes been called impulsive but the impulse . . . is only secondary and takes place against the periodic crisis of mood.
>
> Labile [persons] present a picture of shiftless, social instability. They develop sudden dislikes and distastes. They experience sudden restlessness. . . . Many . . . are socially shiftless and inconstant.
>
> As a social group . . . the more irritable ones are apt to get into trouble through impulsive violence, and the more inconstant ones have all sorts of chance lapses.
>
> We may wonder whether the mood shift of our labile personalities is a matter of cyclothymic . . . mood. Clinically everything speaks against cyclothymia. The transience of the mood and the general volatility are the chief contraindications. . . . (1923/1950, pp. 116–120)

Finally, brief note should be made of the contributions of Kasanin (1933), who first coined the label "schizoaffective." Reviewing the atypical premorbid characteristics of several cases of young psychotics who were initially hospitalized with the diagnoses of acute schizophrenic episodes, Kasanin concluded that they appeared to possess social dispositions and affective inclinations more typical of manic–depressives. The acute nature of the disorder and the blend of features portrayed in Kasanin's syndrome are somewhat tangential to the borderline formulation, yet the following quote suggests elements of comparability:

> A subjective review of their . . . personalities reveals that they are very sensitive, critical of themselves, introspective, very unhappy and preoccupied with

their own conflicts, problems, and sometimes with life in general. These
conflicts and problems may go on for years before the patient breaks down. . . .
The fact that there is comparatively little of the extremely bizarre, unusual
and mysterious, is what perhaps gives these cases a fairly good chance of
recovery. They do not exhibit any profound regression socially. . . . Their
reaction is one of protest, or a fear, without the ready acceptance of the
solution offered by the psychosis. (1933, p. 101)

CONTEMPORARY PERSPECTIVES

Given the brevity of this chapter, I must bypass numerous theoretical viewpoints
that deserve mention, if not careful review; several are discussed and elaborated
in subsequent chapters. For purposes of introduction, the present survey is
limited to viewpoints representing the three major sources from which personality disorders originate—namely, the biogenic, psychogenic, and sociogenic.
Thoughtful scholars and experienced clinicians acknowledge that behavior
patterns are an interactive product of each of these three spheres of influence
acting in concert; differences in theoretical perspective usually reflect matters
of emphasis, and not attempts at exclusivity. Hence, most recognize that
borderline personality disorder (BPD) derives from a matrix of biopsychosocial
causes, the particular weightings and combinations being unique to each
clinical case.

    In the sections that follow, I have chosen a representative and prominent
theoretical perspective on BPD from each of these three sources of developmental
influence.

The Biological Thesis: BPD as an Affective
Spectrum Disorder

Conceiving of the borderline syndrome as a personality variant that falls
within the spectrum of affective disorders parallels recent views of the schizotypal
personality syndrome, which has increasingly been conceived of as fitting
within the schizophrenic spectrum. The major exponents of this view are
found most prominently among researchers of a biological persuasion, but
a number of psychoanalytically oriented theorists have offered suggestions
of a similar cast; a number of these analytic theorists are mentioned briefly
here.

    Although referring only tangentially to Kraepelin's views, which address
the same thesis directly and cogently, Jacobson (1953) recorded her experiences
with a group of "cyclothymic depressives" who gave evidence of "simple
depression . . . without psychotic symptoms, yet belong[ing] to the manic–

depressive group" (p. 52). As would be anticipated, Jacobson sought to interpret the behavior of these "borderline" cyclothymics in psychoanalytic terms. To her, their behaviors reflected an effort to find solutions to psychosexual conflicts through regressive maneuvers. An "inherited constitution" might be operative, but, according to Jacobson, these affective borderlines more than likely experienced emotional deprivation; had poor self versus object differentiations; and displayed a "remarkable vulnerability, and intolerance of frustration, hurt and disappointment" (p. 55).

More relevant to current conceptions of the borderline are the affective symptoms that Easser and Lesser (1965) described in their psychoanalytic formulation of the "hysteroid" borderline type. This group of patients exhibits the outward behaviors of the classical hysterical (histronic) personality, but unquestionably constitute a more deeply disturbed variant. Worthy of mention is that the features of Easser and Lesser's hysteroid are akin to the symptoms outlined in Kernberg's (1967, 1970) portrayal of the "infantile personality," a character type he judged structurally at the "lower level" (borderline) of organization. The affinity of the hysteroid to both an affective style and a borderline severity is well portrayed by Easser and Lesser in the following passage:

> In many instances the hysteroid would appear to be a caricature of the hysteric, much as the hysteric has been said to be a caricature of femininity. Each characteristic is demonstrated in even sharper dramatic relief. The bounds of social custom and propriety are breached. The latent aggressivity of the exhibitionism, the competitiveness and the self-absorption becomes blatant, insistent, and bizarre. The chic becomes the mannequin; the casual, sloppy; the bohemian, beat.
>
> The adaptational functioning of the hysteroid is erratic. Inconstancy and irresponsibility cause the patient to suffer realistic rebuffs, injuries, and failure.
>
> The hysteroid starts friendships with great hopes and enthusiasm. The friendship commences with idolatry and ends in bitterness when the expectation of rescue, nurture, and care is not fulfilled. These relational ruptures are often succeeded by detachment, isolation, depression, and paranoid-like trends.
>
> The hysteroid's family life is often . . . disturbed, disorganized, and inconsistent.
>
> Grosser fluctuations of the hysteroid personality are to be anticipated from the more infantile fixation and the consequent weaker integration and synthesis of the ego. Thus we encounter less emotional control, a lessened ability to hold and tolerate tension, and more proneness to action and depression. (1965, pp. 399–400)

Entering from the perspective of differential responsiveness to pharmacological agents, Klein (1975, 1977) has raised serious questions concerning the validity of the borderline syndrome as a unified diagnostic entity. This challenge notwithstanding, he has proposed a series of ostensibly distinct personality disorders that exhibit clinical features frequently associated with recent descriptions of the borderline syndrome. In addition to asserting that the borderline designation subsumes, in effect, several heterogeneous subtypes, he contends further that their characterological and severity-related dimensions are secondary to their shared affective symptomatology. In essence—and in accord with Kraepelin's contention some 80 years earlier to the effect that an endogenous metabolic defect was at the core of the disturbance—Klein has argued that an affective dysfunction lies at the heart of the vulnerability of these syndromes. Three personality types (the phobic–anxious, the emotionally unstable, and the hysteroid dysphoric) are identified as subject to this vulnerability; each displays a long-term and somewhat atypical affective disorder. Worthy of note is the symptomatological affinity between Klein's pharmacologically deduced hysteroid dysphoric type and Easser and Lesser's analytically derived hysteroid portrayal.

Another group of contemporary biological researchers, led by Akiskal (Akiskal, 1981; Akiskal, Djenderedjian, Rosenthal, & Khani, 1977; Akiskal et al., 1985), has studied and marshaled data from a variety of pharmacological and family sources. Their findings support the position that what they term "cyclothymia" is in essence a subclinical or borderline personality condition found in biological relatives of manic–depressives, which predisposes those afflicted to the clinical form of the illness—a view quite reminiscent, once more, of Kraepelin's early thesis, but one only modestly supported in the empirical literature (Gunderson & Phillips, 1991).

The Psychoanalytic Thesis: BPD as Deficient Intrapsychic Organization

The first psychoanalytic attempt to develop the construct of a borderline disorder was formulated by Adolf Stern in 1938. His paper was prompted by the increasing number of patients seen who could not fit readily into standard neurotic or psychotic categories, and who were, in addition, refractory to psychotherapeutic interventions. Stern labeled these patients as comprising a "border line [sic] group of neuroses." Close examination led him to identify 10 symptoms, character traits, and "reaction formations" that, though not unique to the borderline group, were judged to be both more pronounced than in other neurotics and especially resistant to psychoanalytic efforts at resolution. Since a number of these 10 characteristics have remained as criteria for contemporary borderline conceptions, it may be useful to record them briefly: "narcissism," a character trait consequent to deficient maternal affection; "psychic bleeding," a self-protective lethargy or immobility in response to stress; "inordinate hypersensitivity," an undue caution or exquisite awareness of minor slights; "psychic rigidity," a persistent, protectively reflexive body stiffness in anticipation of danger; "negative therapeutic reactions," a quickness to display anger, depression, or anxiety in response to interpretive probes involving self-esteem; "feelings of inferiority," despite demonstrable evidence of self-competence, claiming a personal inadequacy so as to avoid adult responsibilities; "masochism," a depressively toned self-pity, "wound-licking," and self-commiseration; "somatic anxiety," a presumption of one's constitutional inadequacy to function without external assistance; "projection mechanism," a tendency to attribute internal difficulties to ostensive hostile sources in the environment; and "difficulties in reality testing," nonpsychotic deficits in judgment and empathic accuracy.

Although Knight (1953) focused his attention on young adults undergoing schizophrenic-like states or transient psychotic episodes, his paper was a seminal contribution in that he brought to the foreground the importance of "ego weakness" as a crucial element in characterizing the borderline personality structure. In essence, he concluded that psychotic episodes are likely to occur in borderline character structures. Superficial neurotic symptoms provide a "holding position," but the weak ego defenses ultimately display themselves in both microscopic (interview behavior) and macroscopic (life history and behavior) forms. Conceptualizing his incisive and fruitful studies from an ego-analytic perspective, Knight wrote:

> The superficial, clinical picture—hysteria, phobia, obsessions, compulsive rituals—may represent a holding operation in a forward position, while the major portion of the ego has regressed far behind this in varying degrees of disorder.
>
> We conceptualize the borderline case as one in which normal ego functions of secondary process thinking, integration, realistic planning, adaptation to the environment, maintenance of object relationships, and defenses against primitive unconscious impulses are severely weakened.
>
> Other ego functions, such as conventional (but superficial) adaptation to the environment and superficial maintenance of object relationships, may exhibit varying degrees of intactness. And still others, such as memory, calculation, and certain habitual performances, may seem unimpaired.
>
> In addition to these . . . evidences of ego weakness [there is a] . . . lack of concern about the realities of his life predicament; . . . the illness developed in the absence of observably precipitating stress, or under . . . relatively minor stress; . . . the presence of multiple symptoms and disabilities, especially if these are regarded with an acceptance that seems ego-syntonic; . . . lack of achievement over a relatively long period, indicating a chronic and severe failure of the ego to channelize energies constructively; . . . [and] vagueness or unrealism in planning the future with respect to education, vocation, marriage, parenthood, and the like. (1953, pp. 5–8)

Frosch initiated a series of explorations in the 1950s into what he termed the "disorders of impulse control," many of which typify the DSM borderline (e.g., quick-tempered irritability). It was not until his papers on the "psychotic character" (Frosch, 1960, 1964, 1970), however, that he made his contributions more directly relevant to contemporary borderline conceptions. Adhering to a more orthodox psychoanalytic perspective than Knight's ego orientation, Frosch summarized his position as follows:

> We are not dealing with a transitional phase on the way to or back from psychosis, or a latent, or larval psychosis which may become overt. We are dealing with characterological phenomena peculiar to persons who may never show psychosis and who establish a reality-syntonic adaptation. . . .
>
> The psychotic character is dominated by psychotic processes and modes of adaptation. . . . There is a propensity for regressive dedifferentiation and an underlying fear of disintegration and dissolution of the self. The psychotic reactions of fragmentation, projective identification, ego splitting, etc., can also be observed in the psychotic character, especially during periods of decompensation. . . .
>
> He retains a relative capacity to test reality, albeit with techniques frequently consistent with earlier ego states. Object relations, although at times prone to primitivization, as in psychosis, are nonetheless at a higher infantile level. There appears to be a push toward establishing contact with objects, though the simultaneously existing fear of engulfment by the object frequently leads to complications.
>
> The ego is constantly threatened by breakthroughs of id-derived impulses. (1970, pp. 47–48)

Influenced by the articulate and cogent theses of Stern and Knight, and of the British object relations theorists Klein, Fairbairn, and Winnicott in particular, Kernberg's (1967, 1975, 1980, 1984) writings on the "borderline personality organization" have become a prime force in establishing the status and attention given the syndrome in contemporary literature. Combining the central role assigned by Knight to impaired ego functions and the diverse symptom criteria spelled out by Stern, Kernberg has constructed a complex, multilevel, and multidimensional nosology based on psychoanalytic metapsychology. This schema encompasses not only the borderline ego structure or organization, but a wide range of syndromes that are hierarchically ordered in terms of both specific type and pathological severity. Paralleling a similar nosological matrix (Millon, 1969), which is based on a social learning perspective rather than a psychoanalytic metapsychology, Kernberg's schema depicts the borderline concept as a particular form of significantly weakened personality organization. Neither Kernberg nor I (nor, for that matter, Knight or Frosch) suggest that the "borderline" label be employed as a specific or distinct diagnostic type. Rather, it is best treated as a supplementary diagnosis that conveys the dimension of severity in "ego" functioning and "object" relations.

Despite the diversity of forms this personality organization may take, borderlines do possess certain stable and enduring psychostructural features in common, according to Kernberg (1979). In reviewing the clinical manifestations of the borderline personality, which Kernberg considers intermediary between neurotic and psychotic organizations, he has written:

> Clinically, when we speak of patients with borderline personality organizations, we refer to patients who present serious difficulties in their interpersonal relationships and some alteration in their experience of reality but with essential preservation of reality testing. Such patients also present contradictory characteristics, chaotic co-existence of defenses against and direct expression of primitive "id contents" in consciousness, a kind of pseudo-insight into their personality without real concern for nor awareness of the conflictual nature of the material, and a lack of clear identity and lack of understanding in depth of other people. These patients present primitive defensive operations rather than repression and related defenses, and above all, mutual dissociation of contradictory ego states reflecting what might be called a "nonmetabolized" persistence of early, pathological internalized object relationships. They also show "nonspecific" manifestations of ego weakness. The term "nonspecific" refers to a lack of impulse control, lack of anxiety tolerance, lack of sublimatory capacity, and presence of primary process thinking, and indicates that these manifestations of ego weakness represent a general inadequacy of normal ego functioning. In contrast, the primitive defensive constellation of these patients and their contradictory, pathological character traits are "specific" manifestations of ego weakness. (1975, pp. 161–162)

In Kernberg's view, borderlines' pathology reflects the outcropping of a deep "split" in self and object representations that derives from ambivalent and conflicting experiences in early development. Feeling intense anger at others for having frustrated their infantile wishes, or feeling themselves to be malevolent for having such feelings, the future borderlines vacillate back and forth, unable to maintain a balanced and realistic appraisal of either others or themselves. This schism remains deeply embedded and serves as a disorganizing template that precludes future integrative experiences; hence the borderlines' persistent instabilities of affect, relationship, and self.

Similar analytic formulations concerning the developmental origins of BPD have been presented by Mahler (1971), as well as several of her followers, most notably Masterson and Rinsley (1975). According to them, the psychic split stems from a child's inability to work satisfactorily through the transition from early maternal dependence to increasing autonomy. This struggle ostensibly derives from maternal threats to withdraw love, should the child assert itself by progressing toward separation and individuation. Unresolved, this struggle (and the dilemma it poses for increased maturity) continues to undergird the youngster's development, either persisting or readily reactivated under the slightest of provocations.

The Social Learning Thesis: BPD as a Reflection of Cultural Dissolution

It is clear that the borderline's pathological instability of affect, interpersonal relations, and the self has been identified as a clinical syndrome for some centuries now. Why, then, has it been formulated as a distinct entity only recently? Has its prevalence suddenly increased (i.e., has it achieved "epidemic" proportions in the recent past), or is the profession merely following a fad (i.e., is it disposed to interpret these clinical features in line with a novel and highly popular designation) (Kroll, 1988)? Might we simply be putting old wine in new bottles, relabeling what was well recognized formerly with other terms (Simonsen & Mellergard, 1988)? Although there is little question that contemporary diagnostic fashions and fallibilities have contributed to an increase in BPD labeling, there is reason to believe also that the rapid emergence of both the disorder and the diagnosis is a "real" phenomenon rather than an epiphenomenon. If that is the case, then a question must be posed: Which of several sources of influence that may give rise to the symptoms of BPD— namely, an inability to maintain psychic cohesion in the realms of affect, self-image, and interpersonal relationships—has had its impact heightened over the past three or four decades? Is it an unidentified yet fundamental alteration in the intrinsic biological makeup of present-day youngsters? Is it some significant and specifiable change in the way in which contemporary mothers nurture their infants and rear their toddlers? Or is it traceable to fundamental and rapid changes in Western culture that may have generated divisive and discordant life experiences, while reducing the availability of psychically cohering and reparative social customs and institutions?

Despite the fact that tangible evidence favoring one or another of these possibilities is not accessible in the conventional sense of empirical "proof," it is the contention of social learning BPD theorists (e.g., Millon, 1987a; Segal, 1988) that the third "choice" is probatively more sustainable and inferentially more plausible. I believe it is both intuitively and observationally self-evident that sweeping cultural changes can affect innumerable social practices, including those of an immediate and personal nature, such as patterns of child nurturing and rearing, marital affiliation, family cohesion, leisure style, entertainment content, and so on. It would not be too speculative, according both to my view and Segal's, to assert that the organization, coherence, and stability of a culture's institutions are in great measure reflected in the psychic structure and cohesion of its members. In a manner analogous to the DNA double helix, in which each paired strand unwinds and selects environmental nutrients to duplicate its jettisoned partner, so too does each culture fashion its constituent members to fit an extant template. In societies whose customs and institutions are fixed and definitive, the psychic composition of its citizenry will likewise be structured; and in societies whose values and practices are fluid and inconsistent, so too will its residents evolve deficits in psychic solidity and stability.

This latter, more amorphous cultural state, so characteristic of our modern times, is clearly mirrored in the interpersonal vacillations and affective instabilities that typify BPD. Central to recent Western culture have been the increased pace of social change and the growing pervasiveness of ambiguous and discordant customs to which children are expected to subscribe. Under the cumulative impact of rapid industrialization, immigration, urbanization, mobility, technology, and mass communication, there has been a steady erosion of traditional values and standards. Instead of a simple and coherent body of practices and beliefs, children find themselves confronted with constantly shifting styles and increasingly questioned norms whose durability is uncertain and precarious. Lacking a coherent view of life, maturing youngsters find themselves groping and bewildered, swinging from one set of principles and models to another, unable to find stability either in their relationships or in the flux of events.

I believe, furthermore, that recent cultural changes have led to a loss of key cohering experiences that once protected against problematic parent–child relationships. Traditional societies provided meliorative and reparative relationships (grandparents, aunts, older siblings, neighbors) and institutions (church, school) that offered remedies for parental disaffiliation; such societies provided a backup, so to speak, that insured that those who had been deprived or abused would be given a second chance to gain love and to observe models for developmental coherence. As I have noted elsewhere (Millon, 1987a):

> [The BPD patient's] aimless floundering and disaffiliated stagnation . . . might be substantially lessened if concurrent or subsequent personal encounters and social customs were compensatory or restitutive; that is, if they repaired the intrapsychically destabilizing and destructive effects of problematic experiences. Unfortunately, the converse appears to be the case. Whereas the cultural institutions of most societies have retained practices that furnish reparative stabilizing and cohering experiences, thereby remedying disturbed parent–child relationships . . . the changes of the past two to three decades have not only fostered an increase in intrapsychic diffusion and splintering, but have also resulted in the discontinuation of psychically restorative institutions and customs, contributing thereby to both the incidence and exacerbation of features that typify borderline pathology. Without the corrective

effects of undergirding and focusing social mentors and practices, the diffusing
or divisive consequences of unfavorable earlier experience take firm root and
unyielding form. (p. 367)

As implicit in the final sentence of the preceding passage, the social
learning thesis contends that cultural changes are not sufficient in themselves
to give rise to the BPD; rather, they *add* a final ingredient to the trio of
biopsychosocial influences that coalesce to form the disorder.

EMPIRICAL AND LOGICAL ISSUES

Central to this book is the question of whether contemporary hypotheses
addressing the origins, structure, and treatment of the BPD have a sounder
epistemic or probative foundation than that commonly found among most
notions of psychopathology.

The premise that early experience plays a central role in shaping personality
attributes is one shared by all theorists. To say this, however, is not to agree
as to which specific factors during these developing years are critical in generating
particular attributes, nor is it to agree that known formative influences are
either necessary or sufficient. Analytic theorists almost invariably direct their
etiological attentions to the realm of early childhood experience. Unfortunately,
they differ vigorously among themselves (e.g., Kernberg, Mahler/Masterson,
Erikson) as to which aspects of nascent life are crucial to development. In
the following paragraphs, I should like to examine briefly both the logical
and evidential basis for theses concerning the origins of the BPD.

A few words of a more or less philosophical nature are in order concerning
the concept of "etiology" itself; as in other matters that call for an incisive
explication of the nature of psychopathological constructs, the reader is directed
to the writings of Meehl (1972, 1977). In these essays it is made abundantly
clear that the concept of etiology itself is a "fuzzy notion." Not only does it
require the careful separation of constituent empirical elements, but it calls
for differentiating diverse conceptual meanings—ranging from "strong" influences that are both causally necessary and/or sufficient, through progressively
"weaker" levels of specificity, in which causal factors exert consistent though
quantitatively marginal differences, to those that are merely coincidental or
situationally circumstantial.

To be more concrete, there is reason to ask whether etiological deter-
minations are even possible in psychopathology, in light of the complex and
variable character of developmental influences. Can this most fundamental
of scientific activities be achieved, given that we are dealing with an interactive
and sequential chain of "causes" composed of inherently inexact data of a
highly probabilistic nature, in which even the very slightest variation in

context or antecedent condition (often of a minor or random character) produces highly divergent outcomes? Because this "looseness" in the causal network of variables leading to BPD is unavoidable, are there any grounds for believing that such endeavors will prove more than illusory? Furthermore, will the careful study of individual BPD cases reveal repetitive patterns of symptomatic congruence, much less consistency among the origins of such diverse clinical attributes as overt behavior, intrapsychic functioning, and biophysical disposition? And will etiological commonalities and syndromal coherence prove to be valid phenomena—that is, not merely imposed upon observed data by virtue of clinical expectation or theoretical bias (Millon, 1986a, 1986b, 1987b)?

Inferences drawn concerning past experiences, especially those of early childhood, are of limited (if not dubious) value by virtue of having only the patient as the primary (if not the sole) source of information. Events and relationships of the first years of life are notably unreliable, owing to the lack of clarity of retrospective memories. The presymbolic world of infants and young toddlers comprises fleeting and inarticulate impressions that remain embedded in perceptually amorphous and inchoate forms—forms that cannot be reproduced as the growing child's cognitions take on a more discriminative and symbolic character (Millon, 1981). What is "recalled," then, draws upon a highly ambiguous palette of diffuse images and affects—a source whose recaptured content is readily subject to both direct and subtle promptings from contemporary sources (e.g., a theoretically oriented researcher or therapist).

Arguments pointing to thematic or logical continuities between the character of experience and later behaviors, no matter how intuitively rational or consonant with established principles they may be, do not provide un-equivocal evidence for their causal connections; different and equally convincing developmental hypotheses can be and are posited. Each contemporary ex-plication of the origins of BPD is persuasive, yet remains but one among several plausible possibilities. Unfortunately, most theorists favor one cause, a singular experiential event or process—be it the splitting of good and bad introjects, or fears engendered during the separation–individuation phase—that they view as the sine qua non for borderline development. Causal at-tributions appear no more advanced today then they were in former times. It is rather sad that our current BPD literature abounds with brilliantly rationalized yet "competing" unifactorial conceptions.

Among other troublesome aspects of contemporary proposals are the diverse syndromal consequences attributed to essentially identical causes. Al-though it is not unreasonable to trace different outcomes to similar antecedents, there is an unusual inclination to assign the same "early conflict" or "traumatic relationship" to all varieties of psychological ailment. For example, an almost universal experiential ordeal that ostensibly undergirds such varied syndromes as narcissistic personality disorder and BPD, as well as a host of schizophrenic and psychosomatic conditions, is the splitting or repressing of introjected aggressive impulses engendered by parental hostility. This intrapsychic mechanism is seen as requisite to countering the dangers these impulses pose to dependency security, should they achieve consciousness or behavioral expression. However, not only is it unlikely that singular origins would be as ubiquitous as often posited, but even if they were, their ultimate psychological impact would differ substantially, depending on the configuration of other concurrent or later influences to which individuals were exposed. "Identical" causal factors cannot be assumed to possess the same import, nor can their consequences be traced without reference to the larger context of each individual's life experiences. One need not be a Gestaltist to recognize that the substantive impact of an ostensive process or event, however formidable it may seem in theory—be it explicit parental spitefulness or implicit parental abandonment—will differ markedly as a function of its developmental covariants.

To go one step further, there is good reason, as well as evidence, to believe that the significance of early troubled relationships may inhere less in their singularity or the depth of their impact than in the fact that they are precursors of what is likely to become a recurrent pattern of subsequent encounters. It may be sheer recapitulation and consequent cumulative learning that ultimately fashion and deeply embed the engrained pattern of distinctive BPD attributes we observe. Although early encounters and resolutions may serve as powerful forerunners and substantive templates, the presence of persistent and pervasive clinical symptoms may not take firm root in early childhood, but may stem from continuous replication and reinforcement.

Despite the foregoing, I share the view that unit for unit, the earlier the experience, the greater its impact and durability are likely to be (Millon, 1981). For example, the presymbolic and random nature of learning in the first few years often precludes subsequent duplication, and hence "protects" what has been learned. But I believe it is also true that singular etiological experiences, such as "split introjects" and "separation–individuation" struggles, are often only the earliest manifestation of a recurrent pattern of parent–child relationships. Early learnings may fail to change, therefore, not because they have jelled permanently, but because the same slender band of experiences that helped form them continues and persists for years to come. Furthermore, later experiences, even of a rather different cast, may produce effects that prove comparable to and reinforcing of those of early childhood. And no less significant is the fact that potentially remedial subsequent experiences may not be available to enable a person to *un*learn what has been learned in early life.

Finally, and not among the least of concerns regarding either the origins or structure of BPD, is that the "hard data"—unequivocal findings from well-designed and well-executed research—are sorely lacking. Consistent findings on causal factors for the BPD entity would be extremely useful, were such knowledge only in hand. Unfortunately, our data base is both equivocal and unreliable, despite recent thoughtful reviews on the subject (Gunderson & Phillips, 1991). As noted in prior paragraphs, it is likely to remain so, owing to the obscure, complex, and interactive nature of influences that shape psychopathological phenomena. The yearning among theorists of all persuasions for a neat package of attributes simply cannot be reconciled with the complex philosophical issues, methodological quandaries, and difficult-to-disentangle subtle and random influences that shape mental disorders. In the main, almost all theses today concerning BPD are, at best, perceptive conjectures that ultimately rest on tenuous empirical grounds, reflecting the views of divergent "schools of thought" positing their favorite hypotheses. These speculative notions should be conceived as questions that deserve continued empirical evaluation, rather than promulgated as the gospel of confirmed fact. Perhaps the pages that follow will provide us with such an empirical grounding.

REFERENCES

Akiskal, H. S. (1981). Subaffective disorders: Dysthymic, cyclothymic and bipolar II disorders in the "borderline" realm. *Psychiatric Clinics of North America, 4*, 25–46.

Akiskal, H. S., Chen, S. E., Davis, G. C., Puzantian, V. R., Kashgarian, M., & Bolanger, J. M. (1985). Borderline: An adjective in search of a noun. *Journal of Clinical Psychiatry, 46*, 41–48.

Akiskal, H. S., Djenderedjian, A. H., Rosenthal, T. L., & Khani, M. K. (1977). Cyclothymic disorder: Validating criteria for inclusion in the bipolar affective group. *American Journal of Psychiatry, 134*, 1227–1233.

Baillarger, M. (1854). De la folie à double forme. *Année Médicales Psychologie, 27*, 369–384.

Bonet, T. (1684). *Sepulchretum*. Paris.

Dahl, A. A. (1990). Empirical evidence for a core borderline syndrome. *Journal of Personality Disorders, 4*, 194–202.

Easser, R., & Lesser, S. (1965). Hysterical personality: A reevaluation. *Psychoanalytic Quarterly, 34*, 390–402.

Falret, J. (1890). *Études cliniques sur les maladies mentales*. Paris: Baillière.

Falret, J.-P. (1854). De la folie circulaire. *Bulletin de l'Académie Médicale, 19*, 382–394.

Frosch, J. (1960). Psychotic character. *Journal of the American Psychoanalytic Association, 8*, 544–555.

Frosch, J. (1964). The psychotic character. *Psychiatric Quarterly, 38*, 81–96.

Frosch, J. (1970). Psychoanalytic considerations of the psychotic character. *Journal of the American Psychoanalytic Association, 18*, 24–50.

Gunderson, J. G., & Phillips, K. A. (1991). A current view of the interface between borderline personality disorder and depression. *American Journal of Psychiatry, 148*, 967–975.

Jacobson, E. (1953). Contribution to the metapsychology of cyclothymic depression. In P. Greenacre (Ed.), *Affective disorders*. New York: International Universities Press.

Janet, P. (1901). *The mental state of hystericals: A study of mental stigmata and mental accidents* (English translation). New York: Putnam.

Kahlbaum, K. L. (1882). *Uber zyklisches Irresein, Irrenfreund*. Berlin.

Kasanin, J. (1933). Acute schizoaffective psychoses. *American Journal of Psychiatry, 97*, 97–120.

Kernberg, O. F. (1967). Borderline personality organization. *Journal of the American Psychoanalytic Association, 15*, 641–685.

Kernberg, O. F. (1970). A psychoanalytic classification of character pathology. *Journal of the American Psychoanalytic Association, 18*, 800–822.

Kernberg, O. F. (1975). *Borderline conditions and pathological narcissism*. New York: Jason Aronson.

Kernberg, O. F. (1977). The structural diagnosis of borderline personality organization. In P. Hartocollis (Ed.), *Borderline personality disorders*. New York: International Universities Press.

Kernberg, O. F. (1979). Two reviews of the literature on borderlines: An assessment. *Schizophrenia Bulletin, 5*, 53–58.

Kernberg, O. F. (1980). *Internal world and external reality*. New York: Jason Aronson.

Kernberg, O. F. (1984). *Severe personality disorders*. New Haven, CT: Yale University Press.

Klein, D. F. (1975). Psychopharmacology and the borderline patient. In J. E. Mack (Ed.), *Borderline states in psychiatry*. New York: Grune & Stratton.

Klein, D. F. (1977). Psychopharmacological treatment and delineation of borderline disorders. In P. Hartocollis (Ed.), *Borderline personality disorders*. New York: International Universities Press.

Knight, R. P. (1953). Borderline states. *Bulletin of the Menninger Clinic, 17*, 1–12.

Kraepelin, E. (1896). *Psychiatrie: Ein Lehrbuch* (5th ed.). Leipzig: Barth.

Kraepelin, E. (1909–1915). *Psychiatrie: Ein Lehrbuch* (8th ed.). Leipzig: Barth.

Kraepelin, E. (1921). *Manic–depressive insanity and paranoia* (English translation). Edinburgh: Livingston.

Kretschmer, E. (1921). *Korperbau und Charakter*. Berlin: Springer-Verlag. (English translation, *Physique and character*, W. J. Sprott, Trans., London: Kegan Paul, 1925)

Kroll, J. (1988). *The challenge of the borderline patient*. New York: Norton.

Mahler, M. S. (1971). A study of the separation–individuation process and its possible application to borderline phenomena in the psychoanalytic situation. *Psychoanalytic Study of the Child, 26*, 403–424.

Masterson, J. F., & Rinsley, D. B. (1975). The borderline syndrome: The role of the mother in the genesis and psychic structure of the borderline personality. *International Journal of Psycho-Analysis, 56*, 163–177.

Meehl, P. E. (1972). Specific genetic etiology, psychodynamics, and therapeutic nihilism. *International Journal on Mental Health, 1*, 10–27.

Meehl, P. E. (1977). Specific etiology and other forms of strong influence: Some quantitative meanings. *Journal of Medicine and Philosophy, 2*, 33–53.

Millon, T. (1969). *Modern psychopathology: A biosocial approach to maladaptive learning and functioning*. Philadelphia: W. B. Saunders.

Millon, T. (1981). *Disorders of personality*. New York: Wiley-Interscience.

Millon, T. (1986a). A theoretical derivation of pathological personalities. In T. Millon & G. L. Klerman (Eds.), *Contemporary directions in psychopathology: Toward the DSM-IV*. New York: Guilford Press.

Millon, T. (1986b). Personality prototypes and their diagnostic criteria. In T. Millon & G. L. Klerman (Eds.), *Contemporary directions in psychopathology: Toward the DSM-IV*. New york: Guilford Press.

Millon, T. (1987a). On the genesis and prevalence of the borderline personality disorder: A social learning thesis. *Journal of Personality Disorders, 1*, 354–372.

Millon, T. (1987b). On the nature of taxonomy in psychopathology. In C. Last & M. Hersen (Eds.), *Issues in diagnostic research*. New York: Plenum.

Schneider, K. (1923). *Die psychopathischen Personlichkeiten*. Vienna: Deuticke. (English translation, *Psychopathic personalities*, 1950)

Segal, B. M. (1988). A borderline style of functioning: The role of family, society and heredity. *Child Psychiatry and Human Development, 18*, 219–238.

Simonsen, E., & Mellergard, M. (1988). Trends in the use of borderline diagnoses in Denmark from 1975 to 1985. *Journal of Personality Disorders, 2*, 102–000.

Stern, A. (1938). Psychoanalytic investigation of and therapy in the border line group of neuroses. *Psychoanalytic Quarterly, 7*, 467–489.

PART TWO

ETIOLOGY

CHAPTER 2

The Etiology of Borderline Personality Disorder: Developmental Factors

ELSA MARZIALI

Among clinicians, there is considerable variation as to the etiological and developmental precursors of borderline personality disorder (BPD). Although most acknowledge the possible influence of genetic, constitutional, neuro-behavioral, and early developmental factors, clinicians differ as to the primacy of any one of these features in determining the presence of borderline pathology in adults. Historically, the most persuasive postulates regarding the etiology of the borderline syndrome have come from psychodynamic models of personality development. Here emphasis has been placed on inferring, from the adult patients' reconstructions of past experiences, possible intra- and interpsychic models of separation–individuation and identity formation. In the last decade, clinical investigators have begun to explore the relevance of neurological impairment (minimal brain dysfunction, traumatic brain injury) and early life experiences (parental abuse, neglect, separation, and loss) for explaining onset of the disorder and its behavioral manifestations in the adult borderline patient. It is likely that most of these etiological hypotheses have some application and that there exist multiple causal pathways to BPD. This chapter reviews three pertinent developmental perspectives on borderline pathology: psychodynamic, neurobehavioral, and early childhood neglect/abuse. These theories are discussed in relation to the findings from a number of studies of factors that influence infant and child development.

THE PSYCHODYNAMIC PERSPECTIVE

In psychoanalysis, developmental–diagnostic hypotheses are inferred from observations of the patient, reported symptoms, and interview material, which includes recollections of early life experiences with caregivers. Although different psychoanalytic theorists are at variance as to the specific factors contributing

27

to the development of BPD, most locate the occurrence of developmental failures/conflicts in the first 2 years of life (Kernberg, 1975; Masterson & Rinsley, 1975; Adler, 1985; Gunderson, 1984; Mahler, 1971; Mahler, Pine, & Bergman, 1975).

According to Kernberg, certain constitutional phenomena combined with deficiencies in the environment contribute to the formation of early developmental conflicts that fail to be adequately resolved. An excessive aggressive drive, coupled with a deficiency in the capacity to neutralize aggression and/or a lack of anxiety tolerance, is associated with a failure to integrate good and bad self–other object representations. Primitive defenses (denial, projection, and splitting) are mobilized to keep separate the conflicted perceptions of self and other. Kernberg underemphasizes the role of the parent in determining the pathological outcome of the borderline's identity formation. Rather, his focus is on the progressively integrative aspects of ego development. Kernberg's model presumes that the borderline has acquired the cognitive capacity for object constancy, and that borderline pathology evolves from a failure to acquire emotional object constancy. Kernberg outlines four stages for the development of integrated images of self as separate from other. These range from the undifferentiated self-object (first month) to the coalesced good and bad images of the self and of the object (12–18 months). Emotional object constancy and the accompanying capacity for intimacy accrues from the resolution of Kernberg's fourth developmental stage, which overlaps with the separation–individuation subphase of Mahler et al.'s (1975) rapprochement stage of early development.

Masterson and Rinsley (1975) believe that the etiology of BPD is associated with the mother's withdrawal of libidinal supplies at the developmental stage, when the child attempts to separate from the mother in search of his/her own identity. Again, Mahler et al.'s rapprochement subphase of separation–individuation is used by Masterson and Rinsley to locate the developmental conflict. They describe the mother of the borderline as having a pathological need to cling to her child, in order to perpetuate the gratification experienced earlier when the infant's survival was symbiotically bound to the mother. According to this paradigm, the mother is unable to tolerate her separating child's ambivalence, curiosity, and assertiveness; thus the mother is available if the child clings and behaves regressively, and withdraws if the child attempts to separate and individuate. Masterson and Rinsley describe the child's response to the mother's withdrawal as "abandonment depression." In order to avoid the pain of the depressive experience, the child seeks to preserve the image of the pleasurable mother, and this can only be accomplished by keeping separate the positive and negative affective states experienced in relation to the mother. Reality is distorted and ego development is arrested. The borderline patient manifests the developmental failure in behaviors that deny conflicted images of self and other, in order to preserve the fantasy of a symbiotic, pleasurable bond with the object.

Kernberg (1975) and Masterson and Rinsley (1975) have presented the most complete psychodynamic developmental formulations for BPD. Others partially support these positions. Adler (1985) and Gunderson (1984) believe that the borderline patient has not experienced an environment that could support the development of a stable self-identity in relation to a perception of an independent other. Adler (1985) suggests that the aloneness experienced by borderlines may be associated with the absence of "good enough" mothering during the phases of separation–individuation. Because of the mother's emotional unavailability, the child borderline fails to achieve "evocative memory," represented in Piaget's (1954) sixth stage of cognitive development (age 18 months). Thus, the borderline, in the face of certain stresses, is unable to restore a solid, integrated memory of the object and regresses to the earlier stage of "recognition memory" (age 8 months). Even though Adler agrees with other theorists in locating the developmental failure in Mahler's rapprochement/separation–individuation subphase, he believes that borderlines experience a primary emptiness because of the absence of stable images of positive introjects; that is, in the absence of these positive introjects, a holding, soothing sense of self does not develop. In contrast, Kernberg's developmental model presumes that sufficient positive introjects have been developed and that the defensive undertaking for the borderline is to keep separate positive and negative images of the self and of the object.

Although most psychodynamic hypotheses about borderline pathology draw on Mahler's observational, longitudinal studies of mothers and their children, Mahler (1971) cautioned against drawing inferences about adult psychopathology from observations of childhood developmental phenomena. She suggested some link between the ego fixation problems of the borderline and developmental conflicts during the rapprochement subphase of separation–individuation; however, she also believed that this hypothesis is not specific to BPD. Similarly, Kernberg's dynamic view of the etiology of borderline organization is not unique to BPD, but applies as well to schizotypal, narcissistic, histrionic, and antisocial personality disorders.

The psychodynamic formulations about the etiology of borderline pathology discussed above have not been empirically validated. There is no verifiable association between constitutional predisposition (Kernberg, 1975) and the development of personality disorders in adults. Also, Mahler's observational study of child development yielded results that were interpreted from an ego-psychological perspective, and that would now need to be interpreted in the light of infant observational studies and subsequent longitudinal studies of children in interaction with their caregivers. The infant studies show that the neonate plays a significant role in determining the quality and the quantity of interactions with caregivers (Stern, 1985). The longitudinal studies show the powerful role played by constitutional, biological, and environmental factors in determining the outcome in adults of early childhood experiences (Werner & Smith, 1982).

In a review of studies of early child development, Emde (1981) made the following observations: Infants construct their own reality; therefore, what is reconstructed in the psychoanalytic situation may never have happened. Since discontinuities are prominent throughout, developmental experience is reorganized to fit with new demands. There is a strong tendency in children, even very young children, to recover from trauma; thus, not all traumatic events predispose to psychopathology. The adverse effects of early childhood experiences such as neglect and abuse are reversible and responsive to changes in the environment.

Studies by Chess and Thomas (1984) and by Gaensbauer and Harmon (1982) support Emde's observations, in part. Chess and Thomas found that study subjects interviewed in early adulthood did not recall the conflicted aspects of their childhood experiences that had been observed and recorded by the investigators. Because the early childhood difficulties had been resolved, they were no longer prominent in memory. Gaensbauer and Harmon found that abused infants who were separated from their parents responded with considerable adaptability and resilience when placed with nurturing foster mothers. The infants were also able to transfer their positive attachment behaviors to the parents when reunited.

In general, infant studies and longitudinal studies of child development that postdate Mahler's observational studies of child development effectively challenge all psychodynamic hypotheses about the etiology of BPD. It is likely that for every borderline patient who reconstructs a history confirming the problematic separation–individuation hypothesis, there is a patient/individual with a comparable early history who did not develop the disorder. Chess and Thomas's (1984) longitudinal study of childhood temperament, Werner and Smith's (1982) longitudinal study of children in Hawaii, Rutter's (1980) epidemiological studies of children and their families, and the Harvard Grant longitudinal study (Vaillant, 1977) all showed that although some children and adolescents experienced highly conflicted interactions with their caregivers, they did not develop behavior disorders as adults. For example, Werner and Smith (1982) found that children who were particularly at high risk, because of their exposure to poverty, family instability, and mental health problems in their caregivers, remained "invincible" and developed into competent, autonomous young adults. Thus, a linear association between phase-specific developmental problems and BPD in adults cannot be supported. Rather, recent research studies point to a multidimensional model for explaining the etiology of borderline pathology. The important elements under study include assessments of the interactions between and among genetic, biological, and environmental factors, which converge, diverge, and evolve over time to yield significant variations in the development of the adult personality. Theoretical and clinical hypotheses about developmental "conflicts," "deviations," "deficits," or "fixations" provide information about only one aspect of the complex set of factors that influences the course of psychological growth and development, whether the outcome is one of health or pathology. These findings underscore the need for prospective studies, and indicate a major weakness of retrospective studies wherein the parent–child relationship is depicted through recall (which is clearly subject to distortion).

THE NEUROBEHAVIORAL PERSPECTIVE

The neurobehavioral model suggests a connection between the negative developmental effects of childhood brain dysfunction and the development of borderline symptomatology. In the neurologically impaired child, developmental symptoms appear in the form of hyperactivity, short attention span, distractibility, mood oscillation, and high impulsivity. The resultant behavioral syndrome includes problematic social interactions, academic difficulties, and low levels of achievement. Several authors (Hartocollis, 1968; Murray, 1979) postulate an association between the distorting effects of minimal brain dysfunction (MBD) on the one hand, and the child's perceptions of his/her own behaviors and interactions with caregivers on the other. The outcome is one of confused cognition, affect regulation, and impulse control, which together lead ultimately to borderline ego development and behavior. Some studies have explored the MBD and adult psychopathology hypotheses empirically (Quitkin, Rifkin, & Klein, 1976; Milman, 1979; Weiss, Hechtman, Perlman, Hopkins, & Wener, 1979; Wender, Reimher, & Wood, 1981). Only a few have examined factors specific to the development of borderline pathology (Andrulonis et al., 1981; Andrulonis & Vogel, 1984; Akiskal, 1981; Soloff & Millward, 1983; van Reekum, 1990). Overall, the findings are equivocal.

Although borderlines were not the primary focus of study, Quitkin et al. (1976) examined neurological features in a mixed group of patients identified as having "emotionally unstable character disorders" (EUCD). Their symptomatic behaviors paralleled those of borderlines: They were antisocial, were impulsive, and had "short, nonreactive, bipolar mood swings." This group's responses to tests of "neurological soft signs" were compared with the responses of "schizophrenics with premorbid asociality" (SPA). Both groups were also compared with other personality-disordered patients, including a subgroup with "histrionic character disorders" (HCD) and "schizophrenia of mixed subgroups" (SMS). A very thorough examination of neurological soft signs was conducted, controlling for rater bias (raters of neurological signs were blind to diagnosis). Nine tests assessed speech, body movement and coordination, auditory–visual integration, and intelligence. For the schizophrenics, the results showed that the SPA group had more soft signs than the SMS group overall, and more frequent occurrence of several of the body movement signs and speech abnormality. When the character-disordered subgroups were compared with the schizophrenic subgroups, the EUCD group had more soft signs than the SMS group, but there were no differences in the number of soft signs between the HCD and the SMS groups. On the IQ and auditory–visual tests, the SPA group had lower scores than the SMS group. Similarly, the EUCD group had lower scores than the SMS group, whereas the HCD group did significantly better than the SMS group on performance IQ. The authors conclude that a type of schizophrenia (SPA) and a subgroup of character disorders (EUCD) involve brain damage. However, they do not infer specificity or cause; that is, some diagnostic groups may be more likely to suffer brain damage as a result of behavior secondary to the cause of the disorder.

Milman (1979) conducted a follow-up study of patients she had seen in private practice for various learning, behavioral, and psychological childhood problems. Follow-up interviews were conducted either in person or on the telephone when the subjects were in late adolescence or early adulthood. Although 73 subjects were included, the number of refusers was not given. Milman conducted all of the interviews, and there was no attempt to standardize the procedure or to control for the reliability of the diagnoses made either during childhood contacts or at the time of follow-up. No comparison control group was used. Given these limitations, it is difficult to interpret the findings. According to Milman, 80% of the sample had personality disorders, and 14% were "borderline psychotic." Overall, 62% had organic brain syndromes, and 38% were diagnosed as having "developmental lag." Although Milman found a continuity between minimal neurological impairment in childhood and adult psychopathology, the specificity of this association for borderline character disorders was not established. Of value is the fact that Milman's work underscores the importance of including in psychiatric diagnostic procedures the assessment of multiple neurological soft signs, both in children and in adults.

Weiss et al. (1979) assessed levels of adaptation in a group of 75 young adults who had been diagnosed as hyperactive in childhood. These subjects were compared with a matched group of 45 normal control subjects. Two psychiatrists jointly interviewed a subset of subjects, in order to control for reliability of judgments made on information obtained during the interviews. The findings showed that the hyperactives had less education and were more prone to automobile accidents and instability in their living arrangements. Personality trait disorders (impulsive, immature, obsessive–compulsive, and depressive) were diagnosed more frequently in the hyperactive subjects, but only two were diagnosed as "borderline psychotic." Although the hyperactives reported more difficulties in general adjustment, there was no evidence to support an association between hyperactivity in childhood and the development of BPD in adults.

In a study of MBD in adults, Wender et al. (1981) specifically excluded subjects who met *Diagnostic and Statistical Manual of Mental Disorders*, third edition (DSM-III) criteria for BPD. However, several of their inclusion criteria overlap with descriptors that apply to borderlines (affective lability; hot or explosive temper; impaired interpersonal relationships or inability to sustain relationships over time; impulsivity or stress intolerance). Fifty-one subjects selected for the study were given an extensive battery of tests and then randomly assigned to treatment with premoline versus placebo for a period of 6 weeks. Several outcome measures were used to assess effects. The investigators found improvement in both groups, but when a subgroup with parental ratings of higher levels of childhood hyperactivity was examined, premoline was more effective than placebo for this group. The authors suggest that for the diagnosis and successful drug treatment of adults with attention deficit disorder (ADD), only those subjects who qualify retrospectively for the diagnosis of childhood ADD should be selected. Although the outcome of applying the ADD criteria to the assessment of BPD is unknown, there appears to be some merit in pursuing this line of inquiry, given the overlap in behavioral and psychological manifestations of the two disorders.

A frequently cited study by Andrulonis et al. (1981) was the first of a series of studies that examined neurological factors specific to the development of BPD. A retrospective chart review was conducted of 91 subjects meeting DSM-III criteria for the borderline diagnosis. Andrulonis et al. were able to subdivide the subjects into three groups: a nonorganic group; an MBD group with a history of attention deficits or learning disabilities; and an organic pathology group, comprising subjects with a history of traumatic brain injury, encephalitis, or epilepsy. Overall, 38% of the subjects had a history of organicity (either MBD or organic pathology). The group with the history of organicity differed from the nonorganic group on several dimensions: They had earlier onset of illness, acted out more frequently, and were more apt to report family histories of drug and alcohol abuse. In a subsequent study, Andrulonis and Vogel (1984) identified four subcategories of BPD, two of which included organicity factors: "attentional deficit/learning-disabled," and "organic." Of particular interest were the results that showed differences between male and female borderlines. Forty percent of the males, compared with only 14% of the females, suffered from an attentional deficit and/or learning disabilities. Also, 52% of the males, compared with 28% of the females, had either a current or past history of organic insults (e.g., head trauma, encephalitis, or epilepsy). Andrulonis and Vogel concluded that borderlines with MBD are predominantly male and have an earlier onset of emotional and functional difficulties, based in part on a constitutional deficit.

Akiskal (1981; Akiskal et al., 1985) has conducted several studies to demonstrate the association between BPD and affective disorders. Even though his primary focus was not on the exploration of specific neurological factors in borderlines, Akiskal's study of 100 borderline patients showed that in addition to overlapping affective diagnoses for almost half of the group, 11%

had organic disorders, epilepsy, or ADD. The discrepancy between Andrulonis et al.'s (1981) findings (38% of the subjects had histories of organicity) and Akiskal's findings (11% diagnosed as having neurological problems) can be explained by differences in both the aims and methods of the two studies. Andrulonis and colleagues used chart reviews to obtain "histories" of organicity in borderlines. In contrast, Akiskal and colleagues interviewed subjects to explore comorbidity between the borderline diagnosis and other psychiatric disorders, which included organic syndromes; the subjects' past histories of organicity were not explored.

Soloff and Millward (1983) tested several etiological hypotheses in a cohort of borderline patients. Included was a test of a neurobehavioral model of borderline personality style, which was a partial replication of Andrulonis's study. Forty-five patients who met the criteria for BPD on the Diagnostic Interview for Borderlines (DIB; Gunderson, Kolb, & Austin, 1981) were compared with 32 patients meeting the Research Diagnostic Criteria (RDC) for major depressive disorder and 42 patients meeting the RDC for schizophrenia. Information was obtained from the subjects and for 43% of the cases from family members as well. A neurobehavioral checklist was used. The results showed that more complications of pregnancy were reported in the prebirth histories of borderlines than in the other two groups. The borderlines had more childhood psychopathology, including temper tantrums, rocking, and head banging; however, learning difficulties were more prevalent in the schizophrenic group. Since Soloff and Millward excluded subjects with any known central nervous system abnormality, subjects with such abnormalities who also may have qualified for the borderline diagnosis were excluded. The use of developmental histories to infer neurobehavioral factors in both the Soloff and Millward (1983) and Andrulonis et al. (1981) studies may explain the discrepancies in their findings. Historical methods are limited by inaccuracies and incompleteness of recall, as well as by distortions associated with the patients' psychological state at the time the histories are taken.

Using a study format similar to that of Andrulonis and colleagues, van Reekum (1990) conducted chart reviews on 48 borderlines and 50 nonborderlines. A retrospective version of the DIB adapted for chart review was used to select the borderline group (scores of 7 or greater). The controls consisted of subjects with DIB scores below 7. An instrument was developed to collect information on a number of factors: demographic information; onset of BPD (including childhood form); neurological history and trauma; neurobehavioral syndromes; history of drug and alcohol abuse; hospitalizations; and other psychiatric diagnoses. The results showed that the borderlines and controls were comparable on the demographic variables. The borderline group had a statistically greater prevalence of developmental and acquired brain insults. The neurological markers included developmental delay, epilepsy, traumatic brain injury, and other central nervous system illnesses. The author suggests that there is a parallel between symptoms associated with frontal system dysfunction and borderline symptoms (impulsivity, cognitive inflexibility, poor self-monitoring, and perseveration). The limitations of the study include a sample with only male subjects, a retrospective historical method, and neuropsychological data collected by raters who were not blind to diagnosis.

EARLY CHILDHOOD NEGLECT AND ABUSE

In the last decade, the results of a series of studies have provided some support for an etiological hypothesis that links early childhood neglect and/or abuse with the development of BPD in adults. These studies can be viewed as partial attempts to test psychodynamic developmental theories about borderline pathology: That is, what associations, if any, exist between children's early experiences with their caregivers and the later onset of BPD? As has been the case with the psychodynamic and neurobehavioral models for explaining borderline etiology, studies of childhood neglect and abuse have relied on retrospective reports of developmental histories gleaned from chart reviews or reported by adult borderline patients. However, the results across studies are consistent.

Bradley (1979) obtained histories of early maternal separations from the mothers or significant caregivers of 14 young adolescent borderlines and matched groups of 12 psychotic patients, 33 nonpsychotic psychiatric patients, and 23 nonpsychiatric delinquent controls. Separation was defined as removal of the child from the home for periods greater than 3–4 weeks. The results showed that the borderlines had experienced significantly more early separations than the other groups. Soloff and Millward (1983) used a similar retrospective historical method to compare the early life separation experiences of borderlines with those experienced by schizophrenics and patients with major depressive disorder. The borderline group had experienced more parental loss due to death and divorce, but there were no between-group differences for separations experienced because of either parent or child illnesses. The borderlines reported more problems in coping with normal separations, such as attending school, transferring to a different school, and making normal school transitions (elementary school to high school). Both Bradley (1979) and Soloff and Millward (1983) view their findings as support for psychoanalytic theories that associate borderline pathology in the adult with an arrest during the separation–individuation phase of development in childhood.

Several investigators (Paris & Frank, 1989; Goldberg, Mann, Wise, & Segall, 1985) have examined qualities of parental bonding experienced by borderlines. Paris and Frank (1989) assessed subjects' recollections of the quality of care and protection received from parents during early childhood. Eighteen borderline (DIB scores of 7 or more) and 29 nonborderline (DIB scores of 4 or less) female patients completed Parker's Parental Bonding Instrument (PBI; Parker, Tupling, & Brown, 1979). The PBI yields scores on two dimensions: parental care and parental protection. The results showed that only the degree of perceived maternal care significantly differentiated the two groups. In an earlier study, Goldberg et al. (1985) used the PBI to compare the responses of 22 hospitalized, clinically diagnosed borderline patients with two control groups (22 patients with assorted psychiatric disorders, and 10 nonclinical normal subjects). The borderlines reported lower perceived parental care than the two control groups. The borderlines also perceived their parents to be more overprotective than the nonclinical control group, but did not differ on this dimension from the psychiatric controls. Despite the sampling differences in the Paris and Frank (1989) and the Goldberg et al. (1985) studies, the results could be viewed as providing some support for inferring an association between the quality of early parental bonding and the development of BPD. Alternatively, the disorder may have had a significant influence on the perceptions reported in the bonding instrument. Also, both studies share the methodological problems noted earlier—that is, total reliance on recollective data to infer parental neglect.

Because of a changing social climate that is more receptive to examining the incidence and effects of child sexual abuse, there has been a recent proliferation of studies concerned with these issues. There is increasing evidence for associating sexual abuse trauma in childhood with psychological difficulties in adults (Bryer, Nelson, Miller, & Krol, 1987). Bryer et al. (1987) obtained sexual and physical abuse histories from 68 female psychiatric patients who had been admitted to a private psychiatric hospital. The subjects completed a symptom checklist and received the Millon Clinical Multiaxial Inventory. Overall, 72% of the subjects reported a history of early abuse by family members. In the physically abused group, there was a higher proportion of borderline patients who had experienced sexual abuse.

In a similar study, Briere and Zaidi (1989) reviewed 100 charts of female patients seen in a psychiatric emergency service for histories of sexual abuse. Fifty of the charts were selected randomly from files of cases in which the clinician had not been directed to inquire about sexual abuse. These were compared with 50 charts selected randomly from files of cases written up by a clinician who had been instructed to inquire about early childhood sexual abuse. The charts were coded for demographic variables, incidence of sexual abuse, and the presence–absence of three personality disorder clusters (DSM-III-R). The most revealing finding was the very large discrepancy in the rate of reported abuse between subjects who had not been specifically asked about experiences of sexual abuse (6%) and those who had been asked (70%). For the subjects reporting sexual abuse, the associations with clinical variables were similar to those reported by Bryer et al. (1987). Three times as many abused versus nonabused subjects had been given diagnoses of personality disorder. Also, five times as many of the abused patients had received specific diagnoses of BPD or borderline traits.

Three recently reported studies (Zanarini, Gunderson, Marino, Schwartz, & Frankenburg, 1989; Herman, Perry, & van der Kolk, 1989; Shearer, Peters, Quaytman, & Ogden, 1990) compared reports of childhood trauma provided by borderline patients with those provided by several cohorts of patients with other psychiatric disorders. Zanarini et al. (1989) used the revised version of the DIB to select 50 borderlines. The Diagnostic Interview for Personality Disorders was used to select 29 controls with antisocial personality disorder. A second control group consisted of 26 patients who met the criteria for dysthymia on the Structured Clinical Interview for DSM-III-R (SCID). Two semistructured interviews were used to obtain histories of family pathology and early separation experiences. The reported neglect/abuse experiences were segmented into three childhood periods: early childhood (birth to age 5), latency, and adolescence. A significantly higher percentage of borderlines than controls (antisocial and dysthymic patients) reported being abused (verbally, physically, or sexually) during all three childhood periods. The borderlines were more likely than the dysthymic group to have been sexually abused during latency and adolescence, and to have been physically abused during early childhood. A history of neglect, emotional withdrawal, and disturbed caretaker behavior discriminated the borderlines from the antisocial controls in each of the childhood phases. More borderlines than dysthymics reported prolonged separations in early childhood, but the borderlines did not differ from the antisocial group on this dimension. The authors conclude that although their results lend support to hypotheses linking the development of BPD with early life experiences of abuse, neglect, and loss, there is insufficient evidence to suggest that any one type of childhood experience predicts the development of the disorder.

In a similar study (Herman et al., 1989), childhood trauma reported by subjects in an ongoing study of BPD ($n = 21$) were compared with reports provided by subjects with related diagnoses (schizotypal and antisocial personality disorders, and bipolar II affective disorder; $n = 23$). A 100-item semistructured interview was used to obtain childhood histories. The interview data were scored for positive indices of trauma in three areas: physical abuse, sexual abuse, and witnessing of domestic violence. The frequency of occurrence of each type of trauma was segmented into three childhood stages: childhood (0–6 years), latency, and adolescence. Eighty-one percent of the borderline patients gave histories of major childhood trauma; 17% had been physically abused, 67% had been sexually abused, and 62% had witnessed domestic violence. The borderlines also reported more types of trauma that lasted for longer periods of time. To be noted are the overall gender differences: Women had significantly higher total trauma scores, and they reported more physical and sexual abuse in childhood. For the borderline group, when gender differences were controlled, the total childhood trauma score remained significant when compared with the other two groups. The findings are similar to those reported by Zanarini et al. (1989), and similar cautions must be raised in inferring causes of BPD from retrospective reports of early childhood trauma. Rather, these studies suggest that retrospective data can be used effectively to delineate which variables are to be selected for focus in longitudinal studies of children at risk for the development of the disorder.

In a study of suicidal behavior among 40 female inpatients with a diagnosis of BPD, Shearer et al. (1990) obtained histories of childhood sexual and physical abuse. The patients who reported sexual abuse were more likely to have a concomitant diagnosis of "suspected complex partial seizure disorder," an eating disorder, or a drug abuse disorder. A history of physical abuse was associated with early family disruption, more psychiatric hospital admissions, and a concurrent diagnosis of antisocial personality disorder. Because of the small sample size, the authors are cautious in interpreting the significance of their findings. However, they hypothesize that the subjects may have had neurological problems at birth and that the accompanying deficits may have made them more vulnerable to family neglect, abuse, and disruption.

RELEVANCE OF RESEARCH FINDINGS FOR PRACTICE

The research on developmental factors attributed to the onset of BPD underscores the fact that a "pure" borderline type does not exist. Not all borderlines have neurological deficits; not all borderlines have early life experiences of sexual/physical abuse, neglect, or loss; and not all borderlines show evidence of unresolved early developmental conflicts associated with Mahler's rapprochement subphase of separation–individuation. Of equal importance is the fact that not all neurological deficits; instances of early life experiences of sexual/physical abuse, neglect, or loss; or unresolved early developmental conflicts lead to symptoms of BPD. Rather, the research evidence suggests multiple etiological pathways to several, if not numerous, subgroups of BPD. If this hypothesis has currency, it follows that the approaches to treatment and management of the disorder must be as flexible and as varied as the subtypes of the disorder. For example, clinicians need to be alerted to the possibility that some borderlines may have central nervous system deficits. Assessments of neurolgical soft signs would be essential for the proper selection of treatment modalities (e.g., psychoeducational, rehabilitative, or pharmacological approaches).

The developmental etiological hypotheses that arise from the studies of abuse and neglect, and psychodynamic formulations about psychological models of separation–individuation and identity formation, inform clinicians about possible self-object schemas that impinge on the borderline patient's observations of interpersonal transactions. From a social-cognitive perspective, borderlines may be restricted in their capacity to process information because of self-schemas that persevere despite inherent inaccuracies and distortions. Clearly, self-object schemas that contain elements of early life trauma with caregivers will be reflected in the way information is acknowledged and processed in the treatment relationship. Possibly the most therapeutic factor in any treatment encounter with a borderline patient is the therapist's understanding of the affective components of the patient's self-object schemas. When these are understood in the context of the treatment relationship, then the therapist is better equipped to avoid therapeutic error and disruption of the treatment—a frequent outcome with borderline patients.

SUMMARY AND IMPLICATIONS FOR FUTURE RESEARCH

Both the theoretical and empirical explorations of the etiology of BPD are inconclusive. Psychodynamic formulations about early psychic development of borderlines have not been validated. The reliability and validity of adult reconstructions of the past are readily challenged. Even though more recent studies of parental bonding and of caretaker neglect, loss, and abuse lend some support to psychodynamic formulations of borderline pathology (especially those proposed by Masterson and Rinsley), there is no conclusive evidence to support a linear association between any early childhood experience and the development of the disorder. The results of the neurological studies of borderline behavior suggest that there may be a subset of borderlines who also have ADD and other disorders of the central nervous system. Table 2.1 summarizes the most important studies in all three theoretical areas.

The major methodological problem with all of the studies reviewed is the reliance on retrospective, historical methods for obtaining information about early life experiences. In addition, several studies relied on chart reviews for generating both diagnostic and historical data. Even within the limitations of these methods, some investigators failed to control for bias of judgments made, and frequently the judges were not blind to diagnosis when comparison control groups were used. The most carefully controlled study, that by Zanarini et al. (1989), currently represents the best model for generating and comparing data about early life experiences across several cohorts of patients. Even though this study also relied on retrospective self-report, a number of procedures were used to control for bias. Standardized systems for determining the diagnoses of all study groups were used. In addition, two interview questionnaires were designed to reflect recent clinical and theoretical perspectives of salient early childhood experiences. The interviewers were blind to diagnoses, and the questionnaires and other data collection procedures insured uniformity and completeness of data collected.

TABLE 2.1. Summary of Studies

Focus	Authors	Populations	Methods	Findings
Psychodynamic	Kernberg (1975); Masterson & Rinsley (1975); Gunderson (1984); Adler (1985)	BPD; schizotypal, antisocial, narcissistic, histrionic personality disorders; major depression	Case study	Problems with separation–individuation in early childhood; arrest in ego development
Neurobehavioral	Quitkin, Rifkin, & Klein (1976); Milman (1979); Wender, Reimher, & Wood (1981); Andrulonis et al. (1981); Akiskal (1981); Soloff & Millward (1983)	BPD; emotionally unstable personality disorders; schizophrenia	Single group; comparison groups; retrospective chart review; structured interview	Neurological soft signs; organicity in childhood; attention deficit disorder; brain insults
Early childhood neglect and abuse	Bradley (1979); Soloff & Millward (1983); Bryer, Nelson, Miller, & Krol (1987); Briere & Zaidi (1989); Herman, Perry, & van der Kolk (1989); Shearer, Peters, Quaytman, & Ogden (1990)	BPD; other personality disorders; dysthymia	Single group; comparison groups; chart review; interview and questionnaire	Separations from early caregivers; low parental care; early physical and sexual abuse; history of neglect; disturbed caretaker behavior

40

An important alternative approach to the study of borderline etiology is the development and testing of measurement systems of personality dimensions from which levels of early childhood development can be inferred. Three measures of object relations constructs show promise in terms of variables measured and their discriminating power with various psychiatric groups (Bell, Billington, & Becker, 1986; Bell, Billington, Cichetti, & Gibbons, 1988; Burke, Summers, Selinger, & Polonus, 1986; Marziali & Oleniuk, 1990). Preliminary studies of their psychometric properties show that these tests successfully differentiate borderlines from affective, schizoaffective, and schizophrenic groups (Bell et al., 1988); from neurotics and schizophrenics (Burke et al., 1986); and from a nonpsychiatric group (Marziali & Oleniuk, 1989). Concurrent validity tests might include measures that tap parallel dimensions but that are not developmentally based—for example, Horowitz, Rosenberg, Baer, Ureno, and Villaseñor's (1988) Inventory of Interpersonal Problems, and Bond, Gardner, Christian, and Segal's (1983) measure of defensive style. Even though each measurement system differs in structure and interpretation (self-report vs. semiprojective), the aim of each is to determine, in adults, perceptual, attitudinal, and behavioral factors that reflect a developmental continuum. Thus these tests, when combined with historical methods for reconstructing borderline patients' early childhood experiences, could be used to test etiological hypotheses. Furthermore, all of the suggested measures could be used to predict change in borderlines following a course of treatment; this is especially important for those treatments (e.g., long-term psychoanalytic psychotherapy) that are designed to effect changes in the structure of the personality.

An alternative methodology would include the use of a retrospective cohort design—a design often used in epidemiological studies to establish the possible cause(s) of a disease. In this design, the presence or absence of the putative etiological (risk) factor is ascertained from past documentation of events occurring at some point prior to the possible existence of the outcome of interest. On the basis of this documentation, subjects are grouped as exposed or nonexposed and sought out in the present classification as cases or noncases. A measure of the effect or estimate of relative risk is then calculated, to examine increased odds of having the disorder if exposed to the suspected risk factor. The higher the relative risk, the greater the support for the role of the risk factor in influencing the outcome.

The retrospective cohort design can lessen the time and expense of prospective studies if good documentation of early exposure status exists. With respect to examining the etiology of BPD, earlier records from a child welfare agency might be utilized to develop a cohort of subjects with documented early abuse, and a control group of subjects with no documented experiences of abuse (but with records on file at the agency for other reasons). Although tracing these two groups into adulthood would pose challenges, these would be minimal in comparison with those of conducting a prospective study. Also, the quality of data would be infinitely superior to that of data collected in retrospective studies, which are dependent upon adult subjects' selective recall of childhood experiences.

The ideal design for empirically isolating the developmental precursors of borderline pathology is a longitudinal study of children at risk. As is well known, this type of study is difficult to implement and economically unfeasible if criteria for an adequate sample size are met. Perhaps longitudinal study methods should be implemented in multicenter research programs, where the demands on resources can be equitably distributed across centers and over time. Children at risk are readily identifiable through child mental health and child welfare service agencies. Offspring of parents with known severe psychiatric disorders would qualify as "children at risk" and could be accessed through adult clinics for inclusion in a prospective study. The study variables in any longitudinal study would need to be comprehensive (biological, neurological, behavioral, and environmental variables). It might then be possible to identify clusters of developmental experiences that differentiate high-risk, good-outcome groups of children from high-risk or vulnerable children who become adult cases of BPD.

REFERENCES

Adler, G. (1985). *Borderline psychopathology and its treatment*. New York: Jason Aronson.

Akiskal, H. S. (1981). Subaffective disorders: Dysthymic, cyclothymic and bipolar II disorders in the borderline realm. *Psychiatric Clinics of North America, 4,* 28–46.

Akiskal, H. S., Chen, S. E., Davis, G. C., Puzantian, V. R., Kashgarian, M., & Bolinger, J. M. (1985). Borderline: An adjective in search of a noun. *Journal of Clinical Psychiatry, 46,* 41–48.

Andrulonis, P. A., Glueck, B. C., Stroebel, C. F., Vogel, N. G., Shapiro, A. L., & Aldrige, D. (1981). Organic brain dysfunction and the borderline syndrome. *Psychiatric Clinics of North America, 4,* 47–66.

Andrulonis, P. A., & Vogel, N. G. (1984). Comparison of borderline personality subcategories to schizophrenic and affective disorders. *British Journal of Psychiatry, 144,* 358–363.

Bell, M., Billington, R., & Becker, B. (1986). A scale for the assessment of object relations: Reliability, validity and factorial invariance. *Journal of Clinical Psychology, 42,* 733–741.

Bell, M., Billington, R., Cichetti, S., & Gibbons, J. (1988). Do object relation deficits distinguish BPD from other psychiatric groups? *Journal of Clinical Psychology, 44,* 511–516.

Bond, M., Gardner, S. T., Christian, E., & Segal, J. J. (1983). Empirical study of self-rated defense styles. *Archives of General Psychiatry, 40,* 333–338.

Bradley, S. J. (1979). The relationship of early maternal separation to borderline personality in children and adolescents: A pilot study. *American Journal of Psychiatry*, *136*, 424–426.

Briere, J., & Zaidi, L. Y. (1989). Sexual abuse histories and sequelae in female psychiatric emergency room patients. *American Journal of Psychiatry*, *146*, 1602–1606.

Bryer, J. B., Nelson, B. A., Miller, J. B., & Krol, P. K. (1987). Childhood sexual and physical abuse as factors in adult psychiatric illness. *American Journal of Psychiatry*, *144*, 1426–1430.

Burke, W. F., Summers, F., Selinger, D., & Polonus, T. W. (1986). The comprehensive object relations profile: A preliminary report. *Psychoanalytic Psychology*, *3*, 173–185.

Chess, S., & Thomas A. (1984). *Origins and evolution of behavior disorders*. New York: Brunner/Mazel.

Emde, R. N. (1981). Changing models of infancy and the nature of early development: Remodeling the foundation. *Journal of the American Psychoanalytic Association*, *29*, 179–219.

Gaensbauer, T. J., & Harmon, R. J. (1982). Attachment behavior in abused/neglected and premature infants. In R. R. Emde & R. J. Harmon (Eds.), *The development of attachment and affiliative systems*. New York: Plenum Press.

Goldberg, R. L., Mann, L. S., Wise, T. N., & Segall, E. A. (1985) Parental qualities as perceived by borderline personality disorders. *Hillside Journal of Clinical Psychiatry*, *7*, 134–140.

Gunderson, J. G. (1984). *Borderline personality disorder*. Washington, DC: American Psychiatric Press.

Gunderson, J. G., Kolb, J., & Austin, V. (1981). The Diagnostic Interview for Borderline Patients. *American Journal of Psychiatry*, *138*, 896–903.

Hartocollis, P. (1968). The syndrome of minimal brain dysfunction in young adult patients. *Bulletin of the Menninger Clinic*, *32*, 102–114.

Herman, L. H., Perry, J. C., & van der Kolk, B. A. (1989). Childhood trauma in borderline personality disorder. *American Journal of Psychiatry*, *146*, 490–495.

Horowitz, L., Rosenberg, S., Baer, B. A., Ureno, G., & Villasenor, V. S. (1988). Inventory of Interpersonal Problems: Psychometric properties and clinical applications. *Journal of Consulting and Clinical Psychology*, *56*, 885–892.

Kernberg, O. (1975). *Borderline conditions and pathological narcissism*. New York: Jason Aronson.

Mahler, M. S. (1971). A study of the separation–individuation process and its possible application to borderline phenomena in the psychoanalytic situation. *Psychoanalytic Study of the Child*, *26*, 403–424.

Mahler, M. S., Pine, F., & Bergman, A. (1975). *The psychological birth of the human infant*. New York: Basic Books.

Marziali, E., & Oleniuk, J. (1990). Object representations in descriptions of significant others: A methodological study. *Journal of Personality Assessment*, *54*, 105–115.

Masterson, J. F., & Rinsley, D. B. (1975). The borderline syndrome: The role of the mother in the genesis and psychiatric structure of the borderline personality. *International Journal of Psycho-Analysis*, *56*, 163–177.

Millman, D. H. (1979). Minimal brain dysfunction in childhood: Outcome in late adolescence and early adult years. *Journal of Clinical Psychiatry*, *40*, 371–380.

Murray, M. E. (1979). Minimal brain dysfunction and borderline personality adjustment. *American Journal of Psychotherapy*, *33*, 391–403.

Paris, J., & Frank, H. (1989). Perceptions of parental bonding in borderline patients. *American Journal of Psychiatry*, *146*, 1498–1499.

Parker, G., Tupling, H., & Brown, L. B. (1979). A parental bonding instrument. *British Journal of Medical Psychology*, *52*, 1–10.

Piaget, J. (1954). *The construction of reality in the child* (M. Cook, Trans.). New York: Basic Books.

Quitkin, F., Rifkin, A., & Klein, D. F. (1976). Neurological soft signs in schizophrenia and character disorders. *Archives of General Psychiatry*, *33*, 845–853.

Rutter, M. (1980). *Scientific foundations of developmental psychiatry*. London: Heinemann.

Shearer, S. L., Peters, C. P., Quaytman, M. S., & Ogden, R. L. (1990). Frequency and correlates of childhood sexual and physical abuse histories in adult female borderline patients. *American Journal of Psychiatry*, *147*, 214–216.

Soloff, P. H., & Millward, J. W. (1983). Developmental histories of borderline patients. *Comprehensive Psychiatry*, *24*, 574–588.

Stern, D. N. (1985). *The interpersonal world of the infant: A view from psychoanalysis and developmental psychology*. New York: Basic Books.

Vaillant, G. E. (1977). *Adaptation to life*. Boston: Little, Brown.

van Reekum, R. (1990). *Neurobehavioral study of borderline personality disorder*. Paper presented at the annual meeting of the Canadian Psychiatric Association, Toronto.

Weiss, G., Hechtman, L., Perlman, T., Hopkins, J., & Wener, A. (1979). Hyperactives as young adults. *Archives of General Psychiatry*, *36*, 675–681.

Wender, P. H., Reimher, F. W., & Wood, D. R. (1981). Attention deficit disorder ("minimal brain dysfunction") in adults. *Archives of General Psychiatry*, *38*, 449–456.

Werner, E. E., & Smith, R. S. (1982). *Vulnerable but invincible*. New York: McGraw-Hill.

Zanarini, M. C., Gunderson, J. G., Marino, M. F., Schwartz, E. O., & Frankenberg, F. R. (1989). Childhood experiences of borderline patients. *Comprehensive Psychiatry*, *30*, 18–25.

CHAPTER 3

Family Environment and Family Psychopathology in the Etiology of Borderline Personality Disorder

PAUL S. LINKS

The discussion of etiological models that predict a complex adult disorder such as borderline personality disorder (BPD) is problematic. First, there is considerable evidence of great heterogeneity within the BPD diagnosis. Clarkin, Widiger, Frances, Hurt, and Gilmore (1983) have shown that, according to accepted *Diagnostic and Statistical Manual of Mental Disorders*, third edition (DSM-III) criteria, 93 different combinations of symptoms can lead to the diagnosis of BPD. Second, most studies have used retrospective reports of adult patients who meet the BPD diagnosis, and have employed case–control designs to compare the occurrence of purported etiological factors across diagnostic groups. What are actually needed for determining the temporal relationship between etiological factors and the onset of BPD are prospective cohort studies of children at risk. Third, focusing on a specific disorder such as BPD implies that etiological factors may be specific to that disorder. It is more likely that certain factors put children at risk for many forms of psychopathology in adulthood. Fourth, determining the etiology of a chronic disorder with an insidious onset is difficult, and future etiological models will probably show that a chain of interacting events predispose, precipitate and perpetuate the development of BPD.

The focus of this chapter is on the examination of evidence for the role of family environment and/or family history of psychopathology in the etiology of BPD. Although family environment and family history studies are discussed under separate headings, the separation of environmental and genetic factors cannot be implied, and the precise etiological contributions of each have not yet been determined. The empirical literature in this area has been summarized elsewhere (Gunderson & Zanarini, 1989; Links & Munroe-Blum, 1990;

45

Links & van Reekum, 1990) and is selectively discussed in this chapter. The implications of this body of work for future studies of the etiology of BPD are highlighted.

STUDIES OF FAMILY ENVIRONMENT

The empirical studies that explore the role of family environmental variables in the etiology of BPD are summarized on Table 3.1 (Links & Munroe-Blum, 1990). The present review shows that multiple factors are associated with the onset of the disorder, rather than a specific factor, such as difficulty with the separation–individuation phase of development. The early family environment of borderline patients seems to be pervaded with chronic stress. This review yields three etiological mechanisms for consideration: early separation and loss, sexual and physical abuse in childhood, and biparental failure.

Early Separation and Loss

Several studies have found empirical evidence that supports the concept of neglect or deprivation resulting from early separation from, or loss of, a primary caretaker (Gunderson, Kerr, & Englund, 1980; Bradley, 1979; Frank & Paris, 1981; Soloff & Millward, 1983; Akiskal et al., 1985; Goldberg, Mann, Wise, & Segall, 1985; Links, Steiner, Offord, & Eppel, 1988; Zanarini, Gunderson, Marino, Schwartz, & Frankenburg, 1989). A similar etiological linkage has been associated with the onset of depressive disorders; despite contrasting views about the significance of this association, Lloyd (1980) concluded that parental bereavement during childhood increases the risk of depression in adulthood by a factor of 2 to 3. The validity of the early loss hypothesis has been challenged by Rutter (1983), due to the fact that few studies have examined other forms of early loss, and observations of family contextual factors and the effects of repeated losses over time have not been recorded. Brown and Harris (1978) have suggested that losses in early life may influence the symptom pattern of depression: Loss by death may predispose individuals to psychotic depression, and loss by separation is more apt to be associated with neurotic depression. Our own study (Links, Steiner, Offord, & Eppel, 1988) suggested that early separation from parental figures was more often due to marital separation in BPD patients, whereas early separations in the comparison group was more often due to death of a parent. Birtchnell (1980) has suggested that early loss in itself may not be a predisposing factor; rather, the adequacy of the protective role assumed by the remaining parent

TABLE 3.1. Empirical Studies of Borderlines' Family Environments

Study	Concept(s) tested	Design	Sample	Measures	Concept(s) supported
Gunderson, Kerr, & Englund (1980)	Marital difficulty Discomfort with parental roles Psychopathology in mother Alliances and splits Turmoil among siblings Nonprotective, unstable family unit	Case–control	12 borderlines 12 paranoid schizophrenics 12 neurotics	Items derived from literature and clinical experience; ratings based on blind chart review	Both mothers and fathers sicker and less functional (biparental failure) Tightness of marital bond, absence of marital conflict (neglect/loss)
Bradley (1979)	Early maternal separation	Case–control	14 borderlines 45 psychiatric controls 23 delinquents	Separations >3 weeks; no control for socioeconomic status; not rated blindly	Early separation greater in borderlines (neglect/loss)
Frank & Paris (1981)	Parental response to dependent and independent childhood strivings	Case–control	Normals Outpatients with neurosis and personality disorder Borderlines (n's not given)	Childhood Experience Scale—10 items; blind ratings	Fathers of borderlines less approving and less interested (biparental failure) Neglect favored overinvolvement
Soloff & Millward (1983)	Neurobehavioral model Separation hypothesis Family dynamic theory	Case–control	45 borderlines 32 depressives 42 schizophrenics	Neurobehavioral checklist, separation and family dynamic questionnaire; not blind	Separation hypothesis upheld (neglect/loss) Negative, conflictual relationships between patients and parents; overinvolvement in all groups more negative in borderlines; fathers underinvolved (biparental failure)

(*continued*)

47

TABLE 3.1. (Continued)

Study	Concept(s) tested	Design	Sample	Measures	Concept(s) supported
Snyder, Pitts, Goodpaster, & Gustin (1984)	Descriptive study of family experience	No control group	Borderlines (24 males, 2 females)	Developmental and social history	Male figure dominant in three-quarters of borderlines' families Experienced abuse or slapping/hitting (abuse)
Akiskal et al. (1985)	Developmental object loss Assortive parental psychopathology	Case–control	100 borderlines 57 schizophrenics 50 patients with nonaffective personality disorders 50 bipolars 40 unipolars		Borderlines > unipolars on developmental loss (neglect/loss) and parental assortive mating (biparental failure)
Goldberg, Mann, Wise, & Segall (1985)	Parental care versus overprotection	Case–control	24 borderlines 22 psychiatric controls 10 normals	Parental Bonding Inventory (reliability and validity discussed)	Perception of less parental care (neglect/loss) and overprotection interact in borderlines

48

Study	Focus	Design	Sample	Measures	Findings
Zanarini, Gunderson, Marino, Schwartz, & Frankenburg (1989)	Disturbed caretakers versus separations from caretakers	Case–control	50 borderlines, 29 antisocials, 26 with other personality disorders	Retrospective Family Pathology Questionnaire, Retrospective Separation Experiences Questionnaire; rating blind	Verbal and sexual abuse most common in borderlines (abuse). Borderlines > antisocial on reported emotional withdrawal; borderlines > other personality disorders on prolonged separation (neglect/loss)
Links, Steiner, Offord, & Eppel (1988)	Evidence of separations from caretaker and abuse	Case–control	88 borderlines, 42 with borderline traits	Questions on separations, foster home placement, nonintact parental marriage, abuse by caretakers	Borderlines had more separation experiences, physical and sexual abuse by caretakers (abuse and neglect/loss)
Herman, Perry, & van der Kolk (1989)	History of childhood trauma	Case–control	21 borderlines, 11 with borderline traits, 23 with schizotypal, antisocial, or bipolar II disorder	Semistructured interview on childhood histories (rated blindly); Impact of Events Scale; Dissociative Experience Scale	History of trauma (physical and sexual abuse, witnessing of violence) in early childhood most common in borderlines (abuse)

Note. Adapted from "Family Environment and Borderline Personality Disorder: Development of Etiologic Models" by P. S. Links and H. Munroe-Blum, 1990, in P. S. Links (Ed.), *Family Environment and Borderline Personality Disorder*. Copyright 1990 by the American Psychiatric Press. Adapted by permission.

may determine onset of borderline psychopathology. Thus, early parental loss that is due to separation rather than death may predispose a child to borderline psychopathology. The magnitude of this impairment may be partly determined by the protection conferred on the child by the remaining parent.

The association of early loss with psychopathology may be too simplistic, and more complex, comprehensive, and testable etiological models are needed. For example, Davis and Akiskal (1986) hypothesized that for some borderlines "early separation and loss may permanently affect the neural pathways of biogenic amines and endorphins that underlie the reinforcement mechanisms. A disruption of such reinforcement mechanisms is an appealing etiology for [many] of the self-destructive and socially inept behaviors that characterize borderline patients" (p. 690).

The disruption of the parent–child relationship may lead to pathological attachment patterns in adulthood. "Attachment" is defined as a close and enduring bond to a significant other, and the expectation of a shared future is a characteristic of adult attachment relationships (Sheldon & West, 1989). Hypothetically, borderline patients' characteristic unstable, intense relationships may be related to the presence of pathological attachment patterns. Currently, we are attempting to investigate whether certain attachment patterns will differentiate BPD from other personality disorders. West (personal communication, January 24, 1991) has hypothesized that borderline patients evidence insecure attachment and show a feared loss of the attachment relationship. To defend against this feared loss, borderline patients may demonstrate patterns of compulsive care-seeking, in which the individuals try to insure the security of an attachment figure by frequent and urgent displays of care-seeking behavior. Alternating with this pattern, borderline patients may evidence angry withdrawal if the attachment figure is perceived as inaccessible. We are currently testing whether these patterns will differentiate BPD from dependent and avoidant personality disorder.

West, Sheldon, and Reiffer (1987) have developed a self-report scale to measure adult attachment, to capture the features of attachment relationships, and to describe pathological patterns of attachment (West & Sheldon, 1988). The eight scales used to define aspects of adult attachment (proximity seeking, secure base effect, separation protest, feared loss of the attachment figure, reciprocity, availability, responsiveness of the attachment figure, and use of the attachment figure) were found to have satisfactory internal consistency and correctly distinguished patients from nonpatients. Scales defining patterns of attachment relationships (compulsive self-reliance, compulsive caregiving, compulsive careseeking, and angry withdrawal) were also shown to be reliable ($r \geq .85$), and the relationships between scales supported theoretical constructs (West & Sheldon, 1988). Finally, West, Sheldon, and Reiffer (1989) have proposed that specific psychotherapy strategies can be developed to change particular pathological patterns of attachment.

Sexual and Physical Abuse in Early Childhood

The occurrence of sexual and physical child abuse as part of the causal chain of events in the development of BPD has been supported by several recent studies (Bryer, Nelson, Miller, & Krol, 1987; Links, Steiner, Offord, & Eppel, 1988; Herman, Perry, & van der Kolk, 1989; Zanarini et al., 1989; Ogata, Silk, & Goodrich, 1990; Stone, 1990). •

Recent evidence suggests that exposure to prolonged and varied abuse, rather than a single abusive event, predicts the onset of adult psychopathology (Herman et al., 1989; Bryer et al., 1987). Bryer et al. (1987) examined the rates of childhood abuse in a sample of 68 female inpatients consecutively admitted to a private psychiatric hospital. They found that subjects who had experienced both physical and sexual abuse had higher mean borderline symptom scores than subjects who had experienced only one type of abuse or subjects who had not been abused at all.

Hostile and conflictual relationships have been reported in the histories of borderline patients. Soloff and Millward (1983) found that overinvolvement with mothers was present in all patient groups studied, but the unique aspect of the borderline patients' environment was the fact that this overinvolvement was perceived negatively by the patients. Goldberg et al. (1985) suggested an interaction between evidence of less caring and overprotectiveness in the parents of borderline patients. Paris and Frank (1989) have re-examined the neglect and overprotection hypotheses, using Parker's Parental Bonding Instrument (PBI; Parker, Tupling, & Brown, 1979) to measure the concepts of care and overprotection. The first factor, "care," is defined by the polarities of affection, emotional warmth, empathy, and closeness versus emotional coldness, indifference, and neglect. The second factor, "overprotection," is defined by the polarities of control, intrusion, excessive contact, infantilization, and prevention of independent behavior versus the ability to allow independence and autonomy.

In their first report, Paris and Frank (1989) compared 18 borderlines defined by the Diagnostic Interview for Borderlines (DIB) to 29 nonborderline control patients. The results indicated that the borderline patients perceived both of their parents as less caring than did the nonborderline controls. Frank and Paris (1989) extended these findings by studying a group of 62 borderlines versus 99 nonborderline controls. The borderline subjects again reported significantly less care from both their parents than did the nonborderline controls. The perceptions were not found to be different for male and female borderline probands. In addition, Frank and Paris (1989) found support for the overprotective hypothesis, as borderline subjects reported their parents as overprotective in comparison to the nonborderline subjects. This finding contradicted earlier findings by these investigators (Frank & Paris, 1981; Frank & Hoffman, 1986).

Another recent report has supported the concept of an interaction between low caring and overprotectiveness. Byrne, Velamoor, Cernovsky, Cortese, and Losztyn (1990) compared 15 borderline patients to 14 schizophrenic patients, using Parker et al.'s PBI. Borderline patients had significantly lower scores for maternal care but higher scores for paternal overprotection than did schizophrenic patients.

These studies suggest that overinvolvement between patient and parent may not be unique to the borderline family; rather, the interaction of ov-erinvolvement with an expression of hostility may create the characteristic environment. Particularly striking is the fact that this hostility appears to indicate a highly malevolent attitude on the part of the parent toward the child. My colleagues and I speculate that the interaction of overinvolvement with this malevolent attitude is singularly characteristic of the childhood environment of the borderline patient. At one extreme, the interaction of overinvolvement and malevolence can be seen in parents who persistently physically or sexually abuse their children from an early age.

In summary, BPD appears to stem at least in part from the early and prolonged effects of physical and sexual abuse on the child's developing personality. The mechanisms by which these traumas act require further examination, but may be a result of the interaction between parental over-involvement and malevolence.

Biparental Failure

At least four studies have shown that both mothers and fathers of borderline patients showed significant impairment and a failure to carry out their parental functions (Gunderson et al., 1980; Frank & Paris, 1981; Soloff & Millward, 1983; Akiskal et al., 1985). Frank and Paris (1981) observed "biparental failure" in borderlines' reports of early family experiences; in particular, the patients' fathers were identified as underinvolved. However, the characterization of the father as underinvolved may be related to the sex of the identified proband. For example, Snyder, Pitts, Goodpaster, and Gustin (1984) found in a study of male borderline patients that the father was typically the dominant figure in a patient's family. This evidence suggests that the parental roles may vary, depending on the sex of the affected offspring. Akiskal et al. (1985) noted that assortive mating was more prevalent in the parents of borderline patients than in the parents of patients with affective disorders; whether this reflected a genetic or an environmental risk, it seemed to be characteristic of the borderline patients' families.

Even when the role of genetic factors is put aside, evidence of significant impairment in borderline patients' parents can have major effects on the exposed offspring. Richters and Weintraub (1989) have reviewed the diathesis—stress model employed in high risk studies to explain the etiology of schizophrenia. They caution that early maladjustment in the offspring of a schizophrenic parent is not necessarily synonymous with vulnerability to the disorder, and that this early maladjustment can be reflective of acquired rather than inherited defects. Rutter and Quinton (1984) have outlined several causal explanations for the association between parental psychopathology and offspring maladjustment. Apart from genetic transmission, the parents' symptoms may have a direct impact on the child's learning and development; the parents' psychopathology may interfere with the parents' functioning; or the parents' psychopathology may lead to marital discord.

The parents of borderlines often evidence severe psychopathology themselves (Links, Steiner, & Huxley, 1988; Zanarini, Gunderson, Marino, Schwartz, & Frankenburg, 1990; Ogata et al., 1990), and the environmental impact of this psychopathology on the offspring may be of great etiological significance. Our own data indicated that parental illness in one or both parents of borderline probands increased the risk of childhood early loss or separation, sexual and physical abuse, and nonintact parental marriage (Links, Boiago, Huxley, Steiner, & Mitton, 1990). Borderline probands having both parents diagnosed with psychiatric illness showed poorer school performance and left school at an earlier age than did probands in the comparison groups. Therefore, parental psychopathology may create a home environment that impairs a child's learning or development, thus placing the child at risk for school failure and adult psychopathology.

Understanding the family environmental factors that precipitate or perpetuate borderline pathology is the next crucial step to explore. Clarifying the causal chain of events leading to BPD should make it possible to develop specific intervention strategies to break the links of this chain.

FAMILY HISTORY STUDIES

Family history studies are used for two scientific purposes: to establish the validity of a psychiatric diagnosis, and to examine etiological relationships between disorders. The validity of a psychiatric diagnosis is supported if an increased prevalence of a disorder is found in the biological relatives of probands with the same disorder (Robins & Guze, 1970). Therefore, like begets like. Etiological relationships can be inferred if another disorder is prevalent among the biological relatives of probands with the first disorder. Family history studies cannot distinguish environmental from genetic factors; this requires other research designs, such as twin or adoptive studies.

Family history studies are reviewed here in relation to the purposes outlined above. The present review is restricted to studies using established diagnostic criteria. Earlier studies have been hampered in their examination of associations between disorders, because explicit diagnostic criteria were not in use (Stone, Kahn, & Flye, 1981). DSM-III diagnostic criteria evolved to separate off those disorders possibly related to schizophrenia, and defined "unstable" personality disorder or BPD as a distinct disorder (Spitzer, Endicott, & Gibbon, 1979). This review has included those studies that present prevalence rates of disorders in first-degree family members, and indicates which studies have adjusted for age of risk of family members. Excluded are studies that have presented family data based on the percentage of probands having at least one relative with the diagnosis of interest (Akiskal, 1981). The studies meeting the inclusion criteria include the following: Loranger, Oldham, and Tulis (1982); Loranger and Tulis (1985); Pope, Jonas, Hudson, Cohen, and Gunderson (1983); Soloff and Millward (1983); Baron, Gruen, Asnis, and Lord (1985); Schulz et al. (1986); Links, Steiner, and Huxley (1988); Zanarini et al. (1990); Silverman et al. (1987); and Schulz et al. (1989).

Establishing Diagnostic Validity

A number of investigators have carried out family studies to examine whether BPD is more frequently found in the families of BPD patients. Loranger et al. (1982) tested the validity of BPD by comparing families of borderline patients to families of schizophrenic and bipolar disorder patients. Only female probands were included in the study. The authors employed a chart review to identify those relatives who had been treated for psychiatric problems. They established their own criteria for BPD to use in the chart review, and required that two of nine criteria be present to establish the BPD diagnosis. The criteria appeared to highlight antisocial behaviors, as four of the nine items were as follows: (1) lying, stealing, truancy, runaway, vandalism, arrest, imprisonment, acting out, or behavior problems; (2) alcohol or drug abuse; (3) assaultive, violent physical fights; and (4) impulsive or reckless behavior, injury-proneness, self-mutilation, or suicidal attempts. Loranger et al. compared the lifetime expectancy of BPD in the three groups and found a highly significant increase in the morbid risk of BPD in first-degree family members of BPD patients, compared to the schizophrenic and bipolar groups (11.65% vs. 1.41% and 0.73%, respectively). The rate of BPD in male relatives of borderline patients did not differ significantly from that in the female relatives of borderline patients. The authors concluded that the first-degree relatives of BPD patients were 10 times more likely to be treated for BPD than were the relatives of schizophrenic or bipolar patients.

Pope et al. (1983), in an attempt to establish the validity of DSM-III BPD, reviewed chart information on 33 hospital inpatients. The investigators blindly reviewed chart information on family history to obtain DSM-III diagnoses on parents and siblings of patients. BPD was found in only 1 of 130 (0.8%) relatives. However, the authors reported that there was a high prevalence of personality disorders in these relatives when they considered BPD together with histrionic and antisocial personality disorders; 10 of 130 (7.5%) parents and siblings received these diagnoses.

Baron et al. (1985) examined the families of BPD and schizotypal personality disorder (SPD) patients for a number of purposes, including that of determining whether SPD and BPD clustered in families of probands with the same diagnosis. Baron et al. recruited 310 college students and hospital employees to identify probands for the study. Only 2 of the probands met definite DSM-III criteria for BPD, and 15 subjects were given the diagnosis of probable BPD. Forty-seven percent of the BPD group were men. A total of 576 first-degree relatives were studied, using family history Research Diagnostic Criteria (RDC) and the family history version of the Schedule for Interviewing Borderlines, based on information from the proband. The rating of families was not blind as to the proband's diagnosis. The authors adjusted their data for the decreased sensitivity of indirect data and obtained a weighted morbid risk for BPD of 17.9% in the first-degree family members of BPD patients. This rate was significantly higher than the rates for BPD in definite SPD probands. The authors concluded that the data supported the notion that BPD is a familial disorder.

Schulz et al. (1986) have directly examined the relatives of 17 borderline patients who met criteria for both BPD and SPD, using the Schedule for Interviewing Borderlines. Complete data on the prevalence of Axis II disorders are still to be published; however, they did report an absence of morbid risk (0.0%) for antisocial personality disorder in the first-degree relatives of borderline patients. The authors indicated that this absence was not anticipated.

My colleagues and I (Links, Steiner, & Huxley, 1988) reported on the occurrence of BPD in first-degree relatives of inpatients meeting DIB criteria for BPD. The study constituted an advance on earlier work by (1) using direct, in addition to indirect, family data; (2) examining probands meeting established criteria for BPD who were representative of patients admitted to acute inpatient psychiatric units; and (3) presenting the demographic characteristics of the family members with BPD. From data obtained on 320 first-degree family members, the morbid risk for BPD was found to be 15.3%. Fifty-four percent of the BPD relatives were female, and 46% were male. The relationship of the BPD family members to the probands was as follows: 40.0% were sisters, 31.4% brothers, 14.3% fathers, 11.4% mothers, and 2.9% daughters. The prevalence rate was felt to be similar to those reported by Loranger et al. (1982) and Baron et al. (1985), thus supporting an increased prevalence of BPD in the first-degree family members of borderline patients. However, this study did not include comparison groups to substantiate this conclusion. These data also suggested that the risk of BPD was not confined to the mothers of borderline patients.

Zanarini et al. (1990) carried out a carefully designed study of the family history of outpatients meeting both DIB and DSM-III criteria for BPD. The study extended the results of previous studies by (1) comparing the familial prevalence of BPD to two "near-neighbor" disorders (antisocial personality disorder and dysthymia) plus other personality disorders; (2) assessing family history blind to the proband's diagnosis; and (3) examining the full range of Axis I and II disorders in the first-degree relatives. Family history data were gathered indirectly from 488 first-degree relatives of probands with the following diagnoses: BPD (relative $n = 240$), antisocial personality disorders (relative $n = 139$), and dysthymia plus other personality disorders (relative $n = 109$). The morbid risk of BPD in the first-degree relatives was significantly greater in the BPD probands (24.9%) than in either the antisocial personality disorder (4.1%) or the dysthymic (9.6%) comparison group. The results of this study were felt to support the validity of BPD even when compared to two very closely related diagnostic groups.

Silverman et al. (1987), focusing on substrates of BPD, examined relatives of BPD patients for increased levels of chronic affective instability and chronic impulsivity. The first-degree relatives of 29 probands with definite BPD were compared to the first-degree relatives of 35 probands with other personality disorders and the first-degree relatives of 43 male schizophrenic patients. The morbid risk of relatives of BPD patients was not significantly different from that of the comparison groups for major affective disorders, schizophrenia-related disorders, alcoholism, drug use disorder, or antisocial personality disorder. However, chronic affective instability and chronic impulsivity were significantly more common in the relatives of BPD patients than in the relatives of a restricted group of patients with other personality disorders or the relatives of schizophrenic patients. The authors suggested future investigations should focus on the traits of BPD that may be candidates for the inherited psychobiological substrates of the genetic disorder, rather than on the diagnosis itself.

Almost all studies reviewed have reported an increased prevalence of BPD in the families of BPD patients; only Pope et al. (1983) failed to find such an increase. Thus the family history studies have provided fairly robust support for the validity of the BPD diagnosis.

Examining Etiological Relationships between Disorders

The history of BPD has been a relentless search to understand the relationship of this syndrome to other psychiatric disorders. Hoch and Polatin (1949) related this syndrome to schizophrenia, while Stone (1977) later drew attention to an association between BPD and affective disorders. Most recently, Gunderson and Zanarini (1989) have related BPD to other disorders of impulse control, suggesting a possible linkage to substance abuse and antisocial personality disorder. Family history studies are one method of examining for associations between disorders.

Most of the relevant studies have been described in the "Establishing Diagnostic Validity" section; however, three more reports are introduced here. Loranger and Tulis (1985) published a second paper related to their sample of 83 women meeting DSM-III criteria for BPD. All 83 patients would still have met BPD criteria even if substance use had been excluded as an example of impulsivity. Of the 100 female bipolar controls, 8 had abused alcohol on occasion; of the 100 schizophrenic controls, 1 had a history of alcoholism and 3 had abused alcohol on occasion. Any chart reference to "alcoholism" or "alcoholic" was accepted as prima facie evidence of alcoholism. There was no requirement that the relative had received treatment for alcoholism.

Soloff and Millward (1983) compared 48 DIB-positive borderlines to 32 depressive and 42 schizophrenic patients diagnosed with the RDC. Family histories were obtained from the patients, from family informants, and through chart review using the Kupfer–Detre system. Data were collected prospectively in 43.2% of cases, and retrospectively (by chart review only) in 56.8% of cases.

Schulz et al. (1989) re-examined the relationship of BPD and combined BPD-SPD to affective disorder and schizophrenia by comparing 26 patients meeting DIB and DSM-III criteria for BPD to 59 DSM-III defined schizophrenic patients. All probands were interviewed using the family history RDC to establish diagnoses for first-degree family members.

The results of these studies are summarized in Table 3.2. Although the studies have varied methodologically, the results indicate many consistencies across studies. First, as summarized above, BPD is more frequently found in the families of BPD patients than in the families of patients with schizophrenia, bipolar disorder, SPD, antisocial personality disorder, and dysthymia. Second, the results of the family studies indicate no increased prevalence of schizophrenia in the families of borderline patients. Soloff and Millward (1983) reported a 14.5% rate of schizophrenia in the impaired relatives of patients meeting criteria for both BPD and SPD. Schulz et al. (1989) found rates of schizophrenia in the relatives of patients with BPD that were similar to those found in the relatives of schizophrenics; however, all the schizophrenic relatives were in the families of patients meeting criteria for both SPD and BPD. Therefore, the relationship between BPD and schizophrenia may be attributed to the co-occurrence of SPD in some borderline patients. Without this coexisting diagnosis, there appears to be no relationship between BPD and schizophrenia.

Alcoholism and drug abuse are frequently diagnosed in the first-degree relatives of borderline patients. Although the prevalence of substance abuse

TABLE 3.2. Comparison of Prevalence Rates across Disorders and Studies

Study[a]	BPD	Schizophrenia	Affective disorders	Schizotypal personality disorder	Antisocial personality disorder	Dysthymia/other personality disorders
					Diagnostic groups	
Familial alcoholism and/or drug abuse						
A[b]	18.5%	6.3%*	6.4%			
B	11.5%	6.6%	7.5%			
C	11.8%	7.9%	6.3%			
D[c]	13.6%			16.7%		
E[b]	16.7%		21.2%	14.3%		
F[b]	21.0%					
G[b]	15.3%	4.5%*				
H[b]	24.3%				27.6%	26.5%
I[b]	17.9%	19.3%				12.7%
Familial depression						
A[b]	6.4%	2.1%*	7.4%			
B	6.2%	0.6%*	7.5%			
C	8.7%	5.0%	15.0%*			
D[c]	13.3%			7.4%		
E[b]	50.0%		34.6%			
F[b]	26.6%					
G[b]	15.3%	6.2%*				
H[b]	31.2%				17.1%	42.9%
I[b]	21.0%	15.8%				22.5%
Familial schizophrenia						
A[b]	0%	2.9%	0.3%			
B	0%	0%	0%			
C	2.6%	4.5%	1.9%			

(*continued*)

disorders in first-degree relatives differentiates borderlines from schizophrenic patients (Loranger & Tulis, 1985; Schulz et al., 1989), the rates of these disorders are similar to those found in the first-degree relatives of patients with other personality disorders or with affective disorders. Antisocial personality disorder is also diagnosed in the first-degree relatives of BPD patients; however, the rate is not significantly different from that found in relatives of patients with schizophrenia, affective disorder, or dysthymia. Zanarini et al. (1990) found that antisocial patients had a significantly higher rate of impaired first-degree relatives who met criteria for antisocial personality disorder than did

TABLE 3.2. (Continued)

Study[a]	BPD	Schizophrenia	Affective disorders	Schizotypal personality disorder	Antisocial personality disorder	Dysthymia/ other personality disorders
			Diagnostic groups			
D[c]	—	—	0%			
E[b]	0%		0%			
F[b]	0%					
G[b]	4.6%	6.6%				
H[b]	0%				2.2%	0%
I[b]	1.0%	2.5%				0.7%
		Familial antisocial personality disorder				
A[b]	—	—	—	—	—	—
B	7.7%	2.2%*	0.6%*			
C	7.0%	3.5%	4.4%			
D[c]	—	—	—	—	—	—
E[b]	0%		13.6%			
F[b]	9.6%					
G[b]	—	—	—	—	—	—
H[b]	13.6%				21.4%	9.6%
I[b]	3.1%	3.2%				2.5%

[a]Key to studies: A, Loranger, Oldham, & Tulis (1982), Loranger & Tulis (1985); B, Pope, Jonas, Hudson, Cohen, & Gunderson (1983); C, Soloff & Millward (1983); D, Baron, Gruen, Asnis, & Lord (1985); E, Schulz et al. (1986); F, Links, Steiner, & Huxley (1988); G, Schulz et al. (1989); H, Zanarini, Gunderson, Marino, Schwartz, & Frankenburg (1990); I, Silverman et al. (1987).

[b]Percentages for this study represent calculated morbid risk.

[c]Percentages for this study adjusted for indirect method.

* Significant difference between groups to the left of asterisk and BPD.

the borderline patients. Again, this suggests that these personality disorders "breed true."

The relationship between major depression and BPD is the most difficult to resolve. High rates of major affective disorders are commonly found in the first-degree relatives of BPD patients, and these rates were significantly higher than those found in relatives of schizophrenic and antisocial personality disorder controls. However, Pope et al. (1983), Zanarini et al. (1990), and Silverman et al. (1987) have attributed the increased familial prevalence of affective disorders to the coexistence of affective disorders in the borderline probands. Zanarini et al. (1990) found a prevalence rate for major depression of 19.8% in depressed BPD subjects versus 1.9% in "pure" borderlines (significant at $p < .01$). Torgersen (1984) studied 44 SPD, 15 SPD-BPD, and 10 BPD same-sex twin probands to determine the relationship between Axis I and Axis II disorders. The results indicated that only for the cotwins of BPD patients with concurrent affective disorders was there evidence of the cotwins' having affective disorders. Schulz et al. (1989) found no difference in the rates of depression in first-degree relatives of depressed (16.8%) and never depressed ("pure") borderline probands (14.5%). However, the majority of evidence supports the hypothesis that here is no specific relationship between BPD and affective disorders except when BPD probands have either concurrent or lifetime histories of major depression.

FUTURE DIRECTIONS

Future research initiatives directed at understanding the etiological significance of the family environment will have to be based on more precise models, to employ measures with proven psychometric properties, and ultimately to have the potential to influence patient management. One example is presented to illustrate these points: The hypothesis of an interaction between hostility and overinvolvement in the family environment as a causal factor in BPD may be used to highlight the direction of future research.

Our hypothesis that hostility rather than indifference or lack of care may characterize the family environment of borderline patients led us to consider measuring the concept of "expressed emotion" (EE) in the family relationships of borderline patients. The index termed EE measures the number of critical remarks, expressions of hostility, and expressions of emotional overinvolvement made by family members during an interview about the index patient. In schizophrenia research, relatives rating high on either critical comments or emotional overinvolvement are considered high on EE. This rating of high EE has been found to have a causal effect on course, strongly predicting relapse in discharged patients (Falloon, 1988). The hypothesis to be tested in borderline patients is that self-report measures recording the patients' recollections of parental abuse, hostility, and overinvolvement will be related to the parents' current measure of EE. In addition, patients from families with high EE scores may demonstrate a worse prognosis than that of patients from families with low EE scores.

The examination of the applicability of the EE concept to borderline patients and their families will have two important future implications. First, the correlation of self-report recollections to current parental attitudes may indicate factors that could be modified to improve the course of BPD. Although parental relationships are frequently identified as clinically relevant, no empirical data exist on the usefulness of family therapy interventions for borderline patients. Second, a clearer delineation of an etiological model incorporating hostility and overinvolvement may lead to the identification of high-risk groups of children, who could be followed prospectively to test this model.

Family history studies have confirmed that major affective disorders, alcoholism, and BPD are frequently found in the families of BPD patients. There is little evidence of specific associations between major affective disorders and BPD, and alcoholism and BPD. However, the strong familial occurrence of BPD in the first-degree family members of BPD subjects is supported by several studies. To clarify whether this is the result of environmental or genetic factors will require other research designs besides family history studies.

Torgersen (1984) has published the only report of a twin study done with the aim of examining the contribution of genetic factors in the development of SPD and BPD. This report was part of a larger Norwegian study of same-sex twins with nonpsychotic functional psychiatric disorders. Twins were diagnosed using DSM-III criteria, and the rater was blind as to the zygosity of the twins. Of the 69 probands receiving personality disorder diagnoses, only 10 were considered to have BPD, and another 15 were diagnosed as having BPD and SPD. The results were not felt to support a genetic etiology for BPD, as none of three monozygotic cotwins and only two of seven dyzygotic cotwins of probands with BPD had BPD. Unfortunately, the prevalence of BPD was low in this sample, leaving the possibility that a type II error may have been committed.

Adoptive studies constitute the other type of research design used to examine the contributions of heredity and environment to abnormal behavior (Bohman, 1981). Several specific designs exist: (1) the "adoptees family study," in which the biological relatives of affected adoptees and unaffected control adoptees are compared (the prevalence of a disorder among relatives of biological and adoptive index and control families allows for an estimation of genetic and environmental factors); (2) the "adoptees study method," in which the prevalence of the disorder among adoptees born to affected and unaffected parents are compared; and (3) "cross-fostering methods," in which adoptees born of affected parents are contrasted with adoptees born to unaffected parents but reared by adoptive parents affected by the disorder under study.

Adoptive studies as summarized by Bohman (1981) have supported the hypothesis that genetic factors are important in the etiology of alcoholism; however, there is less evidence that antisocial behavior is genetically determined. At this writing, there are no published reports of adoptive studies examining parents or adoptees diagnosed with BPD.

Although adoptive status is not uncommon in borderline patients (approximately 10% of our cohort in the Links, Steiner, & Huxley [1988] study were adopted), and borderline mothers may have children removed from their care, adoptive studies focusing on the specific diagnosis may not be as valuable as focusing on specific traits that may be inherited. A crucial question is to determine the phenotype that may be an expression of the inherited defect in BPD. Torgersen (1980) examined heritability of different personality traits in his sample of same-sex twins. As a result, he was able to identify hereditary and environmental factors; for example, the factor named "aggressive impulsiveness" selected as an environmental factor resulting from upbringing, family pattern, and cultural style rather than from genetic factors. Further study of the genetic and environmental origins of impulsivity or other borderline traits would greatly enhance our understanding of BPD.

IMPLICATIONS OF THIS REVIEW

The present review has implications for both research and clinical practice. The next generation of etiological research into BPD will need to consider the following:

1. *Variety of research designs.* To examine the etiological impact of the family environment in greater detail, prospective follow-up studies of children at risk are required. Preventive intervention trials targeted at decreasing the risk of possible etiological factors, with a resultant decrease in the occurrence of BPD, should be developed. Adoptive and twin studies are needed to clarify the role of genetic factors in BPD.

2. *Commitment of more resources and time.* The proposed research designs will require allocation of more research funding to the study of personality disorders. Prospective follow-up studies and intervention programs for high-risk families are expensive and require the commitment of funds over extended periods of time.

3. *Complex conceptual and analytic frameworks.* The exploration of complex conceptual models for explaining the etiology of BPD will need a multidisciplinary approach and will require the expertise of developmental psychologists, sociologists, and epidemiologists (to name but a few). New analytic methods for examining the interactions among a complex and extensive set of factors may need to be developed.

Several implications for clinical practice also arise from this body of work. Although the impact of genetic factors in the development of BPD has not been validated, current evidence shows that environmental factors in the cause and course of BPD need to be considered. Environmental factors that are amenable to change may have importance in our clinical work with these patients and their families. We should consider the following:

1. Patients' experience of abuse and loss need to be accepted, and interventions need to be targeted at resolving the aftermath of the abuse and loss experiences.

2. Family interactions can be distressing and problematic for both the patient and family members, especially when more than one family member

is psychologically impaired. Relationships characterized by hostility and overinvolvement need to be the focus of clinical interventions.

3. The children of borderline patients appear to be at risk of suffering abuse experiences and losses, and of becoming borderlines themselves. Thus, preventive interventions will be needed to "detoxify" the family experiences of children of borderline patients.

The challenges to researchers and clinicians are many, but the importance of the family environment in the etiology of BPD is central to all future endeavors studying the cause and course of borderline pathology.

REFERENCES

Akiskal, H. S. (1981). Subaffective disorders: Dysthymia, cyclothymia and bipolar II disorders in the "borderline" realm. *Psychiatric Clinics of North America, 4,* 25–46.

Akiskal, H. S., Chen, S. E., Davis, G. C., Puzantian, V. R., Kashgarian, M., & Bolinger, J. M. (1985). Borderline: An adjective in search of a noun. *Journal of Clinical Psychiatry, 46,* 41–48.

Baron, M., Gruen, R., Asnis, L., & Lord, S. (1985). Familial transmission of schizotypal and borderline personality disorders. *American Journal of Psychiatry, 142,* 927–934.

Birtchnell, J. (1980). Women whose mothers died in childhood: An outcome study. *Psychological Medicine, 10,* 699–713.

Bohman, M. (1981). The interaction of heredity and childhood environment: Some adoption studies. *Journal of Child Psychology and Psychiatry, 22,* 195–200.

Bradley, S. J. (1979). Relation of early maternal separation to borderline personality in children and adolescents: A pilot study. *American Journal of Psychiatry, 136,* 424–426.

Brown, G. W., & Harris, T. (1978). *Social origins of depression: A study of psychiatric disorder in women.* New York: Free Press.

Bryer, J. B., Nelson, B. A., Miller, J. B., & Krol, P. A. (1987). Childhood sexual and physical abuse as factors in adult psychiatric illness. *American Journal of Psychiatry, 144,* 1426–1430.

Byrne, C. P., Velamoor, V. R., Cernovsky, Z. Z., Cortese, M. D., & Losztyn, S. (1990). A comparison of borderline and schizophrenic patients for childhood life events and parent–child relationships. *Canadian Journal of Psychiatry, 35,* 590–595.

Clarkin, J., Widiger, J., Frances, A., Hurt, S. W., & Gilmore, M. (1983). Prototype typology and the borderline personality disorder. *Journal of Abnormal Psychology, 92,* 263–275.

Davis, G. C., & Akiskal, H. S. (1986). Descriptive, biological, and theoretical aspects of borderline personality disorder. *Hospital and Community Psychiatry, 37,* 685–692.

Falloon, I. R. H. (1988). Expressed emotion: Current status. *Psychological Medicine, 18,* 269–274.

Frank, H., & Hoffman, N. (1986). Borderline empathy: An empirical investigation. *Comprehensive Psychiatry, 27*, 387–395.

Frank, H., & Paris, J. (1981). Recollections of family experience in borderline patients. *Archives of General Psychiatry, 38*, 1031–1034.

Frank, H., & Paris, J. (1989, September). *Emotional neglect and overprotection in the recollections of borderline patients.* Paper presented at the annual meeting of the Canadian Psychiatric Association, St. John's, Newfoundland.

Goldberg, R. L., Mann, L. S., Wise, T. N., & Segall, E. A. (1985). Parental qualities as perceived by borderline personality disorders. *Hillside Journal of Clinical Psychiatry, 7*, 134–140.

Gunderson, J. G., Kerr, J., & Englund, D. W. (1980). The families of borderlines: A comparative study. *Archives of General Psychiatry, 37*, 27–33.

Gunderson, J. G., & Zanarini, M. C. (1989). Pathogenesis of borderline personality. In A. Tasman, R. E. Hales, & A. J. Frances (Ed.), *Review of psychiatry* (Vol. 8). Washington, DC: American Psychiatric Press.

Herman, J. L., Perry, J. C., & van der Kolk, B. A. (1989). Childhood trauma in borderline personality disorder. *American Journal of Psychiatry, 146*, 490–495.

Hoch, P., & Polatin, P. (1949). Pseudoneurotic forms of schizophrenia. *Psychiatric Quarterly, 23*, 248–276.

Links, P. S., Boiago, I., Huxley, G., Steiner, M., & Mitton, J. E. (1990). Sexual abuse and biparental failure as etiologic models in borderline personality disorder. In P. S. Links (Ed.), *Family environment and borderline personality disorder.* Washington, DC: American Psychiatric Press.

Links, P. S., & Munroe-Blum, H. (1990). Family environment and borderline personality disorder: Development of etiologic models. In P. S. Links (Ed.), *Family environment and borderline personality disorder.* Washington, DC: American Psychiatric Press.

Links, P. S., Steiner, M., & Huxley, G. (1988). The occurrence of borderline personality disorder in the families of borderline patients. *Journal of Personality Disorders, 2*, 14–20.

Links, P. S., Steiner, M., Offord, D., & Eppel, A. (1988). Characteristics of borderline personality disorder: A Canadian study. *Canadian Journal of Psychiatry, 33*, 336–340.

Links, P. S., & van Reekum, R. (1990, May). *Constitutional factors in borderline personality disorder.* Paper presented at the annual meeting of the American Psychiatric Association, New York.

Lloyd, C. (1980). Life events and depressive disorder reviewed: I. Events as predisposing factors. *Archives of General Psychiatry, 37*, 529–535.

Loranger, A. W., Oldham, J. M., & Tulis, E. H. (1982). Familial transmission of DSM-III borderline personality disorder. *Archives of General Psychiatry, 39*, 795–799.

Loranger, A. W., & Tulis, E. H. (1985). Family history of alcoholism in borderline personality disorder. *Archives of General Psychiatry, 42*, 153–157.

Ogata, S. N., Silk, K. R., & Goodrich, S. (1990). The childhood experience of the borderline patient. In P. S. Links (Ed.), *Family environment and borderline personality disorder.* Washington, DC: American Psychiatric Press.

Parker, G., Tupling, H., & Brown, L. B. (1979). A parental bonding instrument. *British Journal of Medical Psychology, 52*, 1–10.

Paris, J., & Frank, H. (1989). Perceptions of parental bonding in borderline patients. *American Journal of Psychiatry, 146*, 1498–1499.

Pope, H. G., Jonas, J. M., Hudson, J. I., Cohen, B. M., & Gunderson, J. G. (1983). The validity of DSM-III borderline personality disorder: A phenomenologic, family history, treatment response, and long term follow-up study. *Archives of General Psychiatry, 40*, 23–30.

Richters, J., & Weintraub, S. (1989). Beyond diathesis: Towards an understanding of high risk environments in risk and protective factors. In J. E. Rolf, A. Masten, D. Cicchetti, D. Nuechterlein, & S. Weintraub (Eds.), *Risk and protective factors in the development of psychopathology*. New York: Cambridge University Press.

Robins, E., & Guze, S. B. (1970). Establishment of diagnostic validity in psychiatric illness: Its application to schizophrenia. *American Journal of Psychiatry, 126*, 983–987.

Rutter, M. (1983). Stress, coping and development: Some issues and some questions. In N. Garmezy & M. Rutter (Eds.), *Stress, coping and development in children*. New York: McGraw-Hill.

Rutter, M., & Quinton, D. (1984). Parental psychiatric disorder: Effects on children. *Psychological Medicine, 14*, 853–880.

Schulz, P. M., Schulz, S. C., Goldberg, S. C., Ettigi, P., Resnick, R. J., & Friedel, R. O. (1986). Diagnoses of the relatives of schizotypal outpatients. *Journal of Nervous and Mental Disease, 174*, 457–463.

Schulz, P. M., Soloff, P. H., Kelly, T., Morgenstern, M., DiFranco, R., & Schulz, S. C. (1989). A family history of borderline subtypes. *Journal of Personality Disorders, 3*, 217–229.

Sheldon, A. E. R., & West, M. (1989). The functional discrimination of attachment and affiliation theory and empirical demonstrations. *British Journal of Psychiatry, 155*, 18–23.

Silverman, J. M., Siever, L. J., Coccaro, E. F., Klar, H., Greenwald, S., Rubenstein, K., Mohs, R. C., & Davidson, M. (1987, December). *Risk of affective disorder and personality disorder in the relatives of personality disorder patients*. Paper presented at the meeting of the American College of Neuropsychopharmacology, San Juan, Puerto Rico.

Snyder, S., Pitts, W. M., Goodpaster, W. A., & Gustin, Q. L. (1984). Family structure as recalled by borderline patients. *Psychopathology, 17*, 90–97.

Soloff, P. H., & Millward, J. W. (1983). Psychiatric disorders in the families of borderline patients. *Archives of General Psychiatry, 40*, 37–44.

Spitzer, R. L., Endicott, J., & Gibbon, M. (1979). Crossing the border into borderline personality and borderline schizophrenia: The development of criteria. *Archives of General Psychiatry, 36*, 17–24.

Stone, M. H. (1977). The borderline syndrome: Evolution of the term, genetic aspects and prognosis. *American Journal of Psychotherapy, 31*, 345–365.

Stone, M. H. (1990). Abuse and abusiveness in borderline personality disorder. In P. S. Links (Ed.), *Family environment and borderline personality disorder*. Washington, DC: American Psychiatric Press.

Stone, M. H., Kahn, E., & Flye, B. (1981). Psychiatrically ill relatives of borderline patients: A family study. *Psychiatric Quarterly, 53*, 71–84.

Torgersen, S. (1980). Hereditary–environmental differentiation of general neurotic, obsessive and impulsive hysterical personality traits. *Acta Geneticae Medicae et Gemellologiae, 29,* 193–207.

Torgersen, S. (1984). Genetic and nosological aspects of schizotypal and borderline personality disorders. *Archives of General Psychiatry, 41,* 546–554.

West, M., & Sheldon, A. E. R. (1988). Classification of pathological attachment patterns in adults. *Journal of Personality Disorders, 2,* 153–159.

West, M., Sheldon, A. E. R., & Reiffer, L. (1987). An approach to the delineation of adult attachment: Scale, development and reliability. *Journal of Nervous and Mental Disease, 175,* 738–741.

West, M., Sheldon, A. E. R., & Reiffer, L. (1989). Attachment theory and brief psychotherapy: Applying current research to clinical interventions. *Canadian Journal of Psychiatry, 34,* 369–375.

Zanarini, M. C., Gunderson, J. G., Marino, M. F., Schwartz, E. O., & Frankenburg, F. R. (1989). Childhood experiences of borderline patients. *Comprehensive Psychiatry, 30,* 18–25.

Zanarini, M. C., Gunderson, J. G., Marino, M. F., Schwartz, E. O., & Frankenburg, F. R. (1990). Psychiatric disorders in the families of borderline outpatients. In P. S. Links (Ed.), *Family environment and borderline personality disorder.* Washington, DC: American Psychiatric Press.

CHAPTER 4

Borderline Personality Disorder: Course of Illness

MICHAEL H. STONE

COURSE, OUTCOME, NATURAL HISTORY: DISTINCTIONS

The focus of this chapter is on the course of borderline personality disorder (BPD) as defined in the *Diagnostic and Statistical Manual of Mental Disorders*, third edition (DSM-III; American Psychiatric Association, 1980). I hope also to show the parallels and differences between the course of this personality disorder and the more broadly defined "borderline personality organization" (BPO) of Kernberg (1967).

The information upon which this chapter is based comes from the follow-up studies on borderline conditions that have been reported over the past 25 years. The material from the first 20 of these years is for the most part unsystematic and reflects a less rigorous definition of "borderline" than that currently used. More recently, follow-up reports reflect homogeneity of diagnosis and much longer time periods. The advantages of the latter are clear, inasmuch as the level of adaptation achieved by individuals aged 40 or 45 (as ascertained through long-term evaluation) provides a more accurate picture of the life potential than the level achieved by persons still only in their 20s (as determined by short-term follow-up).

We must also pay attention to distinctions between the "outcome" and the "course" of illness, as well as to the difference between "course" and "natural history." "Outcome," in this context, relates to the status of a former patient at a particular point in time some months or years after initial assessment. The evaluation of "course," in contrast, involves multiple measurements of several key variables, carried out at appropriate intervals throughout the long interval stretching between initial contact and long-term, or even "final" (i.e., up to the time of death), evaluation. The outlining of the typical "course" gives us a handle on the important issue of *quality of life* over a long period, whereas a long-term outcome study does not ordinarily distinguish—in the case, say, of two successful persons now in their 50s—between the one who may have made a dramatic leap upward in function recently after years of a wretched existence, and the one who made a slow and steady uphill climb before ultimately reaching the same level.

The study of outcome and course is further complicated by the question of data reliability. In a retrospective design, for example, the memory of recent events is apt to be superior to that of events from 15 or 20 years ago. Some patients or their families can reconstruct salient features of the remote past well enough for the investigator to map out the course, as well as the current outcome, even within the context of a retrospective study. Usually, however, retrospective analysis permits only a shadowy or blurred image of the life course. On the face of it, a prospective design would seem to have every advantage over its opposite: Re-evaluation of former patients at frequent stages (every 6 months, every year or two) yields much more definitive answers regarding the life course. The accuracy of such studies, however, is purchased at great price, because of the large research team necessary to carry out such work. Even the best prospective study will suffer at least to some degree because of the impossibility of knowing, when the study is in the design stage, all the truly important variables that should be measured. A prospective study begun in 1960, for example, would probably not have inquired carefully into the physical and sexual abuse histories of the participants—histories that play a crucial role in the lives of many borderline patients, as we had begun to realize by 1980. The upshot of all this is that to obtain the clearest view of the course of conditions such as BPD, we must blend information stemming from both retrospective and prospective research.

Clinicians are often interested in the "natural history" of conditions—that is, in their evolution independent of treatment. The "course" of an illness or condition usually implies its evolution under the circumstances of customary treatment. With respect to borderline patients, few ever refrain from getting help in one form or another, so that untreated "control groups" do not occur spontaneously in nature. In fact, people who might be spotted as BPD cases in an epidemiological study—but who never partake of any mental health services—may very well be simultaneously antisocial, or else help-rejecting and chaotic persons who are not really typical of the (presumed) majority of those suffering from this disorder. The fate of the BPD cases identified only epidemiologically may very well be different (in all likelihood, worse) from that of the persons with BPD who seek our help. I noticed, in possible support of this supposition, that patients with BPD hospitalized in the 1960s who signed out of the hospital after a few days had rather uniformly irritable personalities, and, 20 years later, were doing poorly in comparison to the average outcome of the BPD counterparts who remained as long as seemed necessary on the unit. At all events, we cannot speak with any authority about the natural history of (untreated) borderline patients; we can only do so about the course of those treated in the ways most in vogue during the epoch when they were in active treatment.

KEY VARIABLES

Delineation of the key variables in long-term study of course and outcome in borderline conditions is not a process that can be brought to completion before a researcher attempts to trace the former patients. The researcher must begin with a list of variables born of clinical experience and intuition. The variables selected in this fashion may have to suffice for the early phases of the study. But this is, from the perspective of a hypothetical ideal study, only a first step. As the investigator is midway through the work, the responses of the contactees make him think of new variables that were neglected in the original outline. Enumerating the key variables, then, is better seen as a dynamic equilibrium among intuition at the outset; discovery of new variables during the interviewing phase; the creation of an expanded list (adding the new to the old) for use in a more sophisticated future study, the carrying out of which will lead to discovery of hitherto unsuspected variables; and so on.

These remarks notwithstanding, there are certain variables that have to be included in any follow-up study, whether or not they turn out to have discriminating value vis-à-vis life course and outcome. A number of these basic factors are ordinarily subsumed under the rubric of "demographic" variables. The following are essential to the study of borderline patients:

> Age when patient was first seen in consultation, or (in the case of a hospitalized patient) was first admitted to hospital
> Gender
> Socioeconomic status
> Marital status
> Religious background
> Ethnic background
> Regional/cultural background (e.g., rural Midwest, urban New England, etc.)
> Patient's position in sibship
> Was patient a twin? (If so, dizygotic or monozygotic?)
> Was the patient an adoptee? (If so, what is known about the biological parents? Were the latter relatives of the adopting parents?)
> Was the patient born out of wedlock? Are the parents still married, separated, divorced, widowed, dead?

In addition to these demographic variables, several sets of baseline variables are important in the assessment of borderline patients, and hence important also in their eventual follow-up. These may be grouped under the appropriate categories: psychosocial; recent and past symptoms; constitutional; family-related; personality-related; and miscellaneous. Among the pertinent variables I include here are several of whose significance I was not aware until I had completed my own follow-up project and could assess their impact upon outcome. Attractiveness was one such example; a childhood history of fire setting was another. The variables belonging to the above-mentioned six categories are as follows:

Psychosocial
Prior friendships; previous history of intimate relationships
Talent in the areas of music, art, crafts, sports
Positive personality traits (cf. Kolb, 1982: courage, curiosity, flexibility, commitment, perseverance, responsibility, humor, empathy, trust, charm, likeability)
History during childhood and adolescence of verbal, physical, and/or sexual abuse from primary caretakers
History of other traumas, including accidents and sexual molestation by persons outside the family
History of intrafamilial losses (parental death, divorce, abandonment, etc.)
Patterns of recreational/avocational activities
History of antisocial/delinquent tendencies (truancy, vagrancy, shoplifting, imposture, running away, being in jail, being on probation, serious rebelliousness)
History of head trauma, other bodily injuries during childhood (ever lost consciousness?)
History of ever having been raped
Presence of offensive social habits

Constitutional
Somatotype (meso-, ecto-, or endomorphic?)
Attractiveness
Birth weight
History of birth complications
Handedness, laterality
Dyslexia?

Recent and Past Symptoms
Childhood symptoms (tics, imaginary companions beyond the usual age, enuresis past age 3, encopresis, fire setting, hurting animals, violence toward family members)
Abuse of alcohol or illicit drugs
Eating disorder (anorexia nervosa, obesity, bulimia nervosa)

Homosexuality
Sexual disorder (transvestism, fetishism, exposure, pedophilia)
Pathological jealousy
Handicapped? (e.g., polio, cerebral palsy, etc.)
Panic disorder, phobia, other severe anxiety disorder
Obsessions, compulsions, obsessive–compulsive disorder
History of epilepsy, blackout spells, and the like
History of hyperactivity, attention deficit disorder
Dysmorphophobia
Compulsive gambling
Pseudologia fantastica, chronic lying
Hostility, irascibility, abusiveness
Narcolepsy or other sleeping disorders, including night terrors
Dysmenorrhea or premenstrual tension
Psychosomatic conditions
History of self-mutilation, suicidal behavior
Promiscuity/impulsivity/hypersexuality

Family-Related
Family history of mental illness, alcoholism, severe personality disorders,
    antisociality
Notable attributes of the family (e.g., wealth, fame, power, aristocratic
    lineage)

Personality-Related
Prominent personality traits of other personality disorders ("as-if" per-
    sonality, etc.)

Miscellaneous
Academic performance, IQ
Work history
History of previous psychotherapy, hospitalizations

A final set of variables relevant to the assessment of the life course of borderline patients concerns the time span between last contact and follow-up contact. These variables belong to certain overarching dimensions having to do with symptoms and psychiatric help sought (if any), and with Freud's two key measures of love and work. The love factor includes all facets of interpersonal life, especially the sphere of intimacy; the work factor includes the full range of vocational/avocational/academic activities. Briefly set forth, the variables related to a patient's life after last contact are as follows:

Symptoms
Has the patient developed manic–depressive illness in the intervening
    years? Schizophrenia?

Has the patient continued to show, or more recently developed, symptoms such as those mentioned in the "Recent and Past Symptoms" section?

Has the patient ever been rehospitalized? (In the case of an initially hospitalized patient, did the patient elope from the hospital or leave against medical advice?)

Has the patient abused alcohol or drugs in the intervening years? If so, has he joined Alcoholics Anonymous (AA) or a similar organization?

Social and Intimate Life

Intervening history regarding friendships, intimate relationships (marriage, children; any children out of wedlock?)

Has patient joined a religious cult, commune, or the like?

Vocational/Avocational Life

School performance (if applicable)

Recent work history

Recent history with respect to hobbies, sports, other recreational activities

REVIEW AND CRITIQUE OF FOLLOW-UP STUDIES IN THE BORDERLINE DOMAIN

Early Studies

The earliest studies of outcome in patients we would now subsume under the "borderline" label were reported in the 1960s. The term "borderline" itself was not always used. The relationship between some of the older designations and the current concept of BPD was sometimes fairly close, as in the "pseudoneurotic schizophrenic" cases of Hoch and Polatin (1949); at other times it was almost completely disjunctive, as in the "borderline schizophrenic" cases of Nyman (1978). In a recent article (Stone, 1989) I have summarized the results of these studies, which included those of Hoch, Cattell, Strahl, and Pennes (1962) and Gidro-Frank, Peretz, Spitzer, and Winikus (1967), both based on "pseudoneurotic schizophrenic" patients hospitalized at the New York State Psychiatric Institute in the 1950s and 1960s; the Norwegian studies of Holm and Hundevadt (1976, 1981) on "borderline" patients; the Swedish study of Katerina Nyman (1978), contrasting "process schizophrenics" with "borderline schizophrenics," as noted above; and the report of Werble (1970) on the hospitalized "borderline" patients treated several years earlier by Grinker, Werble, and Drye (1968). The Grinker study was the first that reflected a methodical definition of "borderline"—one that acknowledged four subtypes. Grinker's "Type II" signified a "core" borderline patient, whose anger, depressive mood, and impulsivity overlap rather closely with (DSM-defined) BPD. Similarly, Gunderson, Carpenter, and Strauss (1975) used operationalized diagnostic criteria (those of Gunderson & Singer, 1975) in their 2-year follow-up comparison of borderline with schizophrenic patients. At this brief interval, both sets of patients were functioning about equally poorly in the areas of socialization, employment, symptoms, and rate of rehospitalization. Even at 5 years these groups had not begun to diverge in overall function, except that the borderlines were now establishing better social contacts (Carpenter, Gunderson, & Strauss, 1977).

The report of Masterson and Costello (1980) focused on a younger group of patients, whose borderline diagnosis rested on criteria less precise than those used by Grinker et al. and Gunderson et al. Masterson's hospitalized adolescents, followed for up to 7 years, were often well (16%) or only mildly impaired (42%), especially if they had high IQs, supportive families, good peer relations, and hospital stays longer than 6 months. Those with organicity and scholastic underachievement tended to do poorly.

Werble (1970), having traced 80% of the 51 hospitalized patients of the Grinker study, found that most still showed difficulties in maintaining positive object relations. A schizophrenic evolution was rare (only two instances). Despite their impairments in socialization and their tendency not to marry, these borderline patients were now functioning fairly adequately in the occupational arena.

Of the 100 Gunderson-defined borderlines studied by Akiskal (1981) in a 2- to 3-year follow-up, many showed signs of manic–depressive illness, four had already committed suicide, and only one had developed schizophrenia.

The outpatients with BPD studied by Perry (1985) and followed up to 3 years later by Perry and Cooper (1985) characteristically still showed considerable anxiety, hostility, and depression, and were still functioning in the "fair" range (corresponding to Global Assessment Scale [GAS] scores in the 50s; see Endicott, Spitzer, Fleiss, & Cohen, 1976). The hospitalized borderlines followed up to 2 years by Tucker, Bauer, Wagner, Harlam, and Sher (1987) were likewise functioning in the "fair" range—an improvement from the marginal functioning they exhibited at initial evaluation.

The extensive monograph of Wallerstein (1986) provides detailed descriptions of 42 patients (some ambulatory, others hospitalized) treated with analytically oriented psychotherapy at the Menninger Clinic during the 1950s and 1960s. The loose nosological standards of that era make it difficult to situate these patients within a contemporary diagnostic map. But the clinical material is rich enough for the reader to make an educated guess. By my estimate, 18 were originally "borderline," at least by Kernberg criteria; the others were "neurotic." These patients were bright and middle- to upper-class, but they had a high rate of alcoholism. Five of the 18 borderline patients eventually committed suicide; of these, four had abused substances. Only a third of the borderlines, as opposed to four-fifths of the neurotic patients, ended up functioning well (the follow-up intervals varied from brief to over 20 years). An important outgrowth of this study was Wallerstein's observation that the patients whose therapy veered in the direction of "supportive," rather than remaining strictly "expressive," did about as well and made as solid gains as did those whose therapists were able to maintain a more analytically oriented posture throughout.

Apart from Wallerstein's monograph on the Menninger project, the above-cited studies provide little information regarding course of illness or ultimate outcome. The lack of standardized diagnoses makes it difficult to compare Wallerstein's cases with borderline patients of the current era. A more serious drawback to these studies is their generally small sample size. Given the immense number of important prognostic variables (some of which have been outlined in the preceding section), to imagine that one investigator's sample is "matched" adequately to some control group or to another investigator's sample simply because of similarity in age and gender is illusory. As we shall see, the more recent, large-scale, and long-term studies circumvent some of these stumbling blocks, thanks to their more systematic approach to diagnosis, as well as to their larger size and time intervals.

Recent Long-Term Studies

General Outcomes and Suicides

The five long-term studies of outcome in borderline patients thus far reported in the literature are based on material gathered from 454 formerly hospitalized patients adjudged "borderline" either by DSM or by Gunderson's Diagnostic Interview for Borderlines (DIB) criteria. Table 4.1 provides an overview of these studies, mentioning the site of the index admission for each study, the principal investigators reporting the study, the sample size and trace rate, the range of years in the follow-up intervals, and the typical level of functioning at latest contact.

From the standpoint of global functioning, there is a remarkable convergence in these studies: The typical functional level at follow-up was about the same for the borderline patients in each sample. The data in this regard are more convincing for the Chestnut Lodge and New York State Psychiatric Institute (PI-500) studies, where the n's and trace rates were higher; they are less so for the Minneapolis study, because of its small size. At intervals of 10 to 25 years, in other words, about two-thirds of the BPD patients were doing "fair" to "well."

Although there was good agreement as to the usual long-term outcome, each of the investigations noted a wide *range* of outcomes. Accordingly, the standard deviations in the GAS measures were large (11 in Paris's study, 14.5

TABLE 4.1. Overview of the Long-Term Follow-Up Studies of BPD

Site	Principal investigators	No. of traced BPD pts.	% traced of original sample of borderline pts.	Years of follow-up	Outcome
Austin Riggs	Plakun, Burkhardt, & Muller (1985)	63	27%	9–34	60s[b]
Minneapolis	Kroll, Carey, & Sines (1985)	13[a]	87%	20	Fair
Chestnut Lodge	McGlashan (1986)	81	86%	2–32	64[c]
New York State Psychiatric Institute	Stone, Hurt, & Stone (1987)	198	96%	10–25	66[b]
Jewish General Hospital	Paris, Brown, & Nowlis (1987)	100[a]	31%	9–29	63[c]

[a] According to Gunderson's Diagnostic Interview for Borderlines (DIB) criteria (Gunderson, Kolb, & Austin, 1981).
[b] On Global Assessment Scale (GAS; Endicott, Spitzer, Fleiss, & Cohen, 1976).
[c] On Menninger Health–Sickness Rating Scale (Luborsky, 1962).

in Stone's). Indeed, the former patients could be found in any segment of the health–sickness continuum—from suicides to extremely effective individuals in all spheres of life (and asymptomatic).

Despite the generally good outcomes noted at long-term follow-up, the suicide risk in BPD patients—at least in the initially hospitalized groups that were the focus of these studies—was appreciable. Now that 198 BPD patients from the PI-500 have been traced (a slightly larger number than that noted in the earlier reports—Stone, Hurt, & Stone, 1987; Stone, 1989), the 17 suicides constitute 8.6% of those traced. This figure is comparable to the suicide rates noted among the schizophrenic and the manic–depressive patients in the PI-500 (10%), though lower than the 22% rate thus far in the schizoaffectives (62 of 64 having been located). Given the 14-year span of the PI-500 sample (1963–1976, inclusive), the suicide rate translates into a rate per 100,000 per year of 616, or about 55 times higher than the suicide rate in Caucasian persons in the U.S. general population.

As Solomon and Murphy (1984) point out, the annual suicide rate in white males rose steadily between 1950 and 1975 from 11.9 per 100,000 to 25, in those who were in the second half of their 20s (the corresponding rise in females was from 5.1 to 8.0 per 100,00). The factors that underlie these changes may help account for the high rate observed in the PI-500 (in which most of the patients were in their teens or early 20s on admission), in contrast to the lower suicide rate (3%) in the Chestnut Lodge series (where most of the patients were in their late 20s when hospitalized). In effect, the Chestnut Lodge patients were the survivors among a population of borderlines, some of whom had already committed suicide before referral to the Lodge.

With respect to the PI-500 borderlines, many of the suicides were alcohol-related: Concomitant alcohol abuse almost trebled the likelihood of suicide. Incest and sexual entanglements also played a role. The one patient whose death occurred in the hospital had been involved with a staff member. She killed herself when this relationship was about to be exposed to the unit staff. Another borderline patient, whose mother had seduced him into an incestuous relationship and had then killed herself, later killed himself shortly after leaving the unit. Whereas many of the suicides seemed preventable, his appeared unavoidable.

In the PI-500, 93 patients were borderline by Kernberg's (1967) criteria (BPO), but not by DSM-III criteria (BPD). This group included 36 dysthymics (34 traced), none of whom has committed suicide. The remaining 57—of whom 2 have committed suicide—consist of patients with other personality disorders, including schizotypal and antisocial. These data tend to support the impressions of Angst and Clayton (1986) to the effect that irritability and hostility are more important determinants of suicide than mere sadness. This was also the case with the one suicide in my own series of BPD patients seen in private practice and followed from 2 to 24 years (Stone, 1990a): A chronically irascible and vengeful young man of 22, having been rehospitalized after several months of office therapy, killed himself while on pass from the hospital a year later.

Given the bewildering array of factors that influence outcome in psychiatric patients, the question arises: Which factors exert the greatest influence, either for good or for ill? Are there other factors one might have assumed would weigh heavily in the balance that, in the light of follow-up, account for little or none of the variance?

Factors Influencing Outcome

High intelligence emerged as a mitigating factor in both the Chestnut Lodge and the PI-500 series. In the latter, artistic or musical talent, and also attractiveness (in the females), were associated with outcomes superior to the grand average for the whole BPD population. Obsessional traits (though not to the level of obsessive–compulsive *disorder*) were associated with better than average outcome in borderlines. This may have been a reflection of better ability to structure leisure time and to make do even when friends were not readily available (through recourse to hobbies, reading, etc.). Alcohol abuse was common among the PI-500 borderlines, but those who joined and remained with AA in the intervening years were uniformly well at follow-up. This is not only a tribute to AA, but also an index of coexisting personality traits that permitted some BPD × alcoholism patients to persevere, while their more hostile, irresponsible, and denial-prone counterparts persisted in their abuse of alcohol, going steadily downhill or committing suicide.

BPD patients with concomitant major affective disorder (MAD, especially major depression) had a higher suicide rate in the Chestnut Lodge series than did those without MAD (16% vs. 2%); the same was true in the PI-500 series (18% vs. 5%). The Austin Riggs BPD × MAD group was doing worse at follow-up than was the group with pure BPD, though in Pope's shorter-term study (Pope, Jonas, & Hudson, 1983) those with BPD × MAD were doing better. In the PI-500 the BPD × MAD patients also outperformed the pure BPD patients, especially the males. This may be a function of the greater frequency of antisocial traits in the "pure" BPD males, which would tend to impede their social recovery.

Apropos personality traits, BPD patients with irritable/explosive tendencies did almost as poorly as those with antisociality. Most other combinations did not seem to have a strong effect on outcome; prominent narcissistic traits, for example, were not associated with worse than average outcomes at long-term follow-up. Borderlines exhibiting what Kernberg (1988) has called "malignant narcissism"—the confluence of narcissistic and antisocial traits—did uniformly poorly. Some had, in fact, committed murder and were still in jail; others, having had less serious scrapes with the law, were now living as drifters. In a follow-up of 27 private patients with BPD, 26 of whom have been traced (2 to 24 years later), I noted an inverse relationship between general hostility level and successful outcome: The chronically angry patients alienated those upon whom they depended, in such a way as to end up friendless, jobless, and often spouseless as they entered their 40s (Stone, 1990a).

In many of the borderline patients, traumatic life events during childhood and adolescence correlated strongly with worse than average outcomes. The lines of demarcation between life events and personality traits are actually not as easily drawn as these outwardly unrelated terms would suggest. Parental brutality and incest (especially father–daughter), for example, were associated with poor outcome. It was true that more recent events, such as having been jailed and (in women) having been raped, were even more highly correlated with poor outcomes. However, in many instances the latest untoward event (e.g., being jailed) was the outgrowth of antisocial personality trends that were themselves, to every appearance, the consequences of parental brutality and rejection. What is truly relevant, in other words, is not just the linkage between the (proximal) event of jail and the poor outcome, or the (distal) event of the parental brutality; rather, it is the whole chain or pathway leading from the earliest events, through the personality traits they either brought about or intensified, and on to the subsequent untoward events and derailed life course that are the latter-day consequences of those deformations in personality.

Often, the trouble is not so much with unwelcome personality traits per se, but rather with inappropriate object choices made for motives of which the patient is quite unaware. As an example, one of the female PI-500 patients with BPD, whose personality was engaging and pleasant, had been abandoned by her mother and had been struck repeatedly and with some violence by her father. During her 20s she felt drawn to, and became involved with, a whole sequence of rejecting (at best) or violent men. These kinds of linkages—operating via the patient's "inner script" (Stone, 1988)—exert powerful influences on the life course, yet do so in ways totally external to the domain of conventional diagnosis; they easily escape the notice of investigators measuring the more usual variables of follow-up work. Not surprisingly, the more readily assessed variables (e.g., diagnosis, drug abuse, traumatic events) accounted for barely a sixth of the variance when the PI-500 data were subjected to multivariate analysis (Stone, 1990b).

The traits of (DSM-defined) BPD can be found in conjunction with those of most of the other DSM personality disorders (least commonly, perhaps, with schizoid traits). Besides the combinations with the antisocial, narcissistic, or obsessive, as mentioned above, a smaller number of the BPD patients from the follow-up studies had concomitant schizotypal (STP) features. These patients did as well as other borderlines in the Austin Riggs study; in the Chestnut Lodge and PI-500 series, outcomes for BPD × STP patients were usually in the "fair" range (GAS scores of 51–60), rather than in the "good" range (GAS scores of 61–70). In the Chestnut Lodge study, the presence of even three schizotypal items in nonpsychotic, newly admitted patients was associated with a heightened risk for eventual schizophrenia at about a 15-year follow-up, whereas BPD items did not predict this outcome (Fenton & McGlashan, 1989).

In the PI-500 series, BPD × MAD patients, female elopees, and patients with anorexia or bulimia nervosa were all as likely as BPD patients in general to have an outcome GAS score above 60. But those with a history of childhood fire setting, male elopees, and those exhibiting all eight DSM items for BPD were less likely to achieve such levels at follow-up. The most powerful predictor of a poor outcome in this series was a history of parental brutality. The patients least likely to recover (1 out of 10) were the borderlines who had spent even 1 day in jail.

Life Trajectory or Course

Thus far I have concentrated on outcome. Less information is available concerning the life trajectory or course. The patients followed by McGlashan are about 5 years older, on average, than those of the PI-500. Many BPD patients in both series remained dysfunctional (often because of substance abuse) for 5 to 10 years after leaving the hospital, whereupon they began their gradual ascent toward higher levels. A similar number (about a fifth) showed this steady ascent from the moment they were discharged. Although some of the BPD (and more of the Kernberg BPO) patients then showed a level course over 10 to 20 years, for the majority the course was "bumpy," with downturns every few years that were associated with the vicissitudes of close relationships. Ten percent of BPD × MAD patients showed a manic–depressive evolution with a markedly oscillating course, modulated—but not smoothed out perfectly—if they achieved stability in their intimate relations.

Some patients with BPD whose life trajectory had been level, and characterized by good social and occupational function, took a downturn during their 40s (McGlashan, 1986). These were usually patients who had been held together by a sustaining relationship—a marriage or a *de facto* living arrangement of long standing—which, after a certain number of years, had begun to deteriorate. In some instances the borderline patient was the protagonist (or, rather, the antagonist) in sabotaging a relationship through hostile, irritable behavior. In other instances the patient had been by far the more amicable and adaptive partner—but, having been "programmed" to choose destructive mates (usually alcoholic), persevered with such a mate for many years until the inevitable breakup. Once the latter occurred, the borderline patient was alone again and often became symptomatic.

In one such case in the PI-500, a woman of 21 had been hospitalized because of suicide gestures and agoraphobia. Her mother and her alcoholic and agoraphobic father had divorced when she was 15. After a year in the hospital, she recovered, married, and raised two children, but divorced 12 years later when her husband's drinking problem became intolerable. She remarried 4 years later. In the meantime she had worked, and had established herself as an active and well-liked participant in community affairs. Her second husband also turned out to be alcoholic. At the time of follow-up contact (24 years after she had left the unit), she reported that her husband had wrecked the house in a drunken fit. "Something in me," she mentioned, "makes me pick men just like my dad." After her second divorce, she was for a time depressed and discouraged; she was able to return to work, but pessimistic about the future.

In another PI-500 case, a woman in her early 40s had been married for 14 years to a well-to-do and much older man. Histrionic and garrulous in general, she could be generous and abrasive by turns. After having two children, she became extremely moody and petulant. A therapist diagnosed BPD. She quit each of a succession of therapists after a brief time. Self-centered and impatient with motherhood, she became suicidal at times, and made a number of suicidal gestures and attempts. By the time the younger child was 10, she had grown so irascible as to attack her son with a knife and to hurl pottery at her daughter, quite without provocation on their part. This was the "last straw" for her husband, who divorced her and took custody of the children. Intolerant of being alone, and enraged at being "abandoned," she took an overdose and killed herself on her 45th birthday.

Shortcomings of Studies to Date

The studies cited in the foregoing sections represent a significant step forward in our knowledge of the fate of borderline patients. Yet all have obvious shortcomings that either call into question the validity of some of their results or else limit their utility for clinicians.

Given the complexity of studying personality disorders—both because of the huge number of important variables and because of the long time periods necessary before the investigator can harvest any meaningful results—follow-up studies in this domain must ideally be based on large numbers of patients and must make objectified measures of dozens (if not hundreds) of variables. Many of the latter will, of necessity, be "soft" (such as amiability vs. abrasiveness), requiring scales not as yet devised. These "soft" variables account, it would appear, for more of the variance than most of the "hard" variables (e.g., comorbidity of various conditions, family history of mental illness, level of academic achievement, etc.). These considerations in turn raise the issue of reliability, since the more such variables one attempts to assess, the greater the number of blind raters would be necessary, in an ideal design; thus, the greater the expense of the project would be, and so on. In a like vein, the sheer variability in clinical picture of different "borderline" patients (100 borderline patients show much more internal variation than do, say, 100 patients with broken tibias) necessitates ultra-large n's, if the investigator is to have enough of the main types in the sample. Another reason to start with large n's concerns the rarity of certain phenomena of great interest to clinicians; suicide is the most important example.

The advantages of a prospective design over a retrospective design have already been mentioned. Even here problems arise, since prospective studies cannot assess variables whose significance does not come to light until one is about to determine the original patients' long-term outcome.

An ideal follow-up study of borderline patients should begin with a sample reflecting all "portals of entry": clinics, hospitals, private offices. Perhaps it should even include the general population, where some BPD "cases" exist that do not come to the attention of the helping professions.

Finally, an ideal study should shed light on the course of illness, not just on outcome at some fixed time, and should contain reasonably matched control groups (patients with other personality disorders, schizophrenia, etc.) whose fates could be compared to the borderline patients.

Appraised in this light, all of the major long-term studies to date fall well short of the ideal. Those with the larger *n*'s (the Chestnut Lodge, PI-500, and Jewish General Hospital studies) are still too small to have accumulated enough suicides, schizotypal patients, bulimics, and certain other groups of special interest to permit statistical examinations depending on 50 or 100 index cases. The trace rates were adequately high in the Chestnut Lodge and PI-500 studies, but not in the others; the nontraced patients cannot be said to resemble the traced except in the grossest of measures—measures that are not usually the key determinants of outcome.

The PI-500 study (most of which was carried out by one investigator) lacked the advantage of blind rating of many variables, such as could be performed in the Chestnut Lodge study. The studies have almost all concentrated on hospitalized patients—who are easier to assess with scientific rigor, but who do not constitute a representative sample of BPD patients, many of whom are never hospitalized at any point in their life course. The PI-500 study attempted to measure some of the more subjective variables (e.g., talent, attractiveness), but had to leave out may others (e.g., likeability, charm, courage, sense of responsibility, degree of family support), which probably account for more of the variance than was contained in the set of variables that could be looked at.

IMPLICATIONS FOR TREATMENT

Whereas borderline patients were once considered as apt to remain chronically impaired as were (DSM-III) schizophrenics, the long-term follow-up studies paint a more encouraging picture. Though the risk of suicide is not negligible, and though chronic impairment is the lot of some borderline patients, many are able to fly through the turbulence of their 20s and emerge almost whole. They are more brittle under severe stress than the "average person," but they are capable of leading rewarding lives occupationally and socially—and, in many instances, in the sphere of intimate relationships as well. This is all the more true for the non-DSM borderlines who (1) meet the Kernberg criteria for BPO and (2) are dysthymic. This group, in the PI-500, was mostly recovered at follow-up (GAS scores greater than 70) and contained no suicides. Once clinicians became aware of the special vulnerability borderline patients show in their third decade, a program of treatment can be mapped out so that a therapist (either the primary therapist or a colleague) is always "there" (via a session or a phone contact; on an intensive or on an as-needed basis) until a bridge is built up over time, strong enough to sustain the patient even when he/she is attempting to face life alone.

The follow-up studies shed some light on this vexatious question: What is the best type of psychotherapy for borderline patients? To be sure, none of the studies was designed to deal with this question directly; none employed a randomized technique for assigning patients to alternative to alternative methods of treatment, and so on. Still, minute examination of the data makes certain points clear. Although some patients appeared to have responded most favorably to psychoanalytically oriented ("expressive," "exploratory," "insight-oriented") therapy over long periods (3–10 or more years), others did just as well and made just as lasting adjustments through a treatment that was largely or almost wholly supportive (an observation made also by Wallerstein, 1986, in his Menninger study). Several BPD patients in the PI-500 study remained ill until they received lithium or phenelzine, depending on their target symptoms, and have now remained well for 10 or 15 years. One such patient—a woman with severe trichotillomania, depression, drug abuse, promiscuity, and violence from, and toward, her parents—did poorly with psychotherapy of any type; once on phenelzine, however, she was able to calm down, work, marry, and raise a family. Another patient—a man who had been in therapy for 30 years because of severe depression and ago-raphobia—remained dysfunctional all that time until he spent a week in a kind of marathon session with a "Primal Scream" therapist. Since then he has been literally a new man, successful in business as well as in his interpersonal life. Several borderline patients eloped from the Psychiatric Institute because they could not get on with the therapists assigned to them, never re-entered therapy with anyone else, and are now among the best-functioning patients in this study. Meanwhile, 10 of the borderline patients "clicked" both with expressive therapy and with their particular therapists, eventually became PhD psychologists and therapists themselves, and are also among the best outcomes in the study. No one method can claim an exclusive hold on the title "treatment of choice." Instead, this depends a great deal on the cognitive style of the patient, on the culture in which the patient was raised, on the type of therapy most congenial to the training and personality of the therapist, and on the elusive "chemistry" between them. (As a not-so-irrelevant aside, I have become convinced through my own involvement in long-term follow-up work that a "scientific" answer to the question about the ideal type of psychotherapy for borderline patients will never be forthcoming, owing to the staggering number of variables one would have to control for in a matched, randomized study.)

As a final comment on the issue of expressive therapy, I can add that in the 26 traced (out of 27) BPD patients in my private-practice series, beginning in 1966, the 4 who were most amenable to this modality have all done unusually well (GAS scores greater than 80); the 4 next in line have done moderately well (GAS scores of 48–69). The 8 with only fair or inconsistent amenability are now spread out over a range of GAS scores from 42 to 88, and the 10 I considered not suitable for this modality include 7 with a poor outcome—but also 3 who have done surprisingly well.

Looking at the darker side of the borderline domain, we may note from the follow-up studies that perhaps a third of hospitalized BPD patients have a dismal life trajectory. Sometimes this seems related to heavy genetic loading for affective illness (in those with BPD × MAD, BPD × bipolar II disorder etc.). But, more often, the poor outcomes are correlated with early and chronic parental abuse. The latter may reach the proportions noted in cases of multiple personality (Kluft, 1985). These patients exhibit many of the phenomena of post-traumatic stress disorder. The more brutal and dehumanizing the early environment, the more destructive the effects on development, and often the more rageful, vengeful, and irritable the resulting personality. The sorry fate of most such borderline patients should put therapists on warning not to expect "quick" or even gradual recoveries in many patients with histories of extreme cruelty or rejection. This realization has, however, a benefit attached to it: Namely, therapists need not become entangled in countertransference feelings of "failure" when faced with all-but-incurable patients whom they (and usually many therapists before them) have been unable to help. The follow-up studies have delineated the attributes of this unfortunate group better than was hitherto possible. Therapists should also take some comfort in the realization that a proportion of borderline patients, after years of stormy and ultimately unsuccessful relationships, eventually give up the struggle, opting instead for a less fulfilling but much less troublesome life. Such a resolution may represent an optimum, and therapists confronted with borderline patients of this type should feel pride rather than embarrassment at having helped their patients achieve stability in this way (Stone, 1988; Melges & Swartz, 1989).

SUMMARY AND DIRECTIONS FOR FUTURE FOLLOW-UP STUDIES

The consensus of the long-term studies of BPD thus far reported is that borderline patients (whether defined by DSM or by Gunderson criteria) generally come to the attention of the health care system during late adolescence or their early 20s; they continue to show impaired function throughout their 20s (especially in cases where substance abuse is a complicating factor), but begin to improve 8 to 10 years after their original diagnosis. In these studies, which have focused on hospitalized patients, two-thirds have reached levels of functioning consistent with GAS scores above 60. The suicide risk is such that by 15 or 20 years of follow-up, 3–9% have committed suicide (the figures vary in accordance with age on admission, prevalence of alcohol abuse in the original sample, etc.). Those failing to reach GAS scores above 60 have done so for a variety of reasons, including (1) admixture of schizotypal traits, (2) antisocial features, (3) histories of parental abusiveness, (4) concomitant unipolar depression, or (5) persistent negative traits such as chaotic impulsivity or hostility. Anecdotal material concerning clinic and office patients suggests that their long-term course and outcome is at least as favorable as those first identified via a hospitalization, perhaps better. Patients who meet Kernberg criteria for BPO, but who do not meet DSM/Gunderson criteria for BPD, enjoy a lower suicide risk as a group (since the kinds of anger and impulsivity that predispose patients to suicide would tend to place them in the BPD category); on other respects, their fate depends on the nature of their predominant personality traits.

Borderline patients who have made substantial improvement are found to have done so in relation to a variety of therapeutic modalities: expressive–supportive, purely supportive, cognitive, behavioral, and psychopharmacological (singly or in combination). Patients exhibiting optimal amenability to expressive psychotherapy are more apt to be diagnosed as having BPO but not BPD. This may relate to the more dramatic levels of anger and impulsivity in the BPD patients, rendering them less "containable" within the confines of a purely expressive therapy, and more in need of limit setting and other supportive/behavioral interventions.

Future follow-up studies of patients in the borderline domain should ideally be long-term (more than 5 years) in design, in order to give the patients the opportunity to stabilize at a level more truly consistent with their ultimate life trajectory than can be ascertained within a 2- or 3-year "look" at the future. Research design should be prospective rather than retrospective wherever possible, in order to facilitate the mapping out of the life course, rather than just the outcome at some fixed point on the patients' life calendar. Investigators should pay more attention than heretofore to positive personality traits (e.g., likeableness, courage, responsibility) and to areas of strength (e.g., artistic talents, intellectual skills), rather than just to concomitant DSM Axis I or II conditions. Closer attention should also be paid to the precise details of early abusive experiences at the hands of caretakers. Extensive clinical vignettes of each patient (if these can be made available without sacrifice of confidentiality) will also be useful, by way of enhancing communication among investigators.

REFERENCES

Akiskal, H. (1981). Subaffective disorders: Dysthymic, cyclothymic and bipolar II disorders in the "borderline" realm. *Psychiatric Clinics of North America*, 4(1), 25–46.

American Psychiatric Association. (1980). *Diagnostic and statistical manual of mental disorders* (3rd ed.). Washington, DC: Author.

Angst, J., & Clayton, P. (1986). Premorbid personality of depressive, bipolar and schizophrenic patients with special reference to suicidal issues. *Comprehensive Psychiatry*, *27*, 511–532.

Carpenter, W. T., Gunderson, J. G., & Strauss, J. S. (1977). Considerations of the borderline syndrome: A longitudinal comparative study of borderline and schizophrenic patients. In P. Hartocollis (Ed.), *Borderline personality disorders*. New York: International Universities Press.

Endicott, J., Spitzer, R. L., Fleiss, J. L., & Cohen, J. (1976). The Global Assessment Scale. *Archives of General Psychiatry*, *33*, 766–771.

Fenton, W. S., & McGlashan, T. H. (1989). Risk of schizophrenia in character-disordered patients. *American Journal of Psychiatry*, *146*, 1280–1284.

Gidro-Frank, L., Peretz, D., Spitzer, R., & Winikus, W. (1976). A five-year follow-up of male patients hospitalized at Psychiatric Institute. *Psychiatric Quarterly*, *41*, 1–35.

Grinker, R. R., Werble, B., & Drye, R. C. (1968). *The borderline syndrome*. New York: Basic Books.

Gunderson, J. G., Carpenter, W. T., & Strauss, J. S. (1975). Borderline and schizophrenic patients: A comparative study. *American Journal of Psychiatry*, *132*, 1257–1264.

Gunderson, J. G., Kolb, J., & Austin, V. (1981). The Diagnostic Interview for Borderline Patients. *American Journal of Psychiatry*, *138*, 896–903.

Gunderson, J. G., & Singer, M. T. (1975). Defining borderline patients: An overview. *American Journal of Psychiatry*, *132*, 1–10.

Hoch, P. H., Cattell, J. P., Strahl, M. O., & Pennes, H. H. (1962). The course and outcome of pseudoneurotic schizophrenia. *American Journal of Psychiatry*, *119*, 106–115.

Hoch, P., & Polatin, P. (1949). Pseudoneurotic forms of schizophrenia. *Psychiatric Quarterly*, *23*, 248–276.

Holm, K., & Hundevadt, E. (1976). Psykiatrisk pasient—episode eller livs form? En etterundersøkelse. *Tidsskrift for det Norske Laegeforen*, *96*, 1131–1135.

Holm, K., & Hundevadt, E. (1981). Borderline states: Prognosis and psychotherapy. *British Journal of Medical Psychology*, *54*, 335–340.

Kernberg, O. F. (1967). Borderline personality organization. *Journal of the American Psychoanalytic Association*, *15*, 641–685.

Kernberg, O. F. (1988, May 11). *The differential diagnosis of antisocial behavior*. Paper presented at the 140th annual meeting of the American Psychiatric Association, Chicago.

Kluft, R. P. (1985). Childhood multiple personality disorder: Predictors, clinical findings, and treatment results. In R. P. Kluft (Ed.), *Childhood antecedents of multiple personality*. Washington, DC: American Psychiatric Press.

Kolb, L. (1982). Assertive traits fostering social adaptation and creativity. *Psychiatric Journal of the University of Ottawa*, *7*, 219–225.

Kroll, J. L., Carey, K. S., & Sines, L. K. (1985). Twenty-year follow-up of borderline personality disorder: A pilot study. In C. Stragass (Ed.), *IV World Congress of Biological Psychiatry* (Vol. 3). New York: Elsevier.

Luborsky, L. (1962). Clinicians' judgments of mental health: A proposed scale. *Archives of General Psychiatry*, *7*, 407–417.

McGlashan, T. H. (1986). The Chestnut Lodge follow-up study: III. Long-term outcome of borderline personality disorder. *Archives of General Psychiatry, 43,* 20–30.

Masterson, J., & Costello, J. (1980). *From borderline adolescent to functioning adult.* New York: Brunner/Mazel.

Melges, F. T., & Swartz, M. S. (1989). Oscillations of attachment in borderline personality disorder. *American Journal of Psychiatry, 146,* 1115–1120.

Nyman, A. K. (1978). Nonregressive schizophrenia: Clinical course and outcome. *Acta Psychiatrica Scandinavica* (Suppl. 272).

Paris, J., Brown, R., & Nowlis, D. (1987). Long-term follow-up of borderline patients in a general hospital. *Comprehensive Psychiatry, 28,* 530–535.

Perry, J. C. (1985). Depression in borderline personality disorder: Lifetime prevalence at interview and longitudinal course of symptoms. *American Journal of Psychiatry, 142,* 15–21.

Perry, J. C., & Cooper, S. H. (1985). Psychodynamics, symptoms, and outcome in borderline and antisocial personality disorders and bipolar type II affective disorder. In T. H. McGlashan (Ed.), *The borderline: Current empirical research.* Washington, DC: American Psychiatric Press.

Plakun, E. M., Burkhardt, P. E., & Muller, J. P. (1985). 14-year follow-up of borderline and schizotypal personality disorders. *Comprehensive Psychiatry, 26,* 448–455.

Pope, H. G., Jonas, J. M., & Hudson, J. (1983). The validity of DSM-III borderline personality disorder. *Archives of General Psychiatry, 40,* 23–30.

Solomon, M. I., & Murphy, G. E. (1984). Cohort studies in suicide. In H. S. Sudak, A. B. Ford, & N. B. Rushforth (Eds.), *Suicide in the young.* Boston: John Wright/PSG.

Stone, M. H. (1988). The borderline domain: The "inner script" and other common psychodynamics. In J. Howells (Ed.), *Modern perspectives in psychiatry* (Vol. 11). New York: Brunner/Mazel.

Stone, M. H. (1989). The course of borderline personality disorder. In A. Tasman, R. E. Hales, & A. J. Frances (Eds.), *Review of psychiatry* (Vol. 8). Washington, DC: American Psychiatric Press.

Stone, M. H. (1990a). Borderline anger: The border of treatability. Follow-up data and implications for amenability to psychotherapy. *Psychiatria et Neurologia Japonica, 92,* 824–830.

Stone, M. H. (1990b). *The fate of borderline patients.* New York: Guilford Press.

Stone, M. H., Hurt, S. W., & Stone, D. K. (1987). The P.I.-500: Long-term follow-up of borderline inpatients meeting DSM-III criteria. *Journal of Personality Disorders, 1,* 291–298.

Tucker, L., Bauer, S. F., Wagner, S., Harlam, D., & Sher, I. (1987). Long-term hospital treatment of borderline patients: A descriptive outcome study. *American Journal of Psychiatry, 144*(11), 1443–1448.

Wallerstein, R. (1986). *Forty-two lives in treatment.* New York: Guilford Press.

Werble, B. (1970). Second follow-up study of borderline patients. *Archives of General Psychiatry, 23,* 3–7.

PART THREE

DIAGNOSIS

CHAPTER 5

Alternative Perspectives on the Diagnosis of Borderline Personality Disorder

THOMAS A. WIDIGER
GLORIA M. MIELE
SARAH M. TILLY

This chapter is concerned with the diagnosis of borderline personality disorder (BPD). We begin with an overview of the major formulations and the research relevant to assessing their convergent validity. We then discuss the principal controversies concerning the diagnosis, including the identification of the optimal diagnostic criteria, the importance of psychotic symptomatology, and the use of a categorical model of classification. We then conclude with a discussion of applications of this research for clinical practice and recommendations for future research.

ALTERNATIVE FORMULATIONS

Kernberg (1967) provided an early and influential formulation. He distinguished between a "descriptive" and a "structural" diagnosis. The descriptive features included (1) chronic, diffuse, free-floating anxiety; (2) polysymptomatic neurosis; (3) polymorphous perverse sexual trends (i.e., manifest sexual deviation with several paraphilias); (4) prepsychotic personality structures (e.g., *Diagnostic and Statistical Manual of Mental Disorders*, second edition [DSM-II] paranoid, schizoid, hypomanic, or cyclothymic); (5) impulse disorders; and (6) low-level character disorders. None of these alone was considered to be pathognomonic, "but the presence of two, and especially of three, symptoms . . . strongly points to the possibility of an underlying borderline personality organization" (Kernberg, 1967, p. 647). A definitive diagnosis required an analysis of the structural derivatives of internalized object relationships. These included (1) nonspecific manifestations of ego weakness; (2) a shift toward primary-process thinking; (3) specific defense operations; and (4) pathology of internalized object relationships. The nonspecific indicators of ego weakness included lack of anxiety tolerance, impulse control, and/or sublimatory channels. The shift toward primary-process thinking was considered to be fundamental: "The regression toward primary-process thinking is still the most important single structural indicator of borderline personality organization" (p. 663). Kernberg further noted that "its detection through the use of projective tests makes sophisticated psychological testing an indispensable instrument for the diagnosis" (p. 663). The specific defensive operations included splitting (the primary borderline defense), projective identification, denial, omnipotence, and devaluation. The pathology of internalized object relationships was believed to be essentially identity diffusion (i.e., confused, contradictory, vague, or exaggerated perceptions and representations of self and/or others).

Gunderson and Singer (1975) canvassed the literature 8 years later to identify "the most common and distinguishing characteristics" (p. 2). They gleaned six features from their review: (1) intense affect (usually strongly hostile or depressed, with depersonalization and an absence of flatness and pleasure); (2) history of impulsive behavior (e.g., self-mutilation, overdose, drug dependency, or promiscuity); (3) social adaptiveness (e.g., good achievement in school or work, appropriate appearance and manners, and strong social awareness); (4) brief psychotic experiences (likely to have a paranoid quality, with psychosis becoming particularly evident during drug use or in unstructured situations); (5) bizarre or primitive performance on unstructured tests (e.g., the Rorschach), but not on structured tests (e.g., intelligence tests); and (6) vacillation between transient, superficial relationships and intense, dependent relationships marred by devaluation, manipulation, and demandingness.

The effort by Gunderson and Singer (1975) was followed by a comparable review by Perry and Klerman (1978). Perry and Klerman, however, confined themselves to the four descriptions provided by Knight (1953), Kernberg (1967), Grinker, Werble, and Drye (1968), and Gunderson and Singer (1975). They systematically extracted the diagnostic features from each monograph and assessed their congruency: "Of the total of 104 separate criteria, 55, approximately half, are present in only *one* of the four different sets of diagnostic criteria. Conversely, only one criterion was found in all four sets" (p. 149). This lack of congruency is particularly surprising, given that Gunderson and Singer provided features common to the prior descriptions (including those by Kernberg, Knight, and Grinker et al.). The only feature common to all four models was "that the patient's behavior in the interview is usually adaptive and appropriate" (p. 146)—a feature that not only is nonspecific but is no longer associated with BPD in current formulations.

Perry and Klerman (1978) lamented the lack of congruency and suggested that it was due to the presence of subtypes. Nevertheless, in a subsequent paper, Perry and Klerman (1980) abandoned the notion of subtyping and developed a Borderline Personality Scale (BPS) for the diagnosis of one inclusive type. They constructed 129 items to operationalize the 104 criteria. The BPS consisted of the 81 items that successfully differentiated a group of 18 borderlines from patients with neurosis ($n = 13$), schizophrenia ($n = 13$), other personality disorder ($n = 17$), and adjustment reaction ($n = 25$). Space limitations prohibit listing all 81 features, but it is worth noting some that are no longer associated with BPD (e.g., less attractive than other patients, seems bright/intelligent, lacks creative achievement, previous psychiatric hospitalizations, destructive to property or things, sadistic in close relationships, masochistic in close relationships, talks as if omnipotent, suggests grossly inappropriate treatment, narcissistically preoccupied, and not psychotic during time of interview).

A third formulation of BPD was provided by Spitzer, Endicott, and Gibbon (1979): "It appeared to us, from a review of the literature as well as from personal contact with current investigators . . . that there are two major ways in which 'borderline' is currently used" (p. 17). The first referred to a constellation of instability and vulnerability, as exemplified by the formulations of Gunderson and Singer (1975) and Kernberg (1967). The second referred to a set of schizophrenic-like features, as exemplified in the "borderline schizophrenia" research of Kety, Rosenthal, Wender, and Schulsinger (1971). The former became the DSM-III BPD, and the latter became the DSM-III schizotypal personality disorder (American Psychiatric Association [APA], 1980). The initial draft of the BPD criteria consisted of nine items: (1) identity disturbance, manifested by uncertainty about several issues related to identity (e.g., self-image, gender identity, long-term goals or career choice, friendship patterns, values, or loyalties); (2) unstable and intense relationships (e.g., marked shifts of attitude, idealization, devaluation, or manipulation); (3) impulsivity or unpredictability in at least two areas that are potentially self-damaging (e.g., spending, sex, gambling, drug or alcohol use, shoplifting, overeating, or physically self-damaging acts); (4) inappropriate intense anger or lack of control of anger; (5) physically self-damaging acts (e.g., suicidal gestures, self-mutilation, recurrent accidents, or physical fights); (6) work history or school achivement unstable or below intelligence, training, or opportunities; (7) affective instability (marked shifts from normal mood to depression, irritability, or anxiety); (8) chronic feelings of emptiness or boredom; and (9) problems tolerating being alone (e.g., frantic efforts to avoid being alone or depressed when alone) (Spitzer et al., 1979).

There are more similarities than differences between the formulations by Spitzer et al. (1979) and Gunderson and Singer (1975), but it is useful to highlight the differences. A fundamental difference is the inclusion of brief psychotic experiences by Gunderson and Singer (1975) and their exclusion by Spitzer et al. (1979). Spitzer et al. excluded such features because they made a distinction between (1) the "borderline" conditions associated with schizophrenia, such as borderline schizophrenia (Kety et al., 1971), pseudo-neurotic schizophrenia (Hoch & Cattell, 1959), latent schizophrenia (Bleuler, 1911/1950), and ambulatory schizophrenia (Zilboorg, 1941); and (2) "borderline" conditions characterized instead by a history of impulsivity, affective instability, and unstable, intense relationships, as exemplified in the descriptions of Kernberg (1967), Stern (1938), and Grinker et al. (1968). Gunderson and Singer (1975), on the other hand, made no such distinction, including within their formulation of BPD the borderline schizophrenia of Kety et al. (1971), the pseudoneurotic schizophrenia of Hoch and Cattell (1959), and other conditions that would now be diagnosed as schizotypal. It is thus not surprising that Gunderson initially opposed the inclusion of the schizotypal diagnosis in DSM-III (Gunderson, 1983; Siever & Gunderson, 1979) and has argued that the DSM-III (-R) formulation is inadequate in its exclusion of the psychotic-like features.

There are similarities in the formulations by Kernberg (1967, 1975) and Spitzer et al. (1979). The Spitzer et al. item of identity disturbance corresponds to Kernberg's feature of identity diffusion. However, Kernberg (1984) has characterized the features emphasized by Spitzer et al. (1979), Gunderson and Singer (1975), and Perry and Klerman (1980) as essentially nonspecific manifestations. Kernberg's concept of "borderline personality organization" is also broader than the DSM-III-R concept of BPD. Most inpatients with a personality disorder would probably be at a borderline level of personality organization, particularly those with the more dysfunctional personality disorders (such as borderline, schizotypal, schizoid, paranoid, antisocial, and histrionic).

The final formulation to be considered here is that provided by Millon (1969, 1981). Millon (1983) suggested that the DSM-III diagnosis of BPD was "written from a perspective at variance with traditional psychiatric roots" (p. 812). "The Borderline personality was formulated to be a disintegrated Dependent, Histrionic, and Passive–aggressive mix" (Millon, 1983, p. 512). This is somewhat at variance with the discussion by Spitzer et al. (1979). Nevertheless, because of Millon's influence on DSM-III (Gunderson, 1983; Kernberg, 1984) and the popularity of the Millon Clinical Multiaxial Inventory (MCMI; Millon, 1977, 1987), Millon's formulation of BPD is of substantial clinical and theoretical importance.

Millon (1969, 1981) based his formulation on a review of the prior literature, but he also derived the borderline construct from a theoretical model that posits three basic polarities: pleasure–pain, self–other, and active–passive. BPD is considered to be a severe variant of the dependent, histrionic, passive–aggressive, and compulsive personality disorders, sharing with them an ambivalent and/or dependent orientation. Millon's (1969) original term for the borderline was "cycloid," which nicely connotes the emphasis he placed on fluctuating affective symptomatology. "The most striking feature of the cycloid is the intensity of his moods and the frequent changeability of his behaviors" (Millon, 1969, p. 318). In his 1981 formulation, he identified five diagnostic criteria: (1) intense, endogenous moods (including euphoria, as well as anxiety, depression, and anger); (2) dysregulated activation (e.g., irregular sleep–wake cycle); (3) self-condemnatory conscience (e.g., self-mutilation and suicidal thoughts, contrition, and self-derogation); (4) dependency anxiety (preoccupied with securing affection, intense reactions to separation, and haunting fear of isolation or loss); and (5) cognitive–affective ambivalence (conflicting emotions and thoughts regarding others).

The formulations of Millon (1981) and Kernberg (1984) share a distinction from those of Spitzer et al. (1979), Gunderson and Singer (1975), and Perry and Klerman (1980): They refer to a more dysfunctional variant of personality *organization*, rather than to a distinct personality *disorder*. However, an important distinction between them is that Kernberg (1984) gives primary attention to internal structural characteristics, whereas Millon (1981) gives equal emphasis to overt phenomenology.

Revisions

One of the problems cited in the early borderline literature was that descriptions changed over time. Gunderson and Singer (1975), for example, criticized the tendency for "some authors [to] expand or contract their definitions of borderline patients in later publications" (p. 2). Similar concerns have been raised with respect to the pace at which the DSM is being revised (Zimmerman, 1988). It is therefore useful to note any changes that have occurred in the diagnostic formulations. Here, we consider revisions by Kernberg, Gunderson, Millon, and Spitzer.

Kernberg

Kernberg's (1981, 1984) subsequent presentations of his criteria for the borderline diagnosis have not involved substantive changes. The criteria have simply become somewhat more explicit, with a further emphasis on the structural assessment of internalized object relations and primitive defenses. Kernberg now distinguishes among the neurotic, borderline, and psychotic levels of personality organization on the basis of an assessment of identity integration, defensive operations, and capacity for reality testing. The borderline displays identity diffusion, whereas the neurotic displays an integrated and differentiated identity, and the psychotic displays at best a delusional identity. The borderline also relies on the primitive defenses of splitting, denial, idealization, devaluation, and projective identification, whereas the neurotic uses higher-level defenses such as reaction formation, undoing, intellectualization, and repression. The borderline is distinguished from the psychotic on the basis of responding with improved functioning to the interpretation of these defenses, whereas the psychotic tends to regress. Finally, the borderline and neurotic both display adequate reality testing, as this is usually defined. However, one of the more useful aspects of Kernberg's formulation is the recognition that borderlines have inadequate reality testing with respect to their object (interpersonal) relations, tending to perceive and react to others in an exaggerated, distorted, unrealistic, and inappropriate manner.

Gunderson

Table 5.1 lists the criteria for diagnosing BPD by Gunderson and Singer (1975), Gunderson and Kolb (1978), and Gunderson and Zanarini (1987). It is evident from Table 5.1 that there have been substantial changes in the criteria. For example, the criterion of chronic abandonment fears, characterized by "sustained and conscious apprehensions that those on whom they feel dependent will desert them" (Gunderson & Zanarini, 1987, p. 6), was not included in the first two formulations. It is comparable to, but certainly not equivalent to, the Gunderson and Kolb (1978) criterion of high socialization (which included an intolerance of being alone).

The borderline was characterized by Gunderson and Singer (1975) as manifesting "good achievement in school or work, appropriate appearance and manners, and strong social awareness" (p. 8). Gunderson and Kolb

TABLE 5.1. Diagnosis of Borderline by Gunderson and Colleagues

Gunderson & Singer (1975)	Gunderson & Kolb (1978)	Gunderson & Zanarini (1987)
History of impulsive behavior	Impulsivity Manipulative suicide	Impulsivity Repetitive self-destructive acts
Presence of intense affect	Heightened affectivity	Chronic dysphoric affect
Brief psychotic experiences	Mild psychotic experiences	Cognitive distortions
Vacillation of relationships	Disturbed close relationships	Intense, unstable relationships
Social adaptiveness	Low achievement High socialization	Poor social adaptation Chronic abandonment fears
Psychological test performance		

(1978), however, indicated that "the typical level of the school and work achievement . . . was quite low" (p. 794). In Gunderson and Zanarini (1987), "social adaptiveness" became "poor social adaptation," with borderlines having "functional histories fraught with rapid shifts, repeated fights, and failures" (p. 6).

The description of the psychotic symptomatology has also shifted. Gunderson and Singer (1975) emphasized the paranoid quality of the psychotic symptoms and their tendency to "become evident during drug use or in unstructured situations and relationships" (p. 8). Gunderson and Kolb (1978), however, indicated that the psychotic symptoms "most commonly took the form of drug-free paranoid ideation, derealization experiences, and a history of regressions" (p. 795). This description was broadened in some respects and narrowed in others by Gunderson and Zanarini (1987), who indicated "that the cognitive experiences that best discriminate borderline patients are nondelusional, paranoid experiences (e.g., ideas of reference, undue suspiciousness), dissociative experiences, and odd types of thinking, particularly suspiciousness, magical thinking, and a sixth sense" (p. 6).

These revisions are not without a substantive effect on the diagnosis. Table 5.2 provides the sections and items from the Diagnostic Interview for Borderlines (DIB) developed by Gunderson, Kolb, and Austin (1981) (based largely on Gunderson & Kolb, 1978), and the DIB-R developed by Zanarini, Gunderson, Frankenburg, and Chauncey (1989) (corresponding to Gunderson & Zanarini, 1987). The Social Adaptation section and 5 of the remaining 25 items of the DIB were deleted in the DIB-R (i.e., drug-induced psychosis, flat/elated affect, hallucinations or delusions, mania/delusions, and social isolation/loner). Four items were added (i.e., chronic anxiety, odd thinking or unusual perceptual experiences, quasi-psychotic experiences, and abandonment/engulfment/annihilation concerns). The Psychosis section was renamed the Cognition section and revised to include various forms of disturbed but nonpsychotic thought. An empirical comparison of the DIB and DIB-R has not yet been published, but Zanarini et al. (1989) have indicated that the revised measure results in substantially fewer patients' being diagnosed borderline.

Millon

Table 5.3 summarizes the descriptive features of BPD provided by Millon in 1969, 1981, and 1986. Millon (1969) originally used the term "borderline" to refer to all of the personality patterns at a moderately maladaptive level of functioning. These included the schizoid, cycloid, and paranoid, which corresponded roughly to the DSM-II diagnoses of (1) schizoid personality, latent schizophrenia, and simple schizophrenia (detached borderlines), (2)

TABLE 5.2. Diagnostic Interview for Borderlines: Original and Revised

DIB (Gunderson, Kolb, & Austin, 1981)	DIB-R (Zanarini, Gunderson, Frankenburg, & Chauncey, 1989)
Social Adaptation	
1. Unstable school/work achievement	
2. Special abilities/talent	
3. Active social life	
4. Appropriate appearance/ manners	
Impulse Action Patterns	*Impulse Action Patterns*
5. Self-mutilation	1. Self-mutilation
6. Manipulative suicide efforts	2. Manipulative suicide efforts
7. Drug abuse	3. Substance abuse/dependence
8. Sexual deviance	4. Sexual deviance
9. Antisocial impulsivity	5. Other impulsive patterns
Affect	*Affect*
10. Recent/chronic depression	6. Chronic major depression
11. Hostile	7. Chronic anger/frequent angry acts
12. Demanding/entitled	[see Interpersonal Relations section]
13. Dysphoria/anhedonia	8. Chronic loneliness/boredom/emptiness
14. Flat/elated affect	9. Chronic helpless/hopeless/worthless
	10. Chronic anxiety
Psychosis	*Cognition*
15. Derealization	11. Odd thinking/unusual perceptual experiences
16. Depersonalization	
17. Depressive, drug-free psychosis	[see Affect section]
18. Paranoid, drug-free psychosis	12. Nondelusional paranoid experiences
	13. Quasi-psychotic experiences
19. Drug-induced psychoses	
20. Bizarre hallucinations/grandiose delusions	
21. Mania/widespread delusions	
22. Past therapy regressions	[see Interpersonal Relations section]
Interpersonal Relations	*Interpersonal Relations*
23. Avoids being alone	14. Intolerance of aloneness
24. Socially isolated/loner	
25. Anaclitic relations	15. Counterdependency conflicts
26. Intense, unstable relations	16. Stormy relationships
27. Devaluation/manipulation	17. Devaluation/manipulation/sadism
28. Dependency/masochism	18. Dependency/masochism
29. Countertransference problems	19. Countertransference problems
	20. Demandingness/entitlement
	21. Treatment regression
	22. Abandonment/engulfment/annihilation concerns

Note. Order of DIB-R items has been altered to match that of DIB items.

96

TABLE 5.3. Diagnosis of Borderline by Millon (1969, 1981, 1986)

Millon (1969) Cycloid	Millon (1981) Unstable	Millon (1986) Borderline
Intense moods	Intense endogenous moods	Labile mood
Vacillation of behavior	Dysregulated activation	Behaviorally precipitate
Self-devaluing	Self-condemnatory conscience	Uncertain self-image
Dependency conflicts	Dependency anxiety	Interpersonally paradoxical
Distrustful and hostile		
Anxious, insecure		
Cognitive conflicts	Cognitive–affective ambivalence	Cognitively capricious
		Regression mechanism
		Incompatible internalizations
		Diffused intrapsychic organization

Note. The 1969 list is a summary from a narrative description.

cyclothymic personality (dependent and ambivalent borderlines), and (3) paranoid personality (independent and ambivalent borderlines), respectively. All three shared the features of deficient social competence and periodic but reversible psychotic episodes.

The features of the cycloid borderline (presented in Table 5.3) correspond closely to those of BPD. A more specific description was provided in 1981, with the association shifting from the DSM-II cyclothymic personality to the DSM-III BPD (originally labeled "unstable" by Spitzer et al., 1979, and Millon, 1981). The 1981 unstable pattern was again considered to be a severe variant of the dependent and ambivalent personality patterns. Millon (1986) has more recently attempted to include all of the domains of functioning in the formulations of each personality disorder, including the behavioral presentation, interpersonal style, cognitive style, expressive mood, unconscious defense mechanisms, self-image, internalized representations, and intrapsychic organization. A description of BPD (now termed "borderline") with respect to each of these domains is presented in Table 5.3.

The extent to which the 1986 revision represents a shift in diagnosis can be inferred from the respective versions of the MCMI. The original version of the MCMI (Millon, 1977) corresponds to the 1981 formulation, and the MCMI-II (Millon, 1987) corresponds to the 1986 formulation. Millon (1987) indicates that "significant substantive shifts occurred" (p. 91) in the borderline scale. Three items were deleted, six were added, and a new weighting scheme was implemented, with 11 items given a weight of 3 points each, 19 counting for 2 points each, and 32 counting for 1 point. The correlation between the MCMI and MCMI-II borderline scales is .74 (Millon, 1987), which is substantial but also indicates that only 55% of their variance is shared. It also appears that the MCMI-II diagnoses fewer persons as borderline and gives relatively less emphasis to affective features (Millon, 1987). Costa and McCrae (1990) compared the MCMI and the MCMI-II with respect to their coorelations with the five-factor model of personality. The MCMI borderline scale correlated positively with neuroticism, agreeableness, and introversion, whereas the MCMI-II scale correlated positively with neuroticism but negatively with agreeableness and conscientiousness. In other words, the MCMI described the borderline as agreeable, whereas the MCMI-II described the borderline as antagonistic.

Spitzer

Table 5.4 presents the BPD criteria from Spitzer et al. (1979), DSM-III (APA, 1980), and DSM-III-R (APA, 1987). The initial criteria set generated by Spitzer et al. was essentially a working draft for DSM-III. The only substantial revision by DSM-III was the deletion of the work history item, on the basis of its failure to adequately distinguish borderlines from patients with other disorders and its association with the schizotypal rather than the borderline.

The change from DSM-III to DSM-III-R involved revisions of individual items (e.g, deletion of the feature of manipulation from the interpersonal

TABLE 5.4. Diagnosis of Borderline by Spitzer and Colleagues

Spitzer, Endicott, & Gibbon(1979)	DSM-III (APA, 1980)	DSM-III-R (APA, 1987)
Identity disturbance	Identity disturbance	Marked/persistent identity disturbance
Unstable/intense relationships	Unstable/intense relationships	Unstable/intense relationships
Impulsivity/unpredictability	Impulsivity/unpredictability	Impulsivity
Inappropriate/intense anger	Inappropriate/intense anger	Inappropriate/intense anger
Physically self-damaging acts	Physically self-damaging acts	Recurrent suicidal threats/gestures
Affective instability	Affective instability	Affective instability
Chronic emptiness/boredom	Chronic emptiness/ boredom	Chronic emptiness/boredom
Problems tolerating being alone	Intolerance of being alone	Frantic efforts to avoid abandonment
Unstable work/school history		

relationship item; addition of physical fights to anger; deletion of gambling from impulsivity; deletion of a return to normal mood from affectivity; and the deletion of physical fights and accidents from the self-damaging item), as well as the replacement of intolerance of being alone with frantic efforts to avoid real or imagined abandonment. The effect of these revisions appears to be minimal. Morey (1988b) applied the DSM-III and DSM-III-R criteria to the same group of 291 patients and found little disagreement, with a kappa of .97. However, it should be noted that additional revisions are being considered for DSM-IV, including the deletion of boredom; revision of identity disturbance to a persistent and markedly disturbed, distorted, or unstable self-image and/or sense of self; deletion of the alternation between idealization and devaluation from the unstable relationships item; inclusion of marked reactivity in the affective instability item; and addition of an item concerned with cognitive and/or perceptual aberrations (e.g., cognitive or perceptual disturbances that are stress-related, circumscribed, and responsive to external structure).

Empirical Comparisons

An empirical comparison of the various formulations is complicated by the reliance on assessment instruments of questionable reliability and validity. It is not always clear whether poor agreement is due to the measurement instrument or to the constructs, since there is often poor agreement between instruments that measure the same personality disorder construct (Angus & Marziali, 1988; Dubro, Wetzler, & Kahn, 1988; Reich, Noyes, & Troughton, 1987; Skodol, Rosnick, Kellman, Oldham, & Hyler, 1988). Most of the research has concerned a comparison of the DSM-III and Gunderson and Kolb (1978) formulations, for which the concurrent validity has varied from poor to good (Widiger & Frances, 1989). The expectation has been that the DIB would be more inclusive than the DSM-III, given the broadening of the criteria to include psychotic symptomatology. This expectation was confirmed by Angus and Marziali (1988) and Barrash, Kroll, Carey, and Sines (1983), but not by Frances, Clarkin, Gilmore, Hurt, and Brown (1984), Kullgren (1987), or Loranger, Oldham, Russakoff, and Susman (1984), who found only inconsequential differences. McGlashan (1983) and Nelson et al. (1985), in fact, reported the DSM-III to be more inclusive.

The inconsistency in findings is due in part to variation in settings and in researchers' interpretations of the criteria. In settings where there is little psychotic symptomatology (e.g., private practices and outpatient clinics), the differences could be minimized. Researchers will also develop different operationalizations for each criterion, and raters will vary with respect to the threshold for their attribution of each criterion (Angus & Marziali, 1988;

Skodol et al., 1988). Researchers have been successful in obtaining interrater reliability within particular sites, but this has been at the cost of establishing local operational criteria for the attribution of each item that do not always agree well with the criteria being used elsewhere.

The inclusivity of a criteria set is also dependent upon the algorithm for the diagnosis. DSM-III was based on the presence of any five criteria of eight possible, whereas the DIB was based on the scores for 29 items organized into five sections, with each section given a score from 0 to 2 and the final diagnosis based on a total score of 7 out of a possible 10. It is not at all clear whether a score of 7 on the DIB is comparable to a score of 5 on the DSM-III. Dahl (1985) indicates that one can obtain a maximum section score of 10 on the DIB with only 14 of the 29 individual items endorsed. In addition, the Psychosis section of the DIB need not have an impact on the diagnosis at all.

Dahl's (1985) comments concerning the DIB also apply to the DIB-R (described earlier). The DIB-R includes four sections, with the Affect and Cognition sections each providing 0–2 points toward the final diagnosis, and the Impulse Action Patterns and Interpersonal Relationships sections each providing 0–3 points (Zanarini et al., 1989). A score of 8 on the DIB-R is considered to be indicative of BPD, which could be obtained without any disturbance in affect or cognition. In addition, it is possible to obtain the maximum section score of 2 for the Cognition section by endorsing only 2 of its 31 items (similar thresholds are used for the other three sections). In other words, it is again not at all clear whether a score of 8 on the DIB-R is comparable to a score of 5 on the DSM-III-R.

It has also been assumed that Kernberg's (1975, 1984) structural criteria are more inclusive than those of the DSM-III(-R) or the DIB(-R) (Gunderson & Zanarini, 1987; Stone, 1980; Widiger, 1982), but there was only a trend toward this finding in the studies by Kernberg et al. (1981) and Nelson et al. (1985). Kernberg et al., for example, diagnosed 25 of 48 inpatients as borderline by the structural criteria, whereas 21 of 48 were diagnosed as having BPD by the DIB. Kernberg et al. did suggest that the structural diagnosis was more inclusive, considering "many cases borderline that other methods call psychotic" (p. 230). This is somewhat ironic, given that the DIB is said to be more inclusive than the DSM-III because of its consideration of psychotic symptomatology. Kernberg et al. indicated that in a structural interview the psychotic symptomatology is challenged: "If a patient who initially appears bizarre or who exhibits psychotic like thinking is able to improve his perception of reality, most likely that patient will be called borderline" (1981, p. 230).

Koenigsberg, Kernberg, and Schomer (1983) confirmed the expectation that Kernberg's (1984) criteria would be more inclusive than the DIB. They also indicated, however, that the differences are minimized within inpatient settings. They suggested that in an outpatient setting the DIB has a tendency to underdiagnose BPD because of its emphasis on overt and moderately severe symptomatology, and that the DIB is unable to distinguish between borderline and psychotic levels because of the confusion of transient psychotic features (borderlines) with residual psychotic features (bipolar and schizophrenic patients).

An empirical comparison of Millon's (1969, 1981) formulation with the others is complicated by the absence of a semistructured interview. The measurement of Millon's formulation has relied on the self-report MCMI (Millon, 1977, 1987). A consistent finding has been that the MCMI diagnoses more patients as borderline than are diagnosed as such by the DSM-III (Dubro et al., 1988; Piersma, 1987, 1989; Reich et al., 1987). However, it is not clear whether this is a reflection of a broader formulation of the construct by Millon or the effect of state factors on the self-report methodology (Piersma, 1987, 1989). Self-report inventories in general appear to provide inflated estimates of personality trait pathology, as a result of the depressed or anxious state of the subjects (Reich, 1985; Widiger & Frances, 1987). Choca, Bresolin, Okonek, and Ostrow (1988), in fact, suggest using the MCMI borderline scale to diagnose depression. Edell (1984) and Hurt, Hyler, Frances, Clarkin, and Brent (1984) indicate as well that the tendency of patients (and borderlines in particular) to distort and exaggerate their pathology contributes to inflated scores. On the other hand, the MCMI might be providing a valid measure of Millon's (1981) formulation, in that he does appear to give more emphasis to dysregulated mood than either the DSM-III or the DIB does.

Conclusions

The early history of the borderline diagnosis was a confusing array of concepts (Aronson, 1985; Stone, 1980; Widiger, 1982). The diversity in conceptualization substantially hindered clinical communication and replicable research, because there was little assurance that discussions of the borderline patient were referring to the same clinical group (Perry & Klerman, 1978). There has been considerable progress in the development of explicit and relatively specific criteria for the diagnosis of BPD. However, it is also apparent that there still remains substantial diversity in how borderlines are diagnosed, with each formulation continuing to guide different research programs. Additional formulations beyond those considered here are provided by Frosch (1988), Kroll (1988), Sheehy, Goldsmith, and Charles (1980), and others.

The revisions, however, could suggest an increasing convergence and responsivity to empirical research. Millon's (1987) revision of the MCMI was based in part on an effort to increase its congruency with the DSM-III-

R. The DIB-R revision has resulted in a more restrictive diagnosis, which might increase its concordance with the DSM-III-R. Gunderson has the primary responsibility for developing the initial draft of the BPD criteria for DSM-IV, which could suggest that the DSM-IV formulation might be somewhat closer to that of Gunderson and Zanarini (1987).

The diversity, however, can also be beneficial. Given the controversies and uncertainties regarding the diagnosis of personality disorders, it is advantageous to have alternative formulations rather than to encourage premature closure. In any case, one should not assume that the borderlines discussed in one publication are necessarily comparable to the borderlines discussed in another.

DIAGNOSTIC CONTROVERSIES

BPD is one of the more controversial personality disorder diagnoses. Three of the more problematic diagnostic issues are the identification of the optimal criteria for diagnosis, the importance of psychotic symptomatology, and the use of a categorical versus a dimensional model of classification. Each of these issues is discussed in turn.

Diagnostic Criteria

A substantial body of research has been concerned with identifying which of the borderline criteria are optimal in diagnosis (Clarkin, Widiger, Frances, Hurt, & Gilmore, 1983; Dahl, 1986; Jacobsberg, Hymowitz, Barasch, & Frances, 1986; McGlashan, 1987; Modestin, 1987; Morey, 1988a; Nurnberg, Hurt, Feldman, & Suh, 1988; Pfohl, Coryell, Zimmerman, & Stangl, 1986; Plakun, 1987; Rosenberger & Miller, 1989; Widiger, Frances, Warner, & Bluhm, 1986). Averaging across studies suggests that physically self-damaging acts, unstable and intense relationships, and impulsivity are the most useful items for identifying the presence of BPD, whereas the absence of impulsivity or affective instability is optimal for ruling out the presence of BPD (Widiger & Frances, 1989).

However, it is also the case that the diagnostic efficiency of a symptom depends substantially on the setting and the differential diagnosis that is at issue (Plakun, 1987; Widiger, Hurt, Frances, Clarkin, & Gilmore, 1984). For example, intolerance of being alone was deleted from the DSM-III criteria in part because studies had indicated that it was not particularly common to borderlines (e.g., Clarkin et al., 1983; Pfohl et al., 1986; Widiger, Frances et al., 1986), but it may be the best symptom for distinguishing BPD from narcissistic and schizotypal personality disorders. Narcissistic and schizotypal patients display many borderline traits, but not an intolerance of being alone. As a result, intolerance of being alone has obtained substantial positive predictive values in studies that concerned BPD versus schizotypal personality disorder (McGlashan, 1987) and narcissistic personality disorder (Plakun, 1987). Given the problematic overlap of BPD with these two personality disorders, it may have been premature to delete this item from the criteria set.

The setting is important to diagnosis, because the specificity of a symptom will vary across populations. For example, physically self-damaging acts may be more useful for diagnosing BPD in outpatient than in inpatient settings, since physically self-damaging acts will be more common to nonborderlines in an inpatient setting (e.g., Dahl, 1986; Pfohl et al., 1986; Widiger, Frances, et al., 1986) and more specific to borderlines in an outpatient setting (e.g., Clarkin et al., 1983; Jacobsberg et al., 1986). Unstable and intense relationships, on the other hand, may be more specific to borderlines on an inpatient than on an outpatient service, given the increased prevalence of relationship issues among nonborderlines in an outpatient setting (Widiger & Frances, 1989).

Psychotic Symptomatology

An ongoing controversy is whether psychotic symptomatology should be included in the diagnosis of BPD (Frances, 1980; Gunderson, 1983; Gunderson & Zanarini, 1987). An original impetus for the borderline diagnosis was the tendency for some patients to become psychotic during analytic treatment (Bychowski, 1953; Frosch, 1964; Kernberg, 1975; Knight, 1953; Stern, 1938). Several studies have also confirmed the presence of psychotic and psychotic-like symptomatology in borderline patients (Chopra & Beatson, 1986; George & Soloff, 1986; Gunderson, 1984; Nurnberg et al., 1988; O'Connell, Cooper, Perry, & Hoke, 1989; Soloff, 1981). Gunderson and Singer (1975), Perry and Klerman (1980), and Sheehy et al. (1980) have each included psychotic symptomatology in their formulations of BPD, although as we have also indicated, the particular symptomatology that has been emphasized has varied across researchers and across time.

There are two major issues with respect to the psychotic symptomatology. The first is empirical, the second conceptual. Each is discussed in turn.

Empirical Issues

The empirical issue is whether the inclusion of psychotic symptomatology would improve or diminish the validity of the diagnosis. Research on this issue is difficult, in part because of the absence of accepted external validators. However, correlates such as family history, course, and childhood experiences have been researched (e.g., Herman, Perry, & van der Kolk, 1989), and it would then be useful to determine whether correlations with these variations would be improved by the addition of psychotic features. No study, however, has assessed this hypothesis.

The research to date has focused on descriptive validity, particularly with respect to internal consistency, sensitivity, and specificity. Zanarini, Gunderson, and Frankenburg (1990), for example, have suggested that "quasi-psychotic" symptoms (hallucinations or delusions that are atypical, transient, or circumscribed in their effect) are pathognomonic of BPD. However, a pathognomonic symptom is one that is both a perfect inclusion and a perfect exclusion criterion (Meehl, 1986). Its presence indicates that the disorder is present, and its absence indicates that the disorder is absent. No such phenomenological symptom exists for any mental disorder, particularly for the personality disorders. In the study by Zanarini et al. (1990), the quasi-psychotic symptoms occurred in only 40% of the borderlines. Its absence hardly suggested that a borderline disorder was not present, and its presence would identify only 40% of the cases.

It would be unrealistic, though, to require that a symptom be pathognomonic before it can be included in the diagnosis. The diagnosis of personality disorders is inherently imperfect, because one can only provide an approximate match to a hypothetical construct (Widiger & Frances, 1985). The prototypical case rarely occurs, and the diagnosis is only an approximation.

One could assess descriptive validity by determining whether the inclusion of psychotic or psychotic-like symptomatology would increase the differentiation of BPD from "near-neighbor" disorders that are often confused with BPD. BPD is overdiagnosed and difficult to distinguish from other personality disorders, particularly the schizotypal, histrionic, and antisocial (Morey, 1988b; Widiger & Frances, 1989). The research to date, however, has simply been concerned with determining whether psychotic symptomatology occurs more frequently in borderline versus near-neighbor diagnoses, not with the question of whether their inclusion would increase or decrease the differentiation from these disorders.

The inclusion of psychotic symptomatology could either increase or decrease the specificity of the diagnosis. Their inclusion could make the diagnosis more restrictive (if they became an additional requirement for the diagnosis) or more inclusive (if they became an additional option for making the diagnosis). As we have indicated earlier, research comparing the DIB (which includes psychotic features) to the DSM-III (which does not) has in fact been inconsistent with respect to which criteria set is more inclusive.

The potential effect of the inclusion of psychotic features, however, can be inferred from the current research. For example, there are data to suggest that the psychotic features observed in borderlines may be due to a comorbid mood, substance use, or factitious disorder (Jonas & Pope, 1984; Pope, Jonas, Hudson, Cohen, & Tohen, 1985). The overlap and differentiation of

BPD and mood disorders are controversial, in part because the differentiation can at times be illusory. To the extent that BPD involves a characterological variant of mood (and impulse) pathology, in the same sense that schizotypal is a characterological variant of schizophrenic pathology, the differentiation of BPD and mood disorder becomes a moot issue (Widiger, 1989). In any case, the inclusion of psychotic symptomatology is likely to increase the overlap, co-occurrence, and confusion of BPD with mood disorders, rather than their differentiation.

One of the most problematic differential diagnoses is that of BPD versus schizotypal personality disorder (e.g., Jacobsberg et al., 1986; McGlashan, 1987; Rosenberger & Miller, 1989; Serban, Conte, & Plutchik, 1987). If one assumes that it is useful to distinguish these two disorders, then it is important to determine the effect of the inclusion of psychotic features on their differentiation. Psychotic and psychotic-like symptomatology could be more characteristic of the schizotypal than of the borderline patient. Certainly the psychotic-like (cognitive) features cited most recently by Gunderson and Zanarini (1987), such as ideas of reference, undue suspiciousness, superstitiousness, magical thinking, and a sixth sense, would be seen frequently in schizotypal patients, given that they are included in the criteria for the diagnosis of schizotypal personality disorder (APA, 1987).

A proposal for DSM-IV is to add cognitive distortions that are specific to BPD, thereby contributing to the differentiation of BPD and schizotypal personality disorder. One such proposal involves cognitive and/or perceptual disturbances that are stress-related, circumscribed, and responsive to external structure. Presumably, the cognitive distortions seen in schizotypals are not stress-related. However, there are no data to indicate that this type of cognitive distortion can be assessed reliably and is in fact specific to borderlines.

A final consideration is face validity. This is the weakest form of validity, but the extent to which a criteria set represents clinicians' concepts is informative and particularly relevant to a prototypal model of validation (Blashfield, 1989). The original formulations by Spitzer et al. (1979) and Gunderson and Singer (1975) were efforts to represent how clinicians (or at least the published literature) were describing borderlines. However, as we noted earlier, Spitzer and Gunderson reached quite different conclusions with respect to this literature. The approach taken by Perry and Klerman (1978) was in this respect more informative, in that their survey was more explicit, including a systematic coding and tabular summary of each publication reviewed. It would be of interest to provide a cluster analysis of the coding of all publications on borderlines (treating each publication as a "subject"), to determine whether the two types identified by Spitzer et al. (borderline and schizotypal) occur in an empirical analysis of the literature.

An additional face validity approach would be to survey theorists, researchers, and/or clinical practitioners with respect to how they conceive of BPD. Livesley, Reiffer, Sheldon, and West (1987), for example, provided

45 psychiatrists with a list of features associated with BPD and requested that they rate each on a 7-point scale with respect to prototypicality. The most prototypical features were unstable relationships (mean score of 6.3), identity disturbance (6.0), and inappropriate, intense anger (5.9). Brief psychotic episodes received a mean rating of 5.7, which was higher than the ratings for affective instability (5.5), intolerance of aloneness (4.9), self-damaging acts (5.6), emptiness (5.6), and boredom (4.8).

A limitation of the study by Livesley et al. (1987) is that it provided the clinicians with item lists that had been based in part on the researchers' interpretation of the literature. Hilbrand and Hirt (1987) requested 30 clinicians to generate themselves the descriptors associated with BPD. Psychotic and/ or psychotic-like symptomatology were not included. The six most prototypical features were impulsivity, anger, identity disturbance, self-destructive behavior, dysphoria, and disturbed relationships.

To the extent that the DSM-III-R diagnostic constructs are intended to represent the concepts used by clinicians, the face validity of the criteria set is informative (Blashfield, 1989). However, a limitation of the face validity studies is that the subjects' ratings may have been biased by familiarity with the DSM and/or the DIB. It could also be argued that the criteria sets should not be based on what clinicians *think* is associated with each disorder, but rather on the symptoms that are associated *empirically* in patients diagnosed with the disorder.

Conceptual Issues

The conceptual issue is whether psychotic symptoms are diagnostic or simply associated features of BPD. A personality disorder could predispose a person to the development of a psychosis, but this would be comparable to the tendency of psychopathic persons to use drugs, for avoidant persons to develop anxiety disorders, and for dependent persons to become depressed. A personality disorder involves those features that are chronic and pervasive. Conditions that are time-limited are more appropriately characterized as associated Axis I disorders. In fact, the inclusion of psychotic regressions could blur the distinction of the relationship between the personality trait and the clinical state. The distinction between Axis I and Axis II disorders is problematic and at times illusory (Gunderson & Pollack, 1985; Widiger, 1989), and the inclusion of psychotic features in the diagnosis of BPD would serve to blur the boundary further.

Categorical versus Dimensional Classification

The final issue to be considered is whether it is preferable to diagnose BPD as a distinct personality disorder or as a dimension. The approach taken by the DSM-III-R, Gunderson and Zanarini (1987), and Millon (1981) is to diagnose BPD categorically. The clinical decision is to determine whether a person has or does not have BPD. The approach taken by Kernberg (1984) is essentially categorical. The distinction among neurotic, borderline, and psychotic refers to "levels" of personality organization, but each level represents a qualitatively distinct set of syndromal features (e.g., borderline represents primitive defenses, identity diffusion, and intact reality testing).

A categorical diagnosis has a number of disadvantages. For example, it contributes to a variety of classificatory dilemmas, including the differentiation of BPD from mood disorders, other personality disorders, and normality—distinctions that are likely to be arbitrary and at times even illusory (Widiger, 1989). It is not surprising that considerable disagreement and poor interrater reliability exist, given that the threshold for determining when a person has BPD is arbitrary (Hurt, Clarkin, Koenigsberg, Frances, & Nurnberg, 1986; Widiger et al., 1984). The convention adopted by DSM-III-R is to say that the disorder is present when five of the criteria are present, but persons with four, three, and fewer symptoms still display borderline pathology. Those with four features are more similar to those with five than to those with none (Widiger, Sanderson, & Warner, 1986). In fact, 162 different combinations of borderline features are possible in persons who would not be given a DSM-III-R diagnosis of BPD.

A substantial amount of information is also lost by the categorical distinction. Not all borderlines are alike in their expression of borderline symptomatology (Clarkin et al., 1983; Dahl, 1985). DSM-III-R adopted the polythetic format for diagnosis (i.e., multiple, optional criteria) rather than the monothetic, in recognition of the considerable heterogeneity among persons with the same personality disorder (Spitzer, 1987; Widiger & Frances, 1985). However, although it is accepted that there are many different ways in which a person can be borderline (Clarkin et al., 1983), only one diagnosis is given. No coding is provided to record the variation and heterogeneity in symptomatology. Clinicians might well prefer to consider the extent to which a person is borderline, rather than to lump persons together in broad and undifferentiated categories.

If it were the case that additional information did not increase the reliability or the validity of the diagnosis, then a categorical system might be preferable to the dimensional. This would indicate that the finer differentiations were not useful and were perhaps even illusory. However, in the vast majority of studies that have compared directly the categorical and dimensional approaches to diagnosing BPD, the dimensional rating has increased the reliability and/ or the validity of the data (e.g., Hart & Hare, 1989; Heumann & Morey, 1989; Reich et al., 1987; Standage & Ladha, 1988; Zimmerman, Pfohl, Coryell, Stangl, & Corenthal, 1988). Given the difficulties in obtaining reliable and valid personality disorder diagnoses, it is ironic that the less reliable and valid classification is being used.

Another approach to determining whether the categorical or dimensional model is more valid is to apply taxometric statistical techniques that test the assumptions of both models, such as admixture analysis, maximum covariation analysis (MAXCOV), and discontinuous regression (Grove & Andreasen, 1989). The only application of these techniques to BPD has been carried out by Trull, Widiger, and Guthrie (1989). Trull et al. applied MAXCOV to assess the extent to which the distribution of DSM-III-R BPD symptom-atology in a random sample of psychiatric inpatients was consistent with a dimensional or a catgorical model. The correlation between two indicators of a taxon will approach zero (or indeterminancy) as the sample becomes composed entirely of members (or nonmembers) of the taxon; conversely, the correlation will be maximized in an evenly mixed sample. No such effect should occur if the underlying variable is dimensional. Trull et al. assessed the effect on the correlation between BPD diagnostic criteria in samples with varying mixtures of borderline versus nonborderline subjects. The results were more consistent with the dimensional model. Limitations of the study, however, were the fallibility of the DSM-III-R diagnostic criteria and the reliance on chart review. These limitations could have had unanticipated effects on the interitem correlations and resulting distributions.

CLINICAL APPLICATIONS

BPD is often the most prevalent personality disorder diagnosis within clinical settings. However, it is not entirely clear whether clinicians are using the same concept when they are diagnosing their patients as borderline. It is clear that clinical diagnoses often fail to obtain adequate levels of interrater reliability. Mellsop, Varghese, Joshua, and Hicks (1982) reported a reliability of only .29 in their field trial assessment of the DSM-III BPD diagnosis, and it is likely that comparable findings were obtained in the APA field trials and would be obtained in most clinical settings (Widiger & Frances, 1989).

Poor reliability in clinical practice is due in part to the failure to system-atically assess and to adhere closely to the DSM-III(-R) diagnostic criteria. Morey and Ochoa (1989) obtained from 291 clinicians their personality disorder diagnosis of a recent patient and their assessment of the DSM-III personality disorder criteria (presented in a randomized order). Morey and Ochoa obtained a kappa of only .58 with respect to the agreement between the clinicians' diagnoses of BPD and the diagnoses that would be given on the basis of their assessments of the DSM-III criteria. In other words, their clinical diagnoses were not based on their own assessment of the DSM-III criteria.

However, this is not so much a criticism of the clinicians as it is of the DSM-III. A systematic assessment of each of the 104 DSM-III-R personality disorder criteria requires anywhere from 1 to 4 hours. The DSM-III-R categorical taxonomy is simply too cumbersome for applied clinical use. Instead of considering each of the personality disorders, it is likely that clinicians obtain an initial impression and then focus their assessment on the one or two most probable diagnoses. This approach is realistic and efficient, but it is also susceptible to systematic biases. BPD is one of the most overused and misused diagnoses (Aronson, 1985; Kroll, 1988). Morey and Ochoa (1989), for example, suggested that there is a tendency for less experienced, female, and psychodynamic clinicians to overdiagnose BPD, particularly in poor, white, and female patients. The presence of physically self-damaging acts and suicidal gestures may also contribute to a presumptive diagnosis of BPD.

Reliable and valid diagnoses are unlikely to occur if clinicians do not adhere to the diagnostic criteria. However, because adherence is impractical in everyday clinical practice, self-report inventories can be of substantial clinical utility. It is risky to rely on a self-report measure to provide diagnoses (particularly a computer-generated report), but the self-report measures are at least useful as screening devices (Widiger & Frances, 1987). They can indicate which personality disorder diagnoses should receive a more detailed consideration within the clinical interview, thereby diminishing the effect of any presumptive biases of the clinician.

However, if one does focus on BPD, then it is important to consider each of the DSM-III-R criteria systematically. Clinicians are also advised to consider alternative formulations, particularly those by Gunderson and Zanarini (1987), Kernberg (1984), and Millon (1986). The DSM-III-R formulation is an effort to provide a consensus model for which there is really no consensus. Most clinical assessments require the DSM-III-R diagnosis, but clinicians might find it useful to consider other options. In our own clinical practice, we prefer to conceptualize BPD as a degree of personality dysfunction or neuroticism (Costa & McCrae, 1990) or as a level of personality organization (Kernberg, 1984), rather than as a distinct personality disorder.

CONCLUSIONS

There is perhaps as much research on the diagnosis of BPD as there is on its etiology and treatment. This is appropriate, given the controversial status of the concept. There is no doubt that a substantial proportion of persons in clinics, hospitals, and private practice display borderline symptomatology; however, progress in understanding and treating the disorder is hindered by the absence of a consistent, reliable, and valid diagnosis. The most important achievements have been the development of explicit diagnostic criteria and the subjection of the alternative formulations to empirical scrutiny. The convergent and incremental validity of these formulations, the optimal criteria for diagnosis, and the validity of dimensional versus categorical classifications should remain critical topics of future research.

REFERENCES

American Psychiatric Association (APA). (1980). *Diagnostic and statistical manual of mental disorders* (3rd ed.). Washington, DC: Author.

American Psychiatric Association (APA). (1987). *Diagnostic and statistical manual of mental disorders* (3rd ed., rev.). Washington, DC: Author.

Angus, L. E., & Marziali, E. (1988). A comparison of three measures for the diagnosis of borderline personality disorder. *American Journal of Pychiatry, 145,* 1453–1454.

Aronson, T. A. (1985). Historical perspectives on the borderline concept: A review and critique. *Psychiatry, 48,* 209–222.

Barrash, J., Kroll, J., Carey, K., & Sines, L. (1983). Discriminating borderline disorder from other personality disorders. *Archives of General Psychiatry, 40,* 1297–1302.

Blashfield, R. (1989). Alternative taxonomic models of psychiatric classification. In L. Robins & J. Barrett (Eds.), *The validity of psychiatric diagnosis.* New York: Raven Press.

Bleuler, E. (1950). *Dementia praecox or the group of schizophrenias* (J. Ziskin, Trans.). New York: International Universities Press. (Original work published 1911)

Bychowski, G. (1953). The problem of latent psychosis. *Journal of the American Psychoanalytic Association, 4,* 484–503.

Choca, J., Bresolin, L., Okonek, A., & Ostrow, D. (1988). Validity of the Millon Clinical Multiaxial Inventory in the assessment of affective disorders. *Journal of Personality Assessment, 52,* 96–105.

Chopra, H. D., & Beatson, J. A. (1986). Psychotic symptoms in borderline personality disorder. *American Journal of Psychiatry, 143,* 1605–1607.

Clarkin, J. F., Widiger, T. A., Frances, A., Hurt, S. W., & Gilmore, M. (1983). Prototypic typology and the borderline personality disorder. *Journal of Abnormal Psychiatry, 92,* 263–275.

Costa, P. T., & McCrae, R. R. (1990). Personality disorders and the five-factor model of personality. *Journal of Personality Disorders, 4,* 362–371.

Dahl, A. A. (1985). A critical examination of empirical studies of the diagnosis of borderline disorders in adults. *Psychiatric Developments, 3,* 1–29.

Dahl, A. A. (1986). Some aspects of the DSM-III personality disorders illustrated by a consecutive sample of hospitalized patients. *Acta Psychiatrica Scandinavica, 73*(Suppl. 328), 61–66.

Dubro, A. F., Wetzler, S., & Kahn, M. W. (1988). A comparison of three self-report questionnaires for the diagnosis of DSM-III personality disorders. *Journal of Personality Disorders, 2,* 256–266.

Edell, W. (1984). The Borderline Syndrome Index: Clinical validity and utility. *Journal of Nervous and Mental Disease, 172,* 254–263.

Frances, A. (1980). The DSM-III personality disorders sections: A commentary. *American Journal of Psychiatry, 137,* 1050–1054.

Frances, A., Clarkin, J., Gilmore, M., Hurt, S. W., & Brown, R. (1984). Reliability of criteria for borderline personality disorder: A comparison of DSM-III and the DIB. *American Journal of Psychiatry, 141,* 1080–1084.

Frosch, J. (1964). The psychotic character. *Psychiatric Quarterly, 38,* 81–96.

Frosch, J. (1988). Psychotic character versus borderline character. *International Journal of Psycho-Analysis, 69,* 347–357.

George, A., & Soloff, P. H. (1986). Schizotypal symptoms in patients with borderline personality disorder. *American Journal of Psychiatry, 143,* 212–215.

Grinker, R., Werble, B., & Drye, R. (1968). *The borderline syndrome: A behavioral study of ego functions.* New York: Basic Books.

Grove, W. M., & Andreasen, N. C. (1989). Quantitative and qualitative distinctions between psychiatric disorders. In L. Robins & J. Barrett (Eds.), *The validity of psychiatric diagnosis.* New York: Raven Press.

Gunderson, J. G. (1983). DSM-III diagnosis of borderline personality disorder. In J. P. Frosch (Ed.), *Current perspectives on personality disorders.* Washington, DC: American Psychiatric Press.

Gunderson, J. G. (1984). *Borderline personality disorder.* Washington, DC: American Psychiatric Press.

Gunderson, J. G., & Kolb, J. E. (1978). Discriminating features of borderline patients. *American Journal of Psychiatry, 135,* 792–796.

Gunderson, J. G., Kolb, J. E., & Austin, V. (1981). The Diagnostic Interview for Borderline Patients. *American Journal of Psychiatry, 138,* 896–903.

Gunderson, J. G., & Pollack, W. (1985). Conceptual risks of the Axis I–II division. In H. Klar & L. Siever (Eds.), *Biologic response styles: Clinical implications.* Washington, DC: American Psychiatric Press.

Gunderson, J. G., & Singer, M. T. (1975). Defining borderline patients: An overview. *American Journal of Psychiatry, 132,* 1–10.

Gunderson, J. G., & Zanarini, M. C. (1987). Current overview of the borderline diagnosis. *Journal of Clinical Psychiatry, 48*(Suppl.), 5–11.

Hart, S. D., & Hare, R. D. (1989). Discriminant validity of the psychopathy checklist in a forensic psychiatric population. *Psychological Assessment: A Journal of Consulting and Clinical Psychology, 1,* 211–218.

Herman, J. L., Perry, J. C., & van der Kolk, B. A. (1989). Childhood trauma in borderline personality disorder. *American Journal of Psychiatry, 146,* 490–495.

Heumann, K. A., & Morey, L. C. (1989). *The reliability of categorical and dimensional judgments of personality disorder.* Unpublished manuscript, Vanderbilt University.

Hilbrand, M., & Hirt, M. (1987). The borderline syndrome: An empirically developed prototype. *Journal of Personality Disorders, 1,* 299–306.

Hoch, P., & Cattell, J. (1959). The diagnosis of pseudoneurotic schizophrenia. *Psychiatric Quarterly, 33,* 17–43.

Hurt, S. W., Clarkin, J., Koenigsberg, H., Frances, A., & Nurnberg, H. G. (1986). Diagnostic Interview for Borderlines: Psychometric properties and validity. *Journal of Consulting and Clinical Psychology, 54,* 256–260.

Hurt, S. W., Hyler, S., Frances, A., Clarkin, J., & Brent, R. (1984). Assessing borderline personality disorder with self-report, clinical interview, or semistructured interview. *American Journal of Psychiatry, 141,* 1228–1231.

Jacobsberg, L. B., Hymowitz, P., Barasch, A., & Frances, A. J. (1986). Symptoms of schizotypal personality disorder. *American Journal of Psychiatry, 143*, 1222–1227.

Jonas, J. M., & Pope, H. G. (1984). Psychosis in borderline personality disorder. *Psychiatric Developments, 4*, 295–308.

Kernberg, O. F. (1967). Borderline personality organization. *Journal of the American Psychoanalytic Association, 15*, 641–685.

Kernberg, O. F. (1975). *Borderline conditions and pathological narcissism.* New York: Jason Aronson.

Kernberg, O. F. (1981). Structural interviewing. *Psychiatric Clinics of North America, 4*, 169–195.

Kernberg, O. F. (1984). *Severe personality disorders.* New Haven, CT: Yale University Press.

Kernberg, O. F., Goldstein, E. G., Carr, A. C., Hunt, H. F., Bauer, S. F., & Blumenthal, R. (1981). Diagnosing borderline personality: A pilot study using multiple diagnostic methods. *Journal of Nervous and Mental Disease, 169*, 225–231.

Kety, S. S., Rosenthal, D., Wender, P. H., & Schulsinger, F. (1971). Mental illness in the biological and adoptive families of adopted schizophrenics. *American Journal of Psychiatry, 128*, 302–306.

Knight, R. (1953). Borderline states. *Bulletin of the Menninger Clinic, 17*, 1–12.

Koenigsberg, H. W., Kernberg, O. F., & Schomer, J. (1983). Diagnosing borderline conditions in an outpatient setting. *Archives of General Psychiatry, 40*, 49–53.

Kroll, J. (1988). *The challenge of the borderline patient.* New York: Norton.

Kullgren, G. (1987). An empirical comparison of three different borderline concepts. *Acta Psychiatrica Scandinavica, 76*, 246–255.

Livesley, W. J., Reiffer, L. I., Sheldon, A. E. R., & West, M. (1987). Prototypicality ratings of DSM-III criteria for personality disorders. *Journal of Nervous and Mental Disease, 175*, 395–401.

Loranger, A. W., Oldham, J. M., Russakoff, L. M., & Susman, V. (1984). Structured interviews and borderline personality disorder. *Archives of General Psychiatry, 41*, 565–568.

McGlashan, T. H. (1983). The borderline syndrome: II. Is it a variant of schizophrenia or affective disorder? *Archives of General Psychiatry, 40*, 1319–1323.

McGlashan, T. H. (1987). Testing DSM-III symptom criteria for schizotypal and borderline personality disorders. *Archives of General Psychiatry, 44*, 143–148.

Meehl, P. (1986). Diagnostic taxa as open concepts: Metatheoretical and statistical questions about reliability and construct validity in the grand strategy of nosological revision. In T. Millon & G. L. Klerman (Eds.), *Contemporary directions in psychopathology.* New York: Guilford Press.

Mellsop, G., Varghese, F., Joshua, S., & Hicks, A. (1982). The reliability of Axis II of DSM-III. *American Journal of Psychiatry, 139*, 1360–1361.

Millon, T. (1969). *Modern psychopathology.* Prospect Heights, IL: Waveland Press.

Millon, T. (1977). *Millon Multiaxial Clinical Inventory manual.* Minneapolis: National Computer Systems.

Millon, T. (1981). *Disorders of personality: DSM-III, Axis II.* New York: Wiley–Interscience.

Millon, T. (1983). The DSM-III: An insider's perspective. *American Psychologist, 38*, 804–814.

Millon, T. (1986). Personality prototypes and their diagnostic criteria. In T. Millon & G. L. Klerman (Eds.), *Contemporary directions in psychopathology*. New York: Guilford Press.

Millon, T. (1987). *Manual for the MCMI-II*. Minneapolis: National Computer Systems.

Modestin, J. (1987). Quality of interpersonal relationships: The most characteristic DSM-III BPD criterion. *Comprehensive Psychiatry, 28*, 397–402.

Morey, L. C. (1988a). A psychometric analysis of the DSM-III-R personality disorder criteria. *Journal of Personality Disorders, 2*, 109–124.

Morey, L. C. (1988b). Personality disorders in DSM-III and DSM-III-R: Convergence, coverage, and internal consistency. *American Journal of Psychiatry, 145*, 573–577.

Morey, L., & Ochoa, E. (1989). An investigation of adherence to diagnostic criteria: Clinical diagnosis of the DSM-III personality disorders. *Journal of Personality Disorders, 3*, 180–192.

Nelson, H. F., Tennen, H., Tasman, A., Borton, M., Kubeck, M., & Stone, M. (1985). Comparison of three systems for diagnosing borderline personality disorder. *American Journal of Psychiatry, 142*, 855–858.

Nurnberg, H. G., Hurt, S. W., Feldman, A., & Suh, R. (1988). Evaluation of diagnostic criteria for borderline personality disorder. *American Journal of Psychiatry, 145*, 1280–1284.

O'Connell, M., Cooper, S., Perry, J. C., & Hoke, E. (1989). The relationship between thought disorder and psychotic symptoms in borderline personality disorder. *Journal of Nervous and Mental Disease, 177*, 273–278.

Perry, J. C., & Klerman, G. L. (1978). The borderline patient: A comparative analysis of four sets of diagnostic criteria. *Archives of General Psychiatry, 35*, 141–150.

Perry, J. C., & Klerman, G. L. (1980). Clinical features of the borderline personality disorder. *American Journal of Psychiatry, 137*, 165–173.

Pfohl, B., Coryell, W., Zimmerman, M., & Stangl, D. (1986). DSM-III personality disorders: Diagnostic overlap and internal consistency of individual DSM-III criteria. *Comprehensive Psychiatry, 27*, 21–34.

Piersma, H. (1987). The MCMI as a measure of DSM-III Axis II diagnoses: An empirical comparison. *Journal of Clinical Psychology, 43*, 478–483.

Piersma, H. L. (1989). The MCMI-II as a treatment outcome measure for psychiatric inpatients. *Journal of Clinical Psychology, 45*, 87–93.

Plakun, E. M. (1987). Distinguishing narcissistic and borderline personality disorders using DSM-III criteria. *Comprehensive Psychiatry, 28*, 437–443.

Pope, H. G., Jonas, J. M., Hudson, J. I., Cohen, B. B., & Tohen, M. (1985). An empirical study of psychosis in borderline personality disorder. *American Journal of Psychiatry, 142*, 1285–1290.

Reich, J. (1985). Measurement of DSM-III, Axis II. *Comprehensive Psychiatry, 26*, 352–363.

Reich, J., Noyes, R., & Troughton, E. (1987). Lack of agreement between instruments assessing DSM-III personality disorders. In C. Green (Ed.), *Conference on the Millon clinical inventories*. Minnetonka, MN: National Computer Systems.

Rosenberger, P. H., & Miller, G. A. (1989). Comparing borderline definitions: DSM-III borderline and schizotypal personality disorders. *Journal of Abnormal Psychology, 98*, 161–169.

Serban, G., Conte, H. R., & Plutchik, R. (1987). Borderline and schizotypal personality disorders: Mutually exclusive or overlapping? *Journal of Personality Assessment, 51*, 15–22.

Sheehy, M., Goldsmith, L., & Charles, E. (1980). A comparative study of borderline patients in a psychiatric outpatient clinic. *American Journal of Psychiatry, 137*, 1374–1379.

Siever, L. J., & Gunderson, J. (1979). Genetic determinants of borderline conditions. *Schizophrenia Bulletin, 5*, 49–86.

Skodol, A. E., Rosnick, L., Kellman, D., Oldham, J. M., & Hyler, S. E. (1988, May). The validity of structured assessments of Axis II. In J. M. Oldham (Chair), *Axis II: New perspectives on validity*. Symposium conducted at the 141st Annual Meeting of the American Psychiatric Association, Montreal.

Soloff, P. H. (1981). Affect, impulse and psychosis in borderline disorders: A validation study. *Comprehensive Psychiatry, 22*, 337–350.

Spitzer, R. L. (1987). Nosology. In A. E. Skodol & R. L. Spitzer (Eds.), *An annotated bibliography of DSM-III*. Washington, DC: American Psychiatric Press.

Spitzer, R. L., Endicott, J., & Gibbon, M. (1979). Crossing the border into borderline personality and borderline schizophrenia. *Archives of General Psychiatry, 36*, 17–24.

Standage, K., & Ladha, N. (1988). An examination of the reliability of the Personality Disorder Examination and a comparison with other methods of identifying personality disorders in a clinical sample. *Journal of Personality Disorders, 2*, 267–271.

Stern, A. (1938). Psychoanalytic investigation and therapy in the borderline group of neuroses. *Psychoanalytic Quarterly, 7*, 467–489.

Stone, M. H. (1980). *The borderline syndromes*. New York: McGraw-Hill.

Trull, T. J., Widiger, T. A., & Guthrie, P. (1989). The categorical versus dimensional status of borderline personality disorder. *Journal of Abnormal Psychology, 99*, 40–48.

Widiger, T. A. (1982). Prototypic typologies and borderline diagnoses. *Clinical Psychology Review, 2*, 115–135.

Widiger, T. A. (1989). The categorical distinction between personality and affective disorders. *Journal of Personality Disorders, 3*, 77–91.

Widiger, T. A., & Frances, A. J. (1985). The DSM-III personality disorders. *Archives of General Psychiatry, 42*, 615–623.

Widiger, T. A., & Frances, A. J. (1987). Interviews and inventories for the measurement of personality disorders. *Clinical Psychology Review, 7*, 49–75.

Widiger, T. A., & Frances, A. J. (1989). Epidemiology, diagnosis, and comorbidity of borderline personality disorder. In A. Tasman, R. E. Hales, & A. J. Frances (Eds.), *Review of psychiatry* (Vol. 8). Washington, DC: American Psychiatric Press.

Widiger, T. A., Frances, A. J., Warner, L., & Bluhm, C. (1986). Diagnostic criteria for the borderline and schizotypal personality disorders. *Journal of Abnormal Psychology, 95*, 43–51.

Widiger, T. A., Hurt, S. W., Frances, A. J., Clarkin, J. F., & Gilmore, M. (1984). Diagnostic efficiency and DSM-III. *Archives of General Psychiatry, 41*, 1005–1012.

Widiger, T. A., Sanderson, C., & Warner, L. (1986). The MMPI, prototypal typology, and borderline personality disorder. *Journal of Personality Assessment, 50,* 540–553.

Zanarini, M. C., Gunderson, J. G., & Frankenburg, F. R. (1990). Cognitive features of borderline personality disorder. *American Journal of Psychiatry, 147,* 57–63.

Zanarini, M. C., Gunderson, J. G., Frankenburg, F. R., & Chauncey, D. L. (1989). The Revised Diagnostic Interview for Borderlines: Discriminating BPD from other Axis II disorders. *Journal of Personality Disorders, 3,* 10–18.

Zilboorg, G. (1941). Ambulatory schizophrenia. *Psychiatry, 4,* 149–155.

Zimmerman, M. (1988). Why are we rushing to publish DSM-IV? *Archives of General Psychiatry, 45,* 1135–1138.

Zimmerman, M., Pfohl, B., Coryell, W., Stangl, D., & Corenthal, C. (1988). Diagnosing personality disorder in depressed patients. *Archives of General Psychiatry, 45,* 733–737.

CHAPTER 6

Measurement of DSM-III and DSM-III-R Borderline Personality Disorder

JAMES REICH

The development of a nosological category in medicine has no set formula. Often it begins with astute clinicians' making clinical descriptions of constellations of symptoms they feel are important. This is often followed by initial attempts at measurements and later by validation by empirical criteria, such as those suggested by Robins and Guze (1970). Although the fine points, of course, have not been completely researched, most recent work indicates that borderline personality disorder (BPD) is well on its way toward acceptance as a valid disorder (Tarnopolsky & Berelowitz, 1987). A number of instruments, both self-report and interview, have been developed to measure this construct. This chapter first reports on the specific qualities and validation of these instruments. It then describes research that has attempted to compare these different instruments; research on the value of the individual BPD criteria; the problem of overlap with other personality disorders; the concept of "core criteria" for BPD; and suggested directions for future research. This chapter is limited to the definitions of BPD given in the third and revised third editions of the *Diagnostic and Statistical Manual of Mental Disorders* (DSM-III and DSM-III-R).

MEASUREMENT INSTRUMENTS

This section is divided into three parts. Self-report instruments are covered first, interview instruments are discussed second, and family history methods are covered third. In order to help the reader organize this information and compare these instruments, the first two sections are accomplished by tables summarizing specific pertinent details of each instrument.

It should be noted that some instruments covered in this review have been replaced by newer or modified versions. The degree of change varies with each instrument. Often few data are available on the new instruments. The tables report the new instruments. Data on the previous instruments are reported in the table if the versions appear similar enough that these results probably apply.

Although the tables give an estimate of the percentage of each instrument used to diagnose BPD, for those interviews or inventories where these questions are interspersed with questions for other disorders, taking them out of context may alter greatly the psychometric properties of the test.

Self-Report Instruments

Table 6.1 summarizes information on self-report instruments.

Personality Diagnostic Questionnaire—Revised

The Personality Diagnostic Questionnaire—Revised (PDQ-R; Hyler et al., 1987) is a revision of an earlier version of the instrument, the PDQ. Although the PDQ-R differs in several ways from the PDQ (questions for individual personality disorders are arranged together in one section rather than intermixed, and criteria are now those of DSM-III-R instead of DSM-III), it is likely that the instruments will yield similar results. The PDQ-R is a 155-item, forced-choice, yes–no instrument that takes approximately 20–30 minutes to administer.

The PDQ has now been widely used in different centers on different populations, and in general the results are consistent with those found by other personality testing methods (Reich, 1988c, 1989b; Reich, Noyes, & Troughton, 1987a; Reich & Troughton, 1988; Reich, Yates, & Nduaguba, 1989; Yates, Sellini, & Reich, 1989; Hyler et al., 1989; Pfohl, Coryell, Zimmerman, & Stangl, 1987). However, certain disorders are diagnosed more reliably than others (Reich, 1987). The borderline section contains 17 questions. However, for an individual to be scored positive for a personality disorder, two out of five questions in an impairment distress scale must also be scored in a pathological direction.

Data are beginning to accumulate in regard to the ability of the PDQ and PDQ-R to diagnose BPD. The first report was that by Hurt, Hyler, Frances, Clarkin, and Brent (1984) on the PDQ. Subjects in this study were psychiatric outpatients selected for the presence of at least one personality disorder. Here the PDQ was compared to a clinical interview and a semi-structured interview (the Diagnostic Interview for Borderlines, or DIB; Gun-

TABLE 6.1. Characteristics of Self-Report Instruments Measuring DSM-III or DSM-III-R BPD

Characteristic	PDQ-R[a]	MCMI-II	BSI	Bell	WISPI	SNAP
Informant						
Patient	×	×	×	×	×	×
Significant other						
Other personality diagnoses covered	All DSM-III-R	All DSM-III-R	Diagnoses DSM-III BPD and schizotypal without distinguishing between them	—	All DSM-III	Non-DSM-III normal and abnormal personality traits
BPD criteria						
DSM-III			See above	×	×	×[b]
DSM-III-R	×	×				
Assessment of other psychiatric symptoms	No	Yes, numerous dimensional symptom scores	No		Information on interpersonal relationships	
Subjects: Populations studied	Psychiatric inpatients, outpatients, community survey, normals		Psychiatric inpatients, outpatients (including schizophrenic and depressed), normals	Normals, psychiatric patients (depressed, schizophrenic)	Normals, psychiatric patients	Normals, psychiatric inpatients and outpatients
Norms established	Presence or absence of a personality disorder by dimensional scale		"Borderline" normals, schizophrenics	Normals, "borderline psychotics"	Normals, psychiatric patients	Normals, psychiatric patients
Psychometric properties						
Reliability					×	

Joint interview						
Test–retest	×					
Validity						
BPD patients different from normals	×		×	×	×	
BPD patients different from other psychiatric patients	×		×	×		
BPD patients different from patients with other personality disorders						
Psychometric tests or factor analysis	×			×	×	×
Sensitivity	×			×		×
Scoring system	×	×	×	×	×	×
Number of items (total interview)	155	175	52	45	360	375
Percentage of interview on BPD	Approx. 11%	Approx. 9%	Author's intention was 100%	Author feels interview should be given as a whole	Approx. 9%	6%
Completion time	15–20 min.	15–20 min.	25 min.	15 min.	30–50 min.	Approx. 60 min.
Research or clinical (R or C)	R,C	R,C	Neither	R	R	R

[a] The PDQ-R is in development and has not received much reliability or validity testing at present.

[b] A subscale to score DSM-III-R BPD has been developed, but it was not originally devised for that purpose.

derson, 1982a). The sensitivities and specificities were just above the .60 level (exact number differed by comparison interview used). The PDQ tended to overdiagnose. Eight-week test—retest reliability gave a kappa of .63.

My own work with the PDQ (Reich, 1988c, 1989b) involved 73 panic disorder patients who were tested before treatment and 8 weeks later after treatment. The test—retest kappa was .50. This was a somewhat stringent test, since the patients were in active new treatment between testings.

Data are now available on the comparison of the PDQ-R to two semi-structured interview instruments: the first edition of the Personality Disorder Examination (PDE; Loranger, Sussman, Oldham, & Russakoff, 1987), and the Structured Clinical Interview for DSM-III-R Personality Disorders (SCID-II; Spitzer, Williams, & Gibbon, 1987). Patients studied were 87 consecutive admissions to a long-term research ward known for its ability to treat personality disorders (Skodol, Rosnick, Kellman, Oldham, & Hyler, 1988a; Hyler, personal communication, 1988). Prevalence of BPD was 79% as assessed by the PDQ-R, compared to 61% as assessed by the SCID-II and 67% by the PDE. The kappa for agreement of the PDQ-R with the SCID-II was .53 and with the PDE was .46 (this compares with a .53 kappa between the PDE and SCID-II). Using the PDE and SCID-II to form a narrow definition of BPD gave a sensitivity of .98 and a specificity of .41; using a broader definition gave a sensitivity of .95 and a specificity of .63.

It is clear that the PDQ-R is measuring something highly related to DSM-III-R BPD and that it has test—retest kappas as good as those of most DSM-III-R personality instruments. Its tendency to overdiagnose may well make it unsuitable as a sole instrument for a study whose focus is solely on BPD, but it should be a useful adjunct in other studies or studies requiring rapid testing and little demand on clinician time.

Millon Clinical Multiaxial Inventory II

The Millon Clinical Multiaxial Inventory II (MCMI-II; Millon, 1987) is a modification of the original MCMI. It is still a 175-item, forced-choice, computer-scored, yes—no measurement tool. Millon is a sophisticated test developer who developed the MCMI and MCMI-II using appropriate techniques. The original MCMI has been criticized on several grounds. Widiger and Frances (1987) and Widiger and Sanderson (1987) questioned whether all of the diagnoses were close to those of DSM-III (Millon has his own theoretical system, which differs in some respects from DSM-III; Millon, 1981) and whether the overlap in items diagnosing different disorders created artificial overlap between these disorders. The question was also raised as to whether there was a bias of state illness (anxiety and depression) in the diagnosis of personality disorders (Reich, 1987). Furthermore, there is evidence that the borderline diagnosis of the MCMI does not agree will with that of the Structured Interview for DSM-III Personality Disorders (SIDP; Pfohl, Stangl, & Zimmerman, 1982) or the PDQ (Reich, Noyes, & Troughton, 1987b). Although the MCMI has generally received good reviews when compared to other self-report, non-DSM-III inventories (Hess, 1985; Millon, 1982), the MCMI-II was designed to update the instrument to DSM-III-R and to address the questions raised about the instrument. Exactly how well the modified instrument performs will not be clear until the publication of empirical data.

For BPD, I report the MCMI data. Although, as mentioned above, we do not know exactly how well the MCMI compares to the MCMI-II, the borderline concept of the MCMI was not seen as having major differences from that of DSM-III (Widiger & Sanderson, 1987) and received little criticism. Presumably, the MCMI-II BPD is fairly close to that of the original MCMI. The MCMI borderline scale has been reported as having good test–retest reliability—.77 for test–retest at 4 to 6 weeks in a combination of inpatients and outpatients (Millon, 1982), and .89 in an 8-week test–retest of 73 treated panic disorder patients (Reich, 1987). The diagnosis has good correlation with BPD traits as diagnosed by clinicians (95.2); however, there was also significant overlap with clinician-diagnosed avoidant (74.3), dependent (70.7), passive–aggressive (70.7), and paranoid (68.8) traits (Reich, 1987).

In sum, it is very likely that the MCMI-II will be a cost-effective method for diagnosing degree of borderline traits. However, due to the MCMI's disagreement with other personality measures for BPD (cited above) and its new innovation in scoring, it probably should not be used as the primary instrument in BPD studies, pending the publication of further empirical data.

Borderline Syndrome Index

The Borderline Syndrome Index (BSI) was developed by Conte, Plutchik, and Karasu (1980) as one early attempt to measure borderline psychopathology. Unfortunately, the measure was not updated and revised as new empirical data and theories evolved. It cannot differentiate schizotypal personality disorder from BPD, and there is empirical evidence that it may be tapping broad indices of psychopathology that are not necessarily specific to BPD (Edell, 1984). This instrument is probably of historical interest at this time. Other reviewers have come to a similar conclusion (Widiger & Frances, 1987).

Bell Object Relations Scale

The Bell Object Relations Scale (Bell, 1981; Bell, Metcalf, & Ryan, 1979, 1980) is a 45-item, true–false questionnaire developed by Morris Bell. It was derived from factor-analytic techniques and consists of four scales: Alienation, Insecure Attachment, Egocentricity, and Social Competence. Internal consistency is high, with Cronbach's alpha ranging from .78 for Egocentricity to .90 for Alienation.

The instrument is of interest since it has reported a high level of discrimination of BPD from other disorders (Reich, 1987). Unfortunately, as far as I know, Bell's manuscript describing this has never been published, nor has other work published using the instrument. This is an instrument that appears to be highly promising, although at an early state of development. However, if further development and empirical work are not performed on this instrument, it will rapidly be overtaken and become obsolete as far as DSM-III-R BPD research is concerned.

Wisconsin Personality Inventory

The Wisconsin Personality Inventory (WISPI; Klein, 1985) is a 360-item, self-report Axis II measure whose items are rated on a 10-point scale. In addition to DSM-III criteria, items were included to assess personal interaction styles, response bias, and global ratings of work and social adjustment. It is based largely on the theoretical work of Benjamin (1974, 1984). The instrument's most unusual feature is its computer program version, which allows patients to interact directly with the computer. Many validity studies are in progress, including comparison with other instruments and factor analysis; however, none are yet published (Klein, personal communication, 1988). The alpha of consistency for the borderline items is .88. The WISPI can also be hand-scored. This is an interesting instrument from both a theoretical and an application viewpoint. However, it will remain a research instrument until validity studies are published, and most likely until it is updated to DSM-III-R.

Schedule for Normal and Abnormal Personality

The Schedule for Normal and Abnormal Personality (SNAP; Clark, 1988, 1989) is a 375-item, true–false, forced-choice, self-report scale designed to measure normal and abnormal personality traits. It has 13 scales and 3 higher-order personality dimensions. The instrument has gone through fairly extensive development. Although not a DSM-III instrument, it is included here since there are some preliminary data on a DSM-III-R BPD subscale (Clark, personal communication, 1989). This 23-item subscale had a test–retest kappa of .63 at 1 week in diverse psychiatric patients and a kappa value of .67 (hit rate of 81%) when compared to a clinical BPD diagnosis. This is an interesting scale of which we may expect to see more in the future.

Interview Instruments

Table 6.2 summarizes information on interview instruments.

Schedule for Interviewing Borderlines

The Schedule for Interviewing Borderlines (SIB) is a 70-item, semistructured interview in two parts—one for diagnosing BPD (Schedule for Borderline Personalities, or SBR) and one for diagnosing schizotypal personality disorder (Schedule for Schizotypal Personalities, or SSP). It was developed by Baron (1981). The SBR has had no validity testing and has not become widely used. If further development is not forthcoming, the SBR will be superseded by other instruments that have been undergoing continuous development.

Diagnostic Interview for Borderlines

The DIB is a 165-item, semistructured interview with a complete scoring system that takes 60 minutes to administer (Gunderson, 1982a, 1982b; Gunderson & Kolb, 1978; Gunderson, Kolb, & Austin, 1981). The scale measures five areas of presumed importance to the diagnosis of BPD.

Joint reliability was reported as .80 in one study (Perry & Klerman, 1980) and as .90, with a kappa of .62, in another (Kolb & Gunderson, 1980). Other studies confirm these reliability findings (Cornell, Silk, Ludolf, & Lohr, 1983; Frances, Clarkin, Gilmore, Hurt, & Brown, 1984; Hurt et al., 1984; Kroll, Pyle, et al., 1981). The DIB and subsections of the DIB have been validated against established psychiatric tests, including the Minnesota Multiphasic Personality Inventory (MMPI) (Kroll, Sines, et al., 1981; Kroll, Carey, Sines, & Roth, 1982; Loranger, Oldham, Russakoff, & Sussman, 1984; Soloff, 1981a, 1981b) and also by factor-analytic techniques (Gunderson & Kolb, 1978). Moreover, work has been done validating the DIB against clinical diagnosis of BPD (Gunderson et al., 1981), the checklist rating of Soloff (1981a), DSM-III criteria (Soloff, 1981a), and the borderline score of the structural interview method of ascertaining BPD (Kernberg et al., 1981; Koenigsberg, Kernberg, & Schomer, 1983). It appears probable that the DIB can distinguish borderline personality disorders from affective disorders, schizophrenia, and anxiety disorders (Soloff, 1981a).

Two studies that compare DIB scores of borderlines with DIB scores of other personality disorder patients in the inpatient setting show that the DIB does not discriminate between these two groups (Kroll, Sines, et al., 1981; Kroll et al., 1982). Barrash, Kroll, Carey, and Sines (1983) were able to achieve differentiation between BPD and other personality disorders using

TABLE 6.2. Characteristics of Interview Instruments Measuring DSM-III or DSM-III-R BPD

Characteristic	SIB	DIB	BPD Scale	DIPD	SCID-II	PDE	SIDP-R	PAS	PIQ II
Informant									
Patient	×	×	×	×	×	×	×	×	×
Significant other	×	×			×	×	×	×	
Other (records, etc.)					×		×		
Other personality diagnoses covered	DSM-III schizotypal	None	Antisocial	All DSM-III-R	All DSM-III-R	All DSM-III-R	All DSM-III-R	[a]	All DSM-III-R
Criteria for BPD									
DSM-III	×	×							
DSM-III-R		×	×	×	×	×	×	×	×
Other		×	×						
Assessment of other psychiatric symptoms	No	No			No	No	No	No	No
Subjects: Populations studied	Relatives of schizophrenics; other psychiatric patients	Extensive psychiatric inpatients and outpatients	Patients with BPD, borderline traits, antisocial personality disorder, bipolar disorder, major depression, alcoholism, schizophrenia, adjustment disorder	Mostly psychiatric inpatients	Psychiatric inpatients and outpatients	Extensive inpatients, outpatients, normals	Prior version extensively tested	Psychiatric patients, community survey, normals	Psychiatric inpatients
Norms established	No	Extensive	See above						
Psychometric properties									
Reliability									
Joint	×	×	×	×		×		×	
Test–retest	×	×		×		×		×	×

124

	C1	C2	C3	C4	C5	C6	C7	C8
Validity								
BPD patients different from normals		×	×			×		×[c]
BPD patients different from other psychiatric patients		×	×			×		
BPD patients different from patients with other personality disorders			×[b]					
Psychometric tests or factor analysis		×	×					
Sensitivity	×	×	×	×	×	×	Not for BPD	×
Scoring system	×	×	×	×	×	×	×	×
Number of items (total interviews)	70	165	36	101	120	126	164	24
Percentage of interview on BPD	About 50%	100%	100%	About 9%	About 9%	About 9%	N/A	Approx. 9%
Completion time	50 min.	60 min.	90 min.	60–90 min.	60–90 min.	90 min.	60–90 min.[d]	60 min.
Research or clinical (R or C)	R	R,C	R	R	R,C	R,C	R,C	R,C

[a]The PAS uses a non-DSM-III-based diagnostic system. Some of its diagnoses resemble the DSM-III personality disorder clusters. Tyrer has produced a conversion for some disorders to DSM-III-R, including BPD. Exactly how well the conversion works awaits further empirical testing.
[b]Antisocial personality disorder.
[c]By forced choice.
[d]However, a separate informant interview taking 30–45 minutes is recommended.

the DIB. They were able to do so by using a scoring system derived from cluster analysis of DIB items. However, when they tested the system on a second population, this method was not found to be robust (Barrash, Kroll, Sines, & Carey, 1991). A fourth study shows that in an outpatient population the DIB does have some ability to distinguish BPD from other personality disorders; however, this study also indicates that in our patient setting the DIB loses some ability to distinguish between psychotic and BPD patients (Soloff, 1981c). Frances et al. (1984) have also found that the DIB can discriminate between BPD and other personality disorders in the outpatient setting. Using a DSM-III clinical interview as the criterion, they found that a DIB cutoff score of 7 yielded a sensitivity of .73 and a specificity of .80 for this population.

It is not completely clear that the failure to discriminate BPD from other personality disorders is a liability of the instrument. It is clear that many disorders in DSM-III and DSM-III-R overlap clinically. It is not unreasonable that an instrument designed to pick up only one disorder might pick up others as well. This is not to say that efforts should not be continued to increase this differentiation where possible.

The DSM-III and the DIB criteria for BPD were designed to include a large amount of overlap. Three studies report the expected high correlation between DIB scores and DSM-III clinical diagnoses (Kroll et al., 1982; Loranger et al., 1984; Soloff, 1981c). The exact correlation between a DSM-III/DSM-III-R diagnosis and a DIB diagnosis of BPD may not be perfect, but it is clear that these diagnoses can be easily derived from the information collected by the DIB.

The DIB has become a standard of comparison for developing instruments to measure BPD. It has good reliability and validity. As with some other instruments, it appears that the DIB may not be able to distinguish BPD clearly from other personality disorders. There is no specific work on the effect of state on the DIB.

Borderline Personality Disorder Scale

The Borderline Personality Disorder Scale (BPD Scale) is a 36-item, semi-structured interview with questions in nine categories of behavior relevant to BPD, and it takes 90 minutes to administer (Perry, 1982 and personal communication, 1986; Perry & Klerman, 1980). BPD Items correlate .88 with DSM-III criteria. DSM-III-R criteria can also be diagnosed.

A reliability correlation coefficient of .93 was reported using the videotape method (Perry, personal communication, 1986). Norms are available for the following diagnostic groups: BPD, borderline traits, antisocial personality disorder, bipolar affective disease, alcoholism, schizophrenia, neurosis, and adjustment disorders. The scale can discriminate BPD from nonpersonality disorders and also from antisocial personality disorder. These interviews were not blind, however. Specificity for definite BPD does not go lower than 76% in three studies. A factor-analytic study also provided support for the diagnostic criteria used.

The BPD Scale is a well-developed instrument with evidence for its reliability and validity. Work showing the separation of BPD from other diagnostic groups should be repeated blindly and extended to other personality disorders in addition to antisocial. The effects of state anxiety and depression on the scale should be investigated.

The BPD Scale has not achieved more than local usage. This is probably due to its length and need for further validity publications. Its length and detail appear to make it more generally useful as a research than as a clinical tool.

Diagnostic Interview for Personality Disorders

The McLean Hospital psychosocial research group has contributed the Diagnostic Interview for Personality Disorders (DIPD; Zanarini, 1983; Zanarini, Frankenburg, Chauncey, & Gunderson, 1987). Its 101 sections cover all the DSM-III personality disorder criteria. The interview is grouped by personality disorder and subgrouped by criteria. Each criterion has two or three probes that appear to have good face validity.

The instrument was designed to be administered by trained clinicians, and approximately four conjoint interviews are required to reach proficiency. As in all Axis II interviews, Axis I evaluation needs to be given first. The developers estimate that the interview takes 60 to 90 minutes to administer.

The joint reliability kappa for DIPD personality disorder is .94, and the 1-week test–retest kappa is .85 (Zanarini et al., 1987). This work was performed on nonpsychotic inpatients. At present there are no published comparisons with other measures of BPD.

This instrument is largely an expansion of the concept of the DIB, which Gunderson used to pioneer the empirical study of BPD. As with most instruments, the preliminary data are impressive. However, before this instrument can be properly assessed, it needs to be tested on outpatients (among whom most personality disorders are seen) and in a variety of population settings.

Structured Clinical Interview for DSM-III-R Personality Disorders

The SCID-II is a 120-item, comprehensive, semistructured personality interview designed by Spitzer et al. (1987). Each item has a 4-point scoring scale (inadequate information, negative, subthreshold, threshold), and specific probe questions are supplied. All DSM-III-R personality disorders are included.

The SCID-II occupies a separate niche from other instruments reviewed here, for several reasons. First, it is the only comprehensive DSM-III-R personality instrument that, in effect, is designed for the fastest possible delivery. Some criteria are the same in different but related disorders, and therefore do not have to be repeated. If it is clear that a patient will not qualify for a given disorder, there are "skip-outs" to the next disorder. The SCID-II is the instrument to use to determine the presence or absence of a personality disorder, when the personality disorders themselves are not under study. The SCID-II is also unique in that it is the only instrument designed as an extension to an existing Axis I instrument. The SCID-II is designed to be utilized by a skilled clinician.

A third aspect of the SCID-II that makes it unique is its use of a self-report personality measure prior to the interview. This measure is designed to give some false positives, but no false negatives. The idea is that if the personality symptoms are not present in the screening instrument, then they need not be asked about in the interview.

The SCID-II is currently in use in different research centers; however, its use is not as widespread as one would expect from the reputation and expertise of the developers. The reason is no doubt the relative lack of published data on the reliability and validity of the instrument. A recent report that compares the SCID-II to the Longitudinal Expert Evaluation Using All Data gives a positive predictive power of 1.00 and a negative predictive power of .25. From this it appears that the SCID-II may tend to overdiagnose BPD. This study was performed in a long-term inpatient treatment ward specifically geared to treating personality disorders (Skodol, Rosnick, Kellman, Oldham, & Hyler, 1988b).

Personality Disorder Examination

The PDE (Loranger, 1988) is a 128-section semistructured interview that covers all DSM-III-R diagnoses. It is divided into five headings for ease of administration (work, self, interpersonal relations, affect, and impulse control). Each section is scored on a 3-point scale. The PDE comes with a detailed scoring manual. Joint reliability data on a previous version of the instrument were excellent (Loranger, 1989). Loranger recently presented joint and test–retest reliabilities for his instrument for 84 nonpsychotic inpatients in an acute psychiatry ward. Joint reliability for correlation of criteria ranged from .82 to .94. Joint reliability for BPD criteria was .96. Test–retest consisted of comparing testing at admission by one rater with testing just prior to discharge by another. For BPD, the intraclass correlation of criteria was .86 and the kappa was .57 (Loranger, 1989). The current version has been carefully developed, and efforts have been made to avoid distortion due to state effects of anxiety and depression.

Although the latest version of the PDE has not been available long enough to establish as large an empirical data base as would be comfortable, confidence in the developer and in the preceding version of the PDE has made the PDE one of the most popular research instruments. Versions of the PDE are in use in the World Health Organization cross-national study of personality and the Harvard–Brown Longitudinal Study of Anxiety (HARP). It therefore has the advantage of allowing results of studies using the PDE to be easily comparable to findings that will be forthcoming from these studies.

Structured Interview for DSM-III-R Personality
Disorders—Revised

The SIDP-R (Pfohl, 1989) is an update of the SIDP to DSM-III-R criteria. The author has sent me data indicating that similar percentages of personality disorders are diagnosed by both instruments and that the overlap between histrionic and BPD criteria is similar in both instruments (Pfohl, personal communication, 1989). It is likely that the test characteristics are not radically changed from those of the previous instrument. The new instrument uses the same topic format and has worked to clarify the criteria for each rating. (These clarifications are contained within the test itself; there is no separate scoring manual.) I find the developer's lower time range of 60 minutes highly optimistic when patient populations are concerned.

Although the SIDP does not perform equally well for all personality disorders (see previous reviews—Reich, 1987, 1989b; Widiger & Frances, 1987) the data appear very good for BPD. Joint reliability for two people scoring the same interview is .85 (Stangl, Pfohl, Zimmerman, Bowers, & Corenthal, 1985), and there is a 6-month test–retest kappa of .70 (van der Brink, Slooff, Hanhart, & Rouwendall, 1986). Although this latter number might be mildly inflated because of counting "near neighbors" as hits, it still appears to be very good for the current state of the art of personality measurement instruments.

The SIDP and SIDP-R seem to be occupying a middle ground. Although not "designed for speed" like the SCID-II, and not having as widespread research use as the PDE, the SIDP has gained acceptance in a number of research and clinical settings. Certainly it appears very useful for the BPD diagnosis.

Personality Assessment Schedule

The Personality Assessment Schedule (PAS) is a semistructured interview arranged in 24 topic areas that are scored on a 9-point scale. It takes about 60 minutes to administer, and yields personality diagnoses that are roughly equivalent to DSM-III personality disorder clusters. The PAS was developed by Peter Tyrer (Tyrer, 1979; Tyrer & Alexander, 1979; Tyrer, Alexander, Cichetti, Cohen, & Remington, 1979; Tyrer, Casey, & Gall, 1983), who based it on a cluster analysis of personality traits of personality-disordered patients. It is recommended that it be given to both the subject and a knowledgeable informant; in this way it may avoid the pitfalls of state contamination of symptoms. It is not recommended for administration during acute illness states. It is computer-scored, but a hand-scoring technique is currently available. The PAS personality disorder categories are mutually exclusive. One of the major strengths of the PAS is the reliability of the personality disorder diagnosis. A blind 2.75-year test–retest of psychiatric patients yielded a weighted kappa of .64 for the presence or absence of a personality disorder (Tyrer, Strauss, & Cichetti, 1983). A cross-national videotape reliability study demonstrated that the PAS can be as successfully utilized by American psychiatrists as by their British counterparts (Tyrer et al., 1984).

There is some evidence for the validity of the diagnoses made by the PAS. It was a strong predictor of success in a drug trial and of outcome in an alcoholic treatment program, and the various diagnoses were associated differentially with different Axis I disorders (Griggs & Tyrer, 1981; Tyrer, Casey, & Gall, 1983).

This instrument is included in the current review, since in his latest book Tyrer (1988) gives a conversion method for determining DSM-III BPD. Although we do not know how well this conversion will work, it is an interesting option for those who wish to take another route toward measuring personality, but wish still to maintain the measurement of BPD.

Personality Interview Questionnaire II

The Personality Interview Questionnaire II (PIQ II; Widiger, 1987) is a revision of the PIQ I. It is a semistructured interview composed of 106 questions divided into eight content areas (self-description; self-confidence; work; relationships; emotions; social responsibility; interpersonal sensitivity and aberrant behavior; perceptions and beliefs). Each item is scored on a 9-point scale. Originally Widiger felt that it would be possible to use lay interviews for this instrument, but he has since rethought his position and now feels that clinically experienced raters are required (Widiger & Freiman, 1988). Kappas for joint reliabilities on a nonpsychotic state hospital population, with graduate students as raters, ranged from .45 to .92. For BPD, the kappa was .58 (Widiger & Freiman, 1988). Although the kappas are lower in some instances than those reported for the PIQ I, Widiger believes that what is being measured with the PIQ II (using graduate students) has greater validity.

Family History Methods

Family history methods for assessing personality disorders are at an early stage of development. Although it is not necessary for an illness to be familial for a family history method to be useful, the indications that many personality traits and disorders may be familial has probably spurred interest in this area (Bohman, Cloninger, Sigvardsson, & von Knorring, 1982; Cadoret, O'Gorman, Troughton, & Heywood, 1985; Cloninger, Sigvardsson, Bohman, & von Knorring, 1982; Sigvardsson, Cloninger, Bohman, & von Knorring, 1982; Reich, 1988b, 1989a).

To date there have been four attempts at developing family history measurements in the BPD—dramatic personality disorder cluster. The first I am aware of was by Baron, Gruen, Asnis, and Lord (1985); the second by myself and colleagues (Reich, Andreason, Crowe, & Noyes, 1986; Reich, 1988a); the third by Links and Steiner (1989); and the fourth by Zanarini, Gunderson, and Frankenburg (1989). Of these methods, that of Baron et al. (1985) is not currently in use, and those of Link and Steiner (1989) and Zanarini et al. (1989) have not been validated by interview measures. Our instrument, the Family History for DSM-III Anxiety and Personality Disorder Clusters, has been validated by comparing information obtained from interviews with relatives to information obtained with the instrument. It is also beginning to become more accepted in use. However, it only measures the DSM-III dramatic cluster and not BPD specifically. It is clear that this is a new area with much work yet to be done.

COMPARISON OF DIFFERENT INSTRUMENTS

It has been no secret among researchers that various instruments designed to measure the same DSM-III or DSM-III-R constructs often did not have perfect agreement. Until recently, however there have been few published empirical studies comparing these instruments. Table 6.3 lists the salient points of seven such studies. In general, the agreements are low. Agreement improves in populations where more severely ill borderlines are studied (e.g., inpatients, and outpatients selected for probable presence of a personality disorder) and appears to worsen with milder cases (unselected outpatients). Even in more severely ill cases the kappas of agreement are at best mediocre.

TABLE 6.3. Empirical Studies Comparing DSM-III or DSM-III-R Diagnoses of BPD

Study	Instruments compared	Population	Prevalence of BPD	Results of comparison
Hurt, Hyler, Frances, Clarkin, & Brent (1984)	PDQ, DIB, clinical interview	40 outpatients selected to have at least one personality disorder	PDQ: 18/40 Interview: 13/40 DIB: 19/40	PDQ vs. clinical interview: sensitivity, .69; specificity, .63. PDQ vs. DIB: sensitivity, .63; specificity, .62. Some tendency of the PDQ to overreport is noted.
Loranger, Oldham, Russakoff, & Sussman (1984)	DIB, modified SADS	30 acute psychiatry inpatients without organic brain syndrome	10/30 by final diagnosis	Correlation of DIB (cutoff of 7) and modified SADS = .93
Nelson et al. (1985)	Clinical interview (DSM-III), DIB	51 inpatients in psychiatry; those with organic brain syndrome excluded	DIB cutoff of 7: 15/51 DSM-III interview: 20/51	Fairly high concordance between DSM-III and DIB: 12 of the 15 DIB borderlines were also borderline by DSM-III clinical interview.
Reich, Noyes, & Troughton (1987a)	PDQ, MCMI, SIDP	131 nonpsychotic psychiatric outpatients	Approximately 12%	Kappas of agreement: SIDP vs. MCMI = .32 SIDP vs. PDQ = .43 MCMI vs. PDQ = .35

Study	Instruments	Sample	Agreement	Results
Angus & Marziali (1988)	DIB, PDQ, PDE	22 outpatients referred with a DSM-III diagnosis of BPD	PDQ: 80% DIB: 60% PDE: 45%	Concordance of all three measures, 35%; kappa = .05 Concordance of DIB and PDE, 35%; kappa = .08 Concordance of DIB and PDQ, 50%; kappa = −.33 Concordance of PDE and PDQ, 45%; kappa = .25
Widiger & Freiman (1988)	PIQ, MCMI	84 patients selected from state hospital inpatients who were thought to have personality disorders and did not have schizophrenia or organic brain syndrome	PIQ: 63%	Correlation of PIQ and MCMI = .51
Skodol, Rosnick, Kellman, Oldham, & Hyler (1988a); Hyler, Skodol, Kellman, Oldham, & Rosnick (1990)	PDQ-R, SCID-II, PDE	87 patients in a psychiatry ward used for long-term treatment of personality disorders	PDQ-R: 79% SCID-II: 61% PDE: 67%	Kappas: PDQ-R vs. SCID-II = .53 PDQ-R vs. PDE = .46 SCID-II vs. PDE = .53

It is clear that although all of these instruments are measuring something in the BPD realm, they are not measuring exactly the same thing. This does not mean that meaningful research cannot proceed, but it does raise several areas of caution for investigators. First, direct comparison of results of studies using different instruments may have a high degree of instrument-related variance. Second, investigators should be careful in their selection of instruments to assure that these instruments are well validated for their disorders of interest and in their populations of interest. Third, other sources of variance should be minimized to the greatest extent possible. Although this could involve many procedural aspects, one of the most important on interview instruments would be training of interviewers. Most interview developers agree that the value of an instrument's results are not better than the skill and training of the interviewers who give them.

One interesting side finding from these comparisons is that in one instance a self-report instrument (PDQ) agreed with two interview instruments (PDE, SCID-II) as well as they agreed with each other (Skodol et al., 1988a; Hyler, Skodol, Kellman, Oldham, & Rosnick, 1990). Although the PDQ did tend to overdiagnose, the finding raises the possibility that in some circumstances self-report measures may be capable of providing valid personality diagnoses. This is important, since these instruments are often quick and save expensive clinician time. Another small finding is the report of Loranger et al. (1984) that the Schedule for Affective Disorders and Schizophrenia (SADS) can be easily modified to produce a BPD diagnosis.

There is an article in the literature comparing Kernberg's structural interview technique with clinicians' ratings. Although Kernberg's technique is not reviewed in this chapter (it is a technique and not an instrument), this seems an appropriate point to mention the comparison. In this data reanalysis, the structural interview technique appeared to be picking up more general aspects of personality disorder, rather than a specific personality syndrome (Reich & Frances, 1984). However, to be fair, it appears that many other methods of diagnosing BPD may also be somewhat nonspecific.

THE RELATION OF SPECIFIC CRITERIA TO THE DIAGNOSIS OF BPD

Any psychiatric diagnosis in development requires a period of empirical testing before its criteria are definitively established. Initially, a set of prospective criteria is established from the literature, from theory, from factor-analytic studies, or by skilled clinicians. These criteria must then be empirically evaluated. The criteria for the personality disorders are at such a stage of development now; the question then arises as to how to evaluate them. There are many different approaches from many different disciplines. Baldessarini, Finkelstein, and Arana (1983), and subsequently Widiger, Hurt, Frances, Clarkin, and Gilmore (1984), have described a technique taken from psychology for formally proceeding with this process. This is to calculate sensitivity, specificity, predictive power positive (PPP), and predictive power negative (PPN) for proposed criteria and combinations of proposed criteria (with special emphasis on PPP and PPN). Criteria that appear important across multiple studies and populations may be "core criteria." (By "core criteria," I mean criteria that are necessary or sufficient factors for diagnosis of the disorder.) Criteria can vary in their degree of importance in defining a disorder. For example, although transient depression is often associated with many Axis I and Axis II disorders (i.e., high sensitivity, prevalence), it is seldom sufficiently pathognomonic to be included in defining criteria. This section of the chapter reports a set of results from a new population of BPD patients, using the method from psychology, and places the results in the context of existing findings.

First, I briefly review previous findings. Throughout this section I am, unless otherwise specified, referring to DSM-III criteria. In order to prevent unnecessary repetition of the criteria, I refer to them by abbreviation as follows:

IMP: Impulsivity
UIR: Unstable, intense relationships
ANG: Intense, uncontrolled anger
ID: Identity disturbance
AFF: Affective instability
INT: Intolerance of being alone
SD: Physically self-damaging acts
E&B: Feelings of chronic emptiness and boredom

In order to make the descriptions of the studies easier to follow, I have summarized the key findings in Table 6.4.

Widiger et al. (1984), in a sample of 76 outpatients with a primary Axis II diagnosis (BPD base rate = 34%), found that the PPP for the individual DSM-III criteria for BPD ranged from .56 to .73. (I am using PPP, since Widiger feels that the measure best reflects what clinicians are trying to achieve by diagnosis—that is, how many of those who are given the diagnosis actually have it. Since it is influenced by the prevalence of a disorder, a direct comparison of PPP cannot be made across studies.) More interesting, however, was their examination of combinations of two symptoms. Of 28 pairs, 19 had a PPP of greater than .80. They identified some especially valuable pairs (UIR-SD, SD-ID, UIR-ID, IMP-UIR, IMP-ID, AFF-E&B) with PPP's of greater than .90. They concluded that in their population one did not need the five

TABLE 6.4. Summary of Key Points of DSM-III BPD Criteria Studies

Study	Sample size	Number of BPD patients	Description of sample	Description of comparison group	Method of assessment	Best criteria reported
Reich (1990)	159	32 (20%)	Nonpsychotic, randomly selected psychiatric outpatients with BPD; 74.3% female; mean age, 30.9 (SD = 7.7) years	Same, except no BPD diagnosis; 63% female; mean age, 33.8 (SD = 10.2) years	PDQ (self-report), DSM-III (Axis II)	Single criteria: INT, SD, ID Two criteria: IMP-AFF IMP-SD IMP-E&B ANG-ID ID-INT ID-SD Three criteria: Virtually all were good.
McGlashan (1988)	160	50 (31%)	Patients who had been hospitalized at Chestnut Lodge, who were nonpsychotic, and who had a BPD diagnosis	Same, except did not meet BPD diagnosis	Chart review using standardized methods	ANG-SD combination was the best predictor.

Study	N	n (%) BPD	Patient selection	Comparison group	Diagnostic method	Results
Widiger, Hurt, Frances, Clarkin, & Gilmore (1984)	76	26 (34%)	Psychiatric inpatients at a state hospital, selected for presence of an Axis II disorder, who had BPD	Same, except did not meet BPD diagnosis	Semistructured interview given by lay interviewers	Individual criteria: PPP ranged from .56 to .73. Combinations of two criteria with PPP > .90: UIR-SD, ID-SD, UIR-ID, IMP-UIR, IMP-ID, AFF-E&B
Numberg, Hurt, Feldman, & Suh (1987, 1988)	BPD = 17, Controls = 20	17 (46%)	Hospitalized BPD patients selected from consecutive admissions to an acute inpatient ward; these patients were nonpsychotic and did not have a major affective disorder, predominant drug or alcohol problem, or organic brain syndrome	Members of psychiatric institution staff	DIB ≥ 7	Any combination of IMP, UIR, INT and/or E&B, and "acting out." Also good predictors in combinations of two: ID-IMP, ID-UIR, IMP-E&B

symptoms required by DSM-III to make the diagnosis of BPD. Widiger et al.'s (1984) patients were particularly sick as inpatient populations go, so they may not be representative and easily generalizable.

Nurnberg, Hurt, Feldman, and Suh (1987) carefully examined 17 borderline-related symptoms on a population of 17 hospitalized BPD patients and 20 controls. Their study basically confirmed the value of DSM-III criteria. However, when their four best criteria (roughly IMP, UIR, INT and/or E&B, and "acting out") were combined into any combination of two symptoms, their PPP was .94. They reported no appreciable gain using a combination of three criteria. They also concluded that five symptoms were not necessary to make a borderline diagnosis in their population. Nurnberg, Hurt, Feldman, and Suh (1988) also reported what appears to be a further analysis of their data. They obtained their best results for two criteria with IMP-ID, IMP-E&B, and UIR-ID. They also reported that when using their five best criteria, they found a slight *increase* in the total error rate when five criteria were used as the cutoff rate instead of four. (This was due to an increased false-negative rate.)

McGlashan (1988), in examining borderline criteria in his Chestnut Lodge follow-up study, examined combinations of the borderline criteria with sensitivities greater than .50. He found that the combination of ANG and SD was the best predictor for populations that excluded psychotic patients. He found, as did Nurnberg et al., that there was no gain from using more than two criteria. A weakness of this study was that criteria were assessed retrospectively by chart review.

In my own recent work with nonpsychotic psychiatric outpatients (Reich, 1990), the PDQ was used to assess DSM-III-R borderline criteria. Those without BPD were compared to those with BPD. INT, SD, and ID were the best individual criteria. When combinations of these criteria were used, virtually all combinations had high specificity and sensitivity.

In general, it appears that a combination of two borderline symptoms will often give a fairly good clinical estimate as to the presence or absence of BPD. The specific pairs Widiger et al. (1984) found to be especially powerful (UIR-SD, SD-ID, UIR-ID, IMP-UIR, IMP-ID, and AFF-E&B) also were found to be good, but were not best in my own sample (Reich, 1990). Compared with those combinations first predicted by Nurnberg et al. (1987) (IMP-UIR, IMP-INT, IMP-E&B, UIR-INT, UIR-E&B, and INT-E&B), I found several (IMP-INT, IMP-E&B, and UIR-INT) to be better than average predictors. Nurnberg et al's. second set of combinations (IMP-ID, IMP-E&B, and UIR-ID) represented only fair predictors. It is hard to compare the Reich (1990) results for combinations of three criteria with those of Nurnberg et al. (1988), since it appears that very few combinations of three criteria are really poor predictors.

Judging from individual criteria, IMP, INT, and E&B appear to be stronger predictors. Unlike Nurnberg et al. (1987), but similar to Nurnberg et al. (1988), I found (Reich, 1990) that diagnostic accuracy continued to improve when combinations of three criteria were used. It is possible that an effective diagnosis of BPD could be made with three of the DSM-III criteria rather than the existing five.

It is important to try to make sense of the different findings in different studies. The largest differences in these studies appear to be between the nature of the subject and control groups (see Table 6.4). The largest difference between subject and control groups was in Nurnberg et al.'s (1987, 1988) studies, where rigidly selected borderline patients virtually without other disorders were compared to members of the psychiatric staff. It is not surprising that their discriminators were powerful! It appears that for this comparison IMP, UIR, and INT are excellent predictors. The next most stringent comparison was the McGlashan study (1988), which compared former nonpsychotic inpatients with and without BPD. Here the ANG-SD combination appeared to separate the groups best. The next level of difficulty was that of the comparison between nonpsychotic psychiatric outpatients with and without BPD (Reich, 1990). Here INT, SD, and ID appear to work best. Finally, in a comparison between BPD and other personality disorders in inpatients (Widiger et al., 1984), combinations of SD, UIR, ID, and IMP seemed to work best. It is clear that the best-discriminating criteria depend to a large extent on which groups are being compared.

THE CONCEPT OF "CORE DIMENSIONS" FOR BPD

Another way of examining the differences found in different studies is to examine the concept of "core dimensions." This concept consists of the idea that specific criteria are either necessary or sufficient to diagnose the disorder. Thus two different reports could find different criteria important; however, both could be tapping into the same dimension. Hurt et al. (1990), in a study using advanced statistical methods not commonly used in this area of research, have analyzed four previous studies. They feel that the use of explicit criteria now allows the decision rules for making a diagnosis to be examined and derived statistically. Their analyses indicate three core dimensions to BPD: identity disturbance, affective disturbance, and impulse disturbance (or, as they call them, the Identity cluster, the Affect cluster, and the Impulse cluster). They feel that the latter two should be especially effective for identifying BPD. They conclude that a rule requiring three of the following four criteria should be close to optimum: IMP, UIR, AFF, and ID. Limitations of the Hurt et al. (1990) report include their particularly ill populations, many of whom were diagnosed by chart review. The report also covers some of the studies previously cited, so there is the danger of circularity.

The Hurt et al. (1990) report approaches core dimensions from a statistical approach, utilizing statistically generated decision rules. At present, I see these techniques as giving us valuable guidance, but, because of their limitations, not definitive answers. Some of my work (Reich, 1990) seems to confirm the importance of core dimensions. The best individual criteria in my study seem to be IMP, INT, and E&B. However, for the combination-of-three-criteria analysis, one of the combinations (UIR, ANG, and SD) has a sensitivity, specificity, PPP, and PPN of 1.00. This result would become more understandable if we postulate that these criteria represent two of the Hurt et al. (1990) core dimensions that are valuable in diagnosis (affective disturbance and impulse disturbance).

As a preliminary attempt to examine how core dimensions might work, I have tried to arrange the DSM-III criteria into core dimensions that are suggested by the work of Kernberg, Masterson, Adler, Hurt et al., and Millon, and have compared them to available empirical results. Table 6.5 shows this comparison. In contrast to the criterion comparisons, there is broad agreement across studies. Inappropriate aggressiveness, characteristic affective disturbance, and impulse disturbance are positive from all measures in all studies. Fear of abandonment and characteristic interpersonal problems are also in high agreement.

There are, of course, limitations to this comparison. Some proposed core dimensions are represented by more DSM-III criteria and therefore are more likely to be positive in this analysis. The criteria that fit the proposed

TABLE 6.5. Comparison of Potential Core Dimensions with Empirical Findings

Empirical study	Inappropriate aggressiveness[a]		Fear of abandonment[b]		Identity disturbance[c]	Affective disturbance[d]		Impulse disturbance[e]		Interpersonal problems[f]	
Widiger et al. (1984)	$+_S$	$+_D$	$+_S$	$+_D$	$+_D$	$+_S$	$+_D$	$+_S$	$+_D$	$+_S$	$+_D$
Nurnberg et al. (1987, 1988)	$+_S$	$+_D$	$+_S$	$+_D$	$+_S$	$+_S$	$+_D$	$+_S$	$+_D$	$+_S$	$+_D$
McGlashan (1988)[g]		$+_D$					$+_D$		$+_D$		
Reich (1990)	$+_S$	$+_D$	$+_S$	$+_D$	$+_S$	$+_D$	$+_S$	$+_D$	$+_S$	$+_D$	$+_S$	$+_D$

Note. A core dimension is considered present if either an individual DSM-III criterion or one of a combination of two criteria was a good predictor for a study. Since PPP varies with prevalence, those criteria with the highest PPP within a given study were chosen as best predictors. Natural "break points" were used to separate "good" from "less good" predictors. Single criteria are indicated by a subscript "S," while criteria that are part of a combination of two are indicated by a subscript "D."
[a] Criteria UIR, ANG, SD.
[b] Criteria UIR, INT.
[c] Criterion ID.
[d] Criteria ANG, AFF, INT, E&B.
[e] Criteria IMP, UIR, ANG, SD.
[f] Criteria UIR, ID, INT.
[g] McGlashan only reported his best combination of two pairs, so the data are incomplete.

core dimensions were drawn in a broad fashion, since in general the DSM-III criteria are not tailored to reflect these dimensions. Also, it appears that many of these core dimensions would overlap. Nonetheless, such broad agreement, when contrasted with the disagreement when criteria were compared, represents a potential area for new criteria research.

THE PROBLEM OF PERSONALITY DISORDER OVERLAP

When the DSM-III criteria were originally specified, a decision was made about the approach to this relatively unvalidated and underresearched area. This decision was to describe a greater rather than a lesser number of disorders, so that research on less thoroughly researched disorders would not be prematurely cut off (Spitzer, personal communication, 1985). DSM-III-R, although making some modifications to clarify certain points and to help distinguish various personality disorders from each other, left the DSM-III personality section largely intact. A practical result of this system has been to create multiple personality diagnoses in individual subjects. Most researchers using standardized techniques report that a patient who qualifies for one personality disorder will usually qualify for two or three.

For BPD, overlap has been empirically reported for schizotypal, dependent, histrionic, and other personality disorders (Frances, 1980, 1982; Spitzer & Williams, 1980). This creates a problem in interpreting the results of various studies, since it is quite possible that all "borderlines" are not equivalent. A BPD patient without another personality disorder diagnosis could be significantly different in outcome factors, Axis I comorbidity, and demographic factors from a BPD patient comorbid for schizotypal and obsessive–compulsive personality disorders (Clarkin, Widiger, Frances, Hurt, & Gilmore, 1983). If only BPD is measured or reported, important data relevant to diagnosis, treatment, and comparisons with other studies may be missing. It would appear important that measures of other personality disorders be performed and reported, even if the major focus of the report is on BPD. For those studies limited in time or resources, a self-report inventory may be the answer.

DIRECTIONS FOR FUTURE RESEARCH

There are basically four directions for future research in the BPD criteria. The first two are (1) distinguishing which criteria best distinguish different groups of patients, and (2) experimenting with new criteria based on the "core dimensions" model, to understand how they overlap with other personality disorders or personality disorder symptoms and biological markers. The first area would seem to be one in which substantial work has already been performed.

However, as my earlier section on this area indicates, there are actually relatively few empirical studies utilizing standardized measurement techniques. The results of this arm of research would be to determine which criteria or combination of criteria differentiate different population groups (i.e., normals, outpatients, inpatients, patients with personality disorders, etc.); this approach might eventually allow the discrimination of BPD in some situations with far fewer criteria than we use now. The investigation of new criteria representing the hypothesized "core dimensions" could easily be incorporated into this work.

The third direction for future research—studying the effect of overlap of BPD with other personality disorders or traits on the quality of the BPD diagnosis—may not be so much a specific area of research as a suggestion for all researchers in the area. All researchers should report, at a minimum, the other personality disorders present concurrently in their BPD patients. Reporting concurrent significant personality traits present would ideally also be valuable, but possibly could be difficult in practice. Also important to report are complete Axis I diagnoses. Axis I–Axis II interactions have not been completely worked out. There is some indication that this area could be important: One study has reported differences in family history, depending on the comorbidity of a personality disorder in probands (Reich, 1988b). Reporting this information would perform two functions. First, it would allow a clearer interpretation of the results of any individual study; second, it would create a body of literature from which future hypotheses could be drawn.

Relatively little work has been performed to data on biological markers and BPD or criteria for BPD. (There is one report on reduced rapid-eye-movement latency in nondepressed BPD patients; see Akiskal, Yerevanian, & Davis, 1985.) However, the rapid advances in technology in this area make this an interesting area of potential research in the future.

To sum up, it appears that BPD measurement research has passed beyond the infancy period to an exciting middle level of development. There are now many preliminary empirical studies in the literature, as well as an extensive theoretical base to draw upon. This base, combined with a greater understanding of psychiatric nosology, biological markers, and advanced statistical techniques, has given researchers the material for years of valuable and productive research.

ACKNOWLEDGMENT

I would like to acknowledge the help of John Gunderson, MD, and his Boston Personality Study Group. Discussions with that group were helpful in the development of this chapter.

REFERENCES

Akiskal, A. S., Yerevanian, B. I., & Davis, G. C. (1985). The nosologic status of borderline personality: Clinical and polysomnographic study. *American Journal of Psychiatry, 142,* 192–198.

Angus, L. E., & Marziali, E. (1988). A comparison of three measures for the diagnosis of borderline personality disorder. *American Journal of Psychiatry, 145,* 1453–1454.

Baldessarini, R. J., Finkelstein, S., & Arana, G. W. (1983). The predictive power of diagnostic tests and the effects of prevalence of illness. *Archives of General Psychiatry, 40,* 569–577.

Baron, M. (1981). *Schedule for Interviewing Borderlines.* New York: New York State Psychiatric Institute.

Baron, M., Gruen, R., Asnis, L., & Lord, S. (1985). Familial transmission of schizotypal and borderline personality disorders. *American Journal of Psychiatry, 142,* 927–934.

Barrash, J., Kroll, J., Carey, K., & Sines, L. (1983). Discriminating borderline disorder from other personality disorders. *Archives of General Psychiatry, 40,* 1297–1302.

Barrash, J., Kroll, J., Sines, L., & Carey, K. (1991). *Diagnostic Interview for Borderlines Schizotypy Checklist: A method for identifying schizotypal borderlines.* Manuscript in preparation.

Bell, M. (1981). *Bell Object Relations Self Report Scale.* West Haven, CT: Psychology Service, Veterans Administration Medical Center.

Bell, M., Metcalf, J., & Ryan, E. (1979). *Reality testing and object relations: A self-report instrument.* Paper presented at the 87th Annual Convention of the American Psychological Association, New York.

Bell, M., Metcalf, J., & Ryan, E. (1980). *Reality Testing–Object Relations Assessment Scale: Reliability and validity studies.* Paper presented at the 88th Annual Convention of the American Psychological Association, New York.

Benjamin, L. S. (1974). Structural Analysis of Social Behavior. *Psychological Review, 81,* 392–425.

Benjamin, L. S. (1984). Principles of prediction using Structural Analysis of Social Behavior (SASB). In R. A. Zucker, S. Aronoff, & A. J. Rabin (Eds.), *Personality and the prediction of behavior.* New York: Academic Press.

Bohman, M., Cloninger, C. R., Sigvardsson, S., & von Knorring, A. L. (1982). Predisposition to petty criminality in Swedish adoptees: I. Genetics and environmental heterogeneity. *Archives of General Psychiatry, 39,* 1233–1241.

Cadoret, R. J., O'Gorman, T. W., Troughton, E., & Heywood, E. (1985). Alcoholism and antisocial personality. *Archives of General Psychiatry, 42,* 161–167.

Clark, L. A. (1988, November 14). *The basic maladaptive traits in the domain of personality disorders.* Paper presented at the National Institute of Mental Health Workshop on Assessment of Personality Disorders, Bethesda, MD.

Clark, L. A. (1989). *Preliminary manual for the Schedule for Normal and Abnormal Personality (SNAP).* Dallas, TX: Department of Psychology, Southern Methodist University.

Clarkin, J. F., Widiger, T. A., Frances, A., Hurt, S. W., & Gilmore, M. (1983).

Prototypic typology and the borderline personality disorder. *Journal of Abnormal Psychology*, *92*, 263–275.

Cloninger, C. R., Sigvardsson, S., Bohman, M., & von Knorring, A. L. (1982). Predisposition to petty criminality in Swedish adoptees: II. Cross-fostering analysis of gene–environmental interaction. *Archives of General Psychiatry*, *39*, 1242–1247.

Cornell, G., Silk, K., Ludolf, P., & Lohr, N. E. (1983). The test–retest reliability of the Diagnostic Interview for Borderlines. *Archives of General Psychiatry*, *40*, 1307–1311.

Conte, H., Plutchik, R., & Karasu, T. (1980). A self-report borderline scale: Discriminative validity and preliminary norms. *Journal of Nervous and Mental Disease*, *168*, 428–435.

Edell, W. S. (1984). The Borderline Syndrome Index: Clinical validity and utility. *Journal of Nervous and Mental Disease*, *172*, 254–263.

Frances, A. (1980). The DSM-III personality disorders section: A commentary. *American Journal of Psychiatry*, *137*, 1050–1054.

Frances, A. (1982). Categorical and dimensional systems of personality diagnosis: A comparison. *Comprehensive Psychiatry*, *23*, 516–527.

Frances, A., Clarkin, J., Gilmore, M., Hurt, S. W., & Brown, R. (1984). Reliability of criteria for borderline personality disorder: A comparison of DSM-III and DIB. *American Journal of Psychiatry*, *141*, 1080–1084.

Griggs, S. M., & Tyrer, P. J. (1981). Personality disorder, social adjustment and treatment outcome in alcoholics. *Journal of Studies on Alcohol*, *42*, 802–805.

Gunderson, J. (1982a). *Diagnostic Interview for Borderline Patients*. Belmont, MA: Harvard Medical School.

Gunderson, J. (1982b). Empirical studies of the borderline diagnosis. In L. Grinspoon (Ed.), *Psychiatry update* (Vol. 2). Washington, DC: American Psychiatric Press.

Gunderson, J., & Kolb, J. (1978). Discriminating features of borderline patients. *American Journal of Psychiatry*, *135*, 792–796.

Gunderson, J., Kolb, J., & Austin, V. (1981). The Diagnostic Interview for Borderline Patients. *American Journal of Psychiatry*, *138*, 896–903.

Hess, A. J. (1985). Review of the Millon Clinical Multiaxial Inventory. In J. Mitchell (Ed.), *The ninth mental measurement yearbook* (Vol. 1). Lincoln: University of Nebraska Press.

Hurt, S. W., Clarkin, J. F., Widiger, T. A., Fyer, M. R., Sullivan, T., Stone, M. H., & Frances, A. (1990). Evaluation of DSM-III decision rules for case detection using joint conditional probability structures. *Journal of Personality Disorders*, *4*, 121–130.

Hurt, S. W., Hyler, S. E., Frances, A., Clarkin, J. F., & Brent, R. (1984). Assessing borderline personality disorder with a self report, clinical interview or semi-structured interview. *American Journal of Psychiatry*, *141*, 1228–1231.

Hyler, S. E., Rieder, R. O., Williams, J. B., Spitzer, R. L., Hendler, J., & Lyons, M. (1987). *Personality Diagnostic Questionnaire—Revised (PDQ-R)*. New York: New York State Psychiatric Institute.

Hyler, S. E., Rieder, R. O., Williams, J. B., Spitzer, R. L., Hendler, J., & Lyons, M. (1989). The Personality Diagnostic Questionnaire: Development and preliminary results. *Journal of Personality Disorders*, *2*, 229–237.

Hyler, S. E., Skodol, A. E., Kellman, D., Oldham, J. M., & Rosnick, L. (1990). The utility of the Personality Diagnostic Questionnaire: A comparison with two structured interviews. *American Journal of Psychiatry, 147*, 1043–1048.

Kernberg, O., Goldstein, E., Carr, A., Hunt, A. C., Bauer, S. F., & Blumenthal, R. (1981). Diagnosing borderline personality: A pilot study using multiple diagnostic methods. *Journal of Nervous and Mental Disease, 169*, 225–231.

Klein, M. (1985). *Wisconsin Personality Inventory (WISPI)*. Madison, WI: Department of Psychiatry, University of Wisconsin.

Koenigsberg, H., Kernberg, O., & Schomer, J. (1983). Diagnosing borderline conditions in an outpatient setting. *Archives of General Psychiatry, 40*, 49–53.

Kolb, J., & Gunderson, J. (1980). Diagnosing borderline patients with a semi-structured interview. *Archives of General Psychiatry, 37*, 37–41.

Kroll, J., Carey, K., Sines, L., & Roth, M. (1982). Are there borderlines in Britain: A cross-validation of U.S. findings. *Archives of General Psychiatry, 39*, 60–63.

Kroll, J., Pyle, R., Zander, J., Martin, F., Larry, S., & Sines, L. (1981). Borderline personality disorder: Interrater reliability of the Diagnostic Interview for Borderlines. *Schizophrenia Bulletin, 7*, 269–272.

Kroll, J., Sines, L., Martin, K., Lari, S., Pyle, R., & Zander, J. (1981). Borderline personality disorder: Construct validity of the concept. *Archives of General Psychiatry, 38*, 1021–1026.

Links, P. S., & Steiner, M. (1989, May 11). Subtyping borderlines by family history. In J. Reich (Chair), *Family history and DSM-III, Axis II*. Symposium presented at the annual meeting of the American Psychiatric Association, San Francisco.

Loranger, A. (1988). *Personality Disorder Examination (PDE) manual*. White Plains, NY: Cornell Medical Center.

Loranger, A. (1989, May 22–23). [Training session given to investigators and staff of the Harvard–Brown Anxiety Research Project (HARP), Boston].

Loranger, A., Oldham, J. M., Russakoff, I. M., & Sussman, V. L. (1984). Structured interviews and borderline personality disorder. *Archives of General Psychiatry, 41*, 565–568.

Loranger, A. W., Sussman, V. L., Oldham, J. M., & Russakoff, L. M. (1987). Personality Disorder Examination (PDE): A structured interview for DSM-III-R personality disorders. *Journal of Personality Disorders, 1*, 1–14.

McGlashan, T. (1988, May 11). Diagnostic efficiency of DSM-III borderline personality disorder and schizotypal disorder. In J. M. Oldham (Chair), *Axis II: New perspectives on validity*. Symposium presented at the 141st Annual Meeting of the American Psychiatric Association, Montreal.

Millon, T. (1981). *Disorders of personality: DSM-III, Axis II*. New York: Wiley–Interscience.

Millon, T. (1982). *Manual for the Millon Clinical Multiaxial Inventory* (2nd ed.). Minneapolis: National Computer Systems.

Millon, T. (1987). *Manual for the Millon Clinical Multiaxial Inventory II (MCMI-II)*. Minnetonka: National Computer Systems.

Nelson, H., Tennen, H., Tasman, A., Borton, M., Kubeck, M., & Stone, M. (1985). Comparison of three systems for diagnosing borderline personality disorder. *American Journal of Psychiatry, 142*, 855–858.

Nurnberg, H. G., Hurt, S. W., Feldman, A., & Suh, R. (1987). Efficient diagnosis of borderline personality disorder. *Journal of Personality Disorders, 1*, 307–315.

Nurnberg, H. G., Hurt, S. W., Feldman, A., & Suh, R. (1988). Evaluation of diagnostic criteria for borderline personality disorder. *American Journal of Psychiatry, 145*, 1280–1283.

Perry, J. (1982). *The Borderline Personality Disorder Scale (BPD Scale)*. Cambridge, MA: Cambridge Hospital.

Perry, J., & Klerman, G. (1980). Clinical features of borderline personality disorder. *American Journal of Psychiatry, 137*, 165–173.

Pfohl, B. (1989). *Structured Interview for DSM-III-R Personality Disorders—Revised (SIDPR)*. Iowa City: Department of Psychiatry, University of Iowa Hospitals and Clinics.

Pfohl, B., Coryell, W., Zimmerman, M., & Stangl, D. (1987). Prognostic validity of self report and interview measures of personality disorder in depressed inpatients. *Journal of Clinical Psychiatry, 48*, 468–472.

Pfohl, B., Stangl, D., & Zimmerman, M. (1982). *The Structured Interview for DSM-III Personality Disorders (SIDP)*. Iowa City: University of Iowa Hospitals and Clinics.

Reich, J. (1987). Instruments measuring DSM-III and DSM-III-R personality disorders. *Journal of Personality Disorders, 1*, 220–240.

Reich, J. (1988a). A family history method for DSM-III and DSM-III-R personality disorders. *Psychiatry Research, 26*, 131–139.

Reich, J. (1988b). DSM-III personality disorders and family history of mental illness. *Journal of Nervous and Mental Disease, 176*, 45–49.

Reich, J. (1988c). DSM-III personality disorders and the outcome of treated panic disorders. *American Journal of Psychiatry, 145*, 1149–1153.

Reich, J. (1989a). Familiality of DSM-III personality disorder clusters. *Journal of Nervous and Mental Disorders, 177*, 96–101.

Reich, J. (1989b). Update on instruments to measure DSM-III and DSM-III-R personality disorders. *Journal of Nervous and Mental Disease, 17*, 366–371.

Reich, J. (1990). Criteria for diagnosing DSM-III-R borderline personality disorder. *Annals of Clinical Psychiatry, 2*, 189–197.

Reich, J., Andreason, N., Crowe, R., & Noyes, R. (1986). *Family History for DSM-III Anxiety and Personality Disorder Clusters (FHPD)*. Boston, MA: Department of Psychiatry, Harvard University.

Reich, J., & Frances, A. (1984). A critique of the structural interview method of diagnosing borderline personality disorders. *Psychiatric Quarterly, 56*, 229–235.

Reich, J., Noyes, R., & Troughton, E. (1987a). Comparison of instruments to measure DSM-III, Axis II. In T. Millon (Ed.), *Proceedings of the Millon Clinical Multiaxial Inventory Conference 1986*. Minnetonka, MN: National Computer Systems.

Reich, J., Noyes, R., & Troughton, E. (1987b). Dependent personality in panic patients with phobic avoidance. *American Journal of Psychiatry, 144*, 323–327.

Reich, J., & Troughton, E. (1988). Frequency of personality disorders in panic, outpatient and normal populations. *Journal of Psychiatric Research, 26*, 89–100.

Reich, J., Yates, W., & Nduaguba, M. (1989). Prevalence of DSM-III personality disorders in the community. *Social Psychiatry, 24*, 12–16.

Robins, E., & Guze, S. G. (1970). Establishment of diagnostic validity in psychiatric illness: Its application to schizophrenia. *American Journal of Psychiatry, 126,* 983–987.

Sigvardsson, S., Cloninger, C. R., Bohman, M., & von Knorring, A. L. (1982). Predisposition to petty criminality in Swedish adoptees: III. Sex differences and validation of the male topology. *Archives of General Psychiatry, 39,* 1248–1253.

Skodol, A. E., Rosnick, L., Kellman, O., Oldham, J. M., & Hyler, S. E. (1988a, May 11). The validity of structured assessments of Axis II. In J. M. Oldham (Chair), *Axis II: New perspectives on validity.* Symposium presented at the 141st Annual Meeting of the American Psychiatric Association, Montreal.

Skodol, A. E., Rosnick, L., Kellman, D., Oldham, J. M., & Hyler, S. E. (1988b). Validating structured DSM-III-R personality disorder assessments with longitudinal data. *American Journal of Psychiatry, 145,* 1297–1299.

Soloff, P. (1981a). A comparison of borderline with depressed and schizophrenia patients on a new diagnostic interview. *Comprehensive Psychiatry, 22,* 291–300.

Soloff, P. (1981b). Affect, impulse, and psychosis in borderline disorders: A validation study. *Comprehensive Psychiatry, 22,* 337–350.

Soloff, P. (1981c). Concurrent validation of a diagnostic interview for borderline patients. *American Journal of Psychiatry, 138,* 691–693.

Spitzer, R. L., & Williams, J. B. W. (1980). Classification of mental disorders and DSM-III. In H. Kaplan, A. Freedman, & B. Sadock (Eds.), *Comprehensive textbook of psychiatry III* (3rd ed., Vol. 1). Baltimore: Williams & Wilkins.

Spitzer, R. L., Williams, J. B. W., & Gibbon, M. (1987). *Structured Clinical Interview for DSM-III-R Personality Disorders (SCID-II).* New York: Biometrics Research Department, New York State Psychiatric Institute.

Stangl, D., Pfohl, B., Zimmerman, M., Bowers, W., & Corenthal, C. (1985). A structured interview for DSM-III personality disorders. *Archives of General Psychiatry, 42,* 591–596.

Tarnopolsky, A., & Berelowitz, M. (1987). Borderline personality: a review of recent research. *British Journal of Psychiatry, 151,* 724–734.

Tyrer, P. (1979). *Personality Assessment Schedule (PAS).* (Available from Mapperley Hospital, Porchester Road, Nottingham NG36AA, England, U.K.)

Tyrer, P. (1988). *Personality disorders.* Bristol, England: Wright.

Tyrer, P., & Alexander, J. (1979). Classification of personality disorder. *British Journal of Psychiatry, 135,* 238–242.

Tyrer, P., Alexander, M. S., Cichetti, D., Cohen, M. S., & Remington, M. (1979). Reliability of a schedule for rating personality disorders. *British Journal of Psychiatry, 135,* 168–174.

Tyrer, P., Casey, P., & Gall, J. (1983). Relationship between neurosis and personality disorder. *British Journal of Psychiatry, 142,* 404–408.

Tyrer, P., Cichetti, D. V., Casey, P. R., Fitzpatrick, K., Oliver, R., & Balter, A. (1984). Cross national reliability study of a schedule for assessing personality disorders. *Journal of Nervous and Mental Disease, 172,* 718–721.

Tyrer, P., Strauss, J., & Cichetti, D. (1983). Temporal reliability of personality in psychiatric patients. *Psychological Medicine, 13,* 393–398.

van der Brink, W., Slooff, C., Hanhart, M., & Rouwendall, M. (1986, May 13). Joint and test–retest reliability of DSM-III Axis II diagnoses. In B. Pfohl (Chair),

DSM-III, Axis II, revisions and assessment. Symposium presented at the annual meeting of the American Psychiatric Association, Washington, DC.

Widiger, T. A. (1987). *Personality Interview Questionnaire II (PIQ II).* White Plains, NY: Department of Psychiatry, Cornell Medical Center, Westchester Division.

Widiger, T. A., & Frances, A. (1987). The convergent and discriminant validity of the MCMI as a measure of the DSM-III personality disorders. *Journal of Personality Assessment, 51,* 228–242.

Widiger, T. A., & Freiman, K. E. (1988, November 14). *Personality Interview Questionnaire II: Reliability and methodologic issues.* Paper presented at the National Institute of Mental Health Workshop on Assessment of Personality Disorders, Bethesda, MD.

Widiger, T. A., Hurt, S. W., Frances, A., Clarkin, J. F., & Gilmore, M. (1984). Diagnostic efficiency and DSM-III. *Archives of General Psychiatry, 41,* 1005–1012.

Widiger, T. A., & Sanderson, C. (1987). Interviews and inventories for the measurement of personality disorders. *Clinical Psychology Review, 7,* 49–73.

Yates, W., Sellini, B., & Reich, J. (1989). Comorbidity of bulimia nervosa and personality disorder. *Journal of Clinical Psychiatry, 50,* 57–59.

Zanarini, M. C. (1983). *Diagnostic Interview for Personality Disorders (DIPD).* Belmont, MA: McLean Hospital.

Zanarini, M. C., Frankenburg, F. R., Chauncey, D. L., & Gunderson, J. G. (1987). The Diagnostic Interview for Personality Disorders: Interrater and test–retest reliability. *Comprehensive Psychiatry, 28,* 467–480.

Zanarini, M. C., Gunderson, J. G., & Frankenburg, F. R. (1989). Diagnostic algorithms for familial borderline personality disorder. In J. Reich (Chair), *Family history and DSM-III, Axis II.* Symposium presented at the annual meeting of the American Psychiatric Association, San Francisco.

CHAPTER 7

Axis I Comorbidity of Borderline Personality Disorder: Clinical Implications

JEFFREY M. JONAS
HARRISON G. POPE

Perhaps more than with any other diagnosis, controversy has surrounded the meaning and use of the diagnosis of borderline personality disorder (BPD). Researchers have argued whether or not BPD is related to schizophrenia or affective disorder, and whether BPD can be distinguished reliably from other personality disorders or even Axis I disorders. Clinicians have been uncertain about the best treatment for BPD, with suggested strategies including psychodynamic psychotherapy, short-term symptom-oriented treatment, and medication.

Some of this confusion has arisen from the fact that BPD frequently coexists with Axis I disorders, such as major depression. In such cases, do both disorders stem from a common underlying pathophysiology, or is one disorder largely a consequence of the other? Clearly, these alternative interpretations might lead to very different strategies for treatment.

In this chapter, we examine recent studies of BPD that have addressed the issues of Axis I comorbidity and diagnostic stability. Although these studies, as will be seen, are at times contradictory and subject to methodological limitations, we attempt to assess their theoretical and clinical implications.

EMPIRICAL STUDIES OF BPD

Do subjects with BPD frequently suffer from other disorders that are present simultaneously with BPD? If they do not, this observation would provide relatively clear evidence that BPD is an independent entity. However, such independence has not been observed in most studies. Instead, as has been the experience of many clinicians, patients with BPD are frequently diagnosed as having other Axis I and Axis II disorders. This has led to speculation by some that BPD is a heterogeneous grouping of assorted affective, organic, and schizotypal disorders (Davis & Akiskal, 1986), whereas other groups have suggested that BPD is an independent entity that frequently coexists with other, largely affective disorders (Pope, Jonas, Hudson, Cohen, & Gunderson, 1983; Tarnopolsky & Berelowitz, 1987).

An initial problem in determining whether BPD is a distinct entity had been the development of uniform operational diagnostic criteria, a difficulty that was addressed with the publication of the *Diagnostic and Statistical Manual of Mental Disorders*, third edition (DSM-III). The DSM-III operational criteria for BPD allowed researchers and clinicians to study and compare subjects who were more likely to be diagnosed similarly. Prior to DSM-III, this was not the case; patients with "as-if personalities," "borderline personality organization," "pseudoneurotic schizophrenia," and so forth were frequently considered "borderlines"—making the various studies difficult to compare.

In recognition of this problem, we have confined our review of studies of comorbidity in BPD to those that have utilized DSM-III criteria. We have reviewed elsewhere (Jonas & Pope, 1984) the earlier studies of BPD that utilized DSM-III and "DSM-III-like" criteria. In that review we found that in most instances, subjects with BPD frequently had concomitant affective disorders or other personality disorders.

Table 7.1 presents major studies in the last 10 years that have examined comorbidity in BPD. We have not included studies that examined subjects with other disorders for the presence of BPD, nor have we included studies that have focused on diagnostic reliability of the syndrome. Most of the studies shown utilized a similar methodology. An index population with a diagnosis of BPD was studied using one of a number of assessment tools, or was studied by chart review and clinical assessment. Ideally, assessment for comorbidity with other disorders was performed blindly (e.g., Pope et al., 1983; McGlashan, 1983; Zanarini, Gunderson, & Frankenburg, 1989), or chart review was quality-controlled by selecting some charts at random (Fyer, Frances, Sullivan, Hurt, & Clarkin, 1988). In a few cases (McGlashan, 1983; McManus, Lerner, Robbins, & Barbour, 1984), subjects with BPD were selected from a mixed group of patients.

A number of findings have emerged from these studies. First, nearly all have found that individuals with BPD frequently suffer from numerous depressive symptoms and often have a diagnosis of a concomitant affective disorder. Only a few investigators (Fyer et al., 1988) have found no particular pattern of overlap; others suggest that affective disorder, when it does occur, is mild (Frances, Clarkin, Gilmore, Hurt, & Brown, 1984; Zanarini et al., 1989). Second, no group has found an overlap of BPD and schizophrenia, and a number of researchers specify that BPD and schizophrenia appear to

TABLE 7.1. Studies of Axis I Comorbidity and Diagnostic Overlap with BPD

Study	Study groups	Assessment tools	Areas of overlap and other findings
Soloff (1981)	BPD, S, D	DIB	BPD were more impulsive, self-destructive, and angry.
Snyder, Sajadi, Pitts, & Goodpaster (1982)	BPD, Dy	Ham, BPRS, MMPI, Zung, POMS	Both groups similarly depressed. Depressed group showed sleep disturbance, diurnal variation. BPD on BPRS tended to be more manipulative, suicidal, impulsive.
Pope, Jonas, Hudson, Cohen, & Gunderson (1983)	BPD	DIB, blind chart reviews	BPD and MAD frequently coexisted. BPD not distinguished from HPD and ASPD.
McGlashan (1983)	Mixed	Chart diagnosis, blind follow-up diagnosis	Subjects with DSM-III BPD were distinct, but overlap suggested with D. On follow-up, D and BPD did not separate out.
McManus, Lerner, Robbins, & Barbour (1984)	Adolescents—mixed	SADS, DSM-III, DIB	BPD frequently overlapped with MAD.
Andrulonis & Vogel (1984)	BPD, MAD, S	DSM-III, chart review	Males with BPD showed a high rate of ADD. BPD showed a higher rate of acting out and substance abuse than comparison groups. Family history in BPD group showed a high rate of MAD.
Baxter, Edell, Gerner, Fairbanks, & Gwirtsman (1984)	BPD	DST, discharge diagnosis	Significant association of D and BPD when compared to non-BPD patients. Positive DST in 73% of BPD patients.
Frances, Clarkin, Gilmore, Hurt, & Brown (1984)	BPD	Clinical interview	Of BPD patients, 38% had MAD, 23% had substance abuse. MAD noted to be mild in most cases.

(continued)

TABLE 7.1. (Continued)

Study	Study groups	Assessment tools	Areas of overlap and other findings
Perry (1985)	BPD, ASPD, bipolar II	DSM-III, RDC, DIS, POMS	High rate of overlap of BPD and MAD.
Grunhaus, King, Greden, & Flegel (1985)	BPD	SADS, Ham	High rate of overlap of BPD and MAD; 37% of MAD-BPD subjects had panic disorder. No panic in absence of MAD.
Rippetoe, Alarcon, & Walter-Ryan (1986)	BPD	Chart review	High rate of overlap et BPD and D. BPD subjects with depression more likely to show splitting and to be suicidal. BPD with Dy more likely to complain of emptiness and to have poor functioning.
Soloff (1987)	BPD	SADS, clinical ratings	Overlap of BPD and D. Subtyped according to type of depression: Hysteroid dysphoria seen in 64%, atypical depression in 41%, RDC depression in 49%.
Fyer, Frances, Sullivan, Hurt, & Clarkin (1988)	BPD	Chart review (23 of 180 done blind to assess reliability)	Of those with BPD, 91% had an additional diagnosis; 42% had two or more diagnoses. No distinctive pattern of overlap found.
Benjamin, Silk, Lohr, & Westen (1989)	BPD, D	DIS, SCL-90, SADS, ASQ	BPD not more anxious than other patient groups.
Zanarini, Gunderson, & Frankenburg (1989)	BPD, ASPD, Dy	SCID, given blindly	BPD significantly more likely than controls to have history of MAD; BPD more likely than dysthymics to have substance abuse.

Note. Abbreviations: S, schizophrenia; D, major depression; Dy, dysthymia; HPD, histrionic personality disorder; ASPD, antisocial personality disorder; MAD, major affective disorders; ADD, attention deficit disorder; SPD, schizotypal personality disorder; Ham, Hamilton Rating Scale for Depression; MMPI, Minnesota Multiphasic Personality Inventory; BPRS, Brief Psychiatric Rating Scale; DIS, Diagnostic Interview Schedule; POMS, Profile of Mood States; SCL-90, Symptom Checklist—90; ASQ, Anxiety Symptom Questionnaire; SCID, Structured Clinical Interview for DSM-III-R; DIB, Diagnostic Interview for Borderlines; Zung, Zung Rating Scale for Depression; SADS, Schedule for Affective Disorders and Schizophrenia; RDC, Research Diagnostic Criteria; DST, dexamethasone suppression test.

be distinct diagnoses. Third, one study suggests that men with BPD suffer from an elevated rate of attention deficit disorder (Andrulonis & Vogel, 1984).

If BPD and affective disorders frequently coexist, can they be distinguished from each other? A number of the studies mentioned here have attempted to do this. Soloff (1981) suggests that subjects with BPD are more impulsive, self-destructive, and angry than depressed subjects. Snyder, Sajadi, Pitts, and Goodpaster (1982) found that subjects with BPD tended to be more manipulative, suicidal, and impulsive, whereas depressed subjects had greater sleep disturbances and diurnal variation of mood. Andrulonis and Vogel (1984) found that subjects with BPD had a higher rate of acting out than subjects with major affective disorder or schizophrenia. Rippetoe, Alarcon, and Walter-Ryan (1986) found that subjects with BPD and depression were more likely to exhibit splitting and to be suicidal, whereas those with BPD and dysthymia were more likely to complain of emptiness. Substance abuse was also seen more commonly among patients with BPD than among those with depression (Andrulonis & Vogel, 1984; Frances et al., 1984; Zanarini et al., 1989). In sum, subjects with BPD tended to be more impulsive and manipulative, displayed more suicidal tendencies, and displayed more substance abuse than did depressed subjects.

However, it remains unclear whether these traits can be reliably used to differentiate BPD from depression. It may be that individuals with depression who are impulsive are sometimes mistakenly diagnosed as having BPD when they are assessed. In fact, many of the DSM-III and DSM-III-R criteria for major depression could easily be construed to resemble the criteria for BPD. In Table 7.2, we have placed several of the DSM-III-R criteria (American Psychiatric Association, 1987) side by side, in order to demonstrate how

TABLE 7.2. DSM-III-R Criteria for Major Depression and BPD That Resemble Each Other

Major depression	BPD
Depressed or irritable mood.	Affective instability and irritability. Inappropriate, intense anger.
Feelings of worthlessness and inappropriate guilt.	Identity disturbance and uncertainty about self-image, long-term goals, or career choice.
Diminished interest or pleasure. Fatigue or loss of energy.	Chronic emptiness or boredom.
Recurrent thoughts of death, recurrent suicidal ideation.	Recurrent suicidal threats, gestures, or behavior.

easily they might be confused in a clinical interview. In many cases, only observation of the time course of symptoms allows one to distinguish these clinical features, and in the case of chronic or treatment-resistant depression, even longitudinal observation may not be useful. Given the extent of potential criterion overlap, even an interviewer using a structured instrument, through his/her interpretations of answers, could profoundly influence what diagnosis a subject receives.

This problem is reflected by others who have pointed out that personality disorders are not reliably diagnosed in individuals with depression (Hirschfeld et al., 1983; Zimmerman & Coryell, 1990). In fact, no study to our knowledge has fully addressed the question of how many patients with major depression are erroneously diagnosed as having BPD in a particular clinical setting. However, in a study with a somewhat similar model, we examined the relationship between bulimia nervosa and BPD (Pope, Frankenburg, Hudson, Jonas, & Yurgelun-Todd, 1987). This study noted that patients meeting DSM-III criteria for bulimia automatically satisfied two of the DSM-III criteria for BPD: poor impulse control and affective instability. Thus, the finding of a high prevalence of BPD in patients with bulimia was hypothesized to be partially an artifact of the overlap in criteria. To allow for this possibility, we administered blindly a revised version of the Diagnostic Interview for Borderlines, which took into account the criterion overlap between BPD and bulimia. Using this method, we found little overlap between the two diagnoses. A similar model might be applied to the study of diagnostic overlap between BPD and depression.

Another model that would help distinguish between "true" BPD and coexisting disorders with similar symptoms is the follow-up study. If, for example, most subjects with putative BPD develop major depression and no longer are diagnosed as having BPD, one might infer that BPD in these cases was not a valid diagnosis, and that the subjects' symptoms were attributable to underlying affective disorder from the beginning. On the other hand, if subjects with BPD maintain their diagnosis, this observation is strong support for diagnostic validity. Finally, if some subjects with BPD develop depression while others do not, and if some or all maintain the diagnosis of BPD, this possibility would suggest that BPD and depression are distinct entities that frequently coexist. This last possibility would not exclude other hypotheses about how BPD and affective disorders are related, such as the notion that chronic depression causes personality changes.

Table 7.3 presents follow-up studies of subjects with BPD, diagnosed with DSM-III criteria. Most of these studies utilized a "retrospective–prospective" design, in which index cases were identified from old admissions by chart review, with follow-up obtained in the present. In follow-up studies, obtaining data blindly is of critical importance. Blind methodology, when used, is noted in the table.

TABLE 7.3. Follow-Up Studies of BPD That Address Issues of Comorbidity and Diagnostic Stability

Study	Study groups	Assessment tools	Findings
Pope et al. (1983)	BPD	DIB, blind follow-up interviews	No subject with DSM-III BPD developed S on follow-up. Substantial overlap of BPD and MAD on follow-up. BPD diagnosis stable over time.
McGlashan (1983)	Mixed	Chart diagnosis, blind follow-up diagnosis	Subjects with BPD displayed changes in diagnosis without any particular direction on follow-up. Up to 50% maintained BPD diagnosis. Large overlap in admission diagnoses noted.
Plakun, Burkhardt, & Muller (1985)	BPD, SPD, S	Chart diagnosis, blind follow-up interviews	BPD functioned better than S on follow-up. BPD with MAD functioned worse than "pure BPD." Diagnostic stability not specifically studied.
Barasch, Frances, Hurt, Clarkin, & Cohen (1985)	BPD	Blind follow-up interviews	BPD showed diagnostic stability over time. During 3-year study interval, 40% of subjects had an episode of D, as did controls with other personality disorders.
McGlashan (1986)	BPD, S, D	Chart diagnosis, follow-up questionnaire	BPD and D showed similar outcomes, both significantly better than S.
McGlashan (1987)	BPD, D, BPD + D	Follow-up interview	36% of D patients diagnosed as having BPD on follow-up. BPD + D group had 45% diagnosed with BPD, 30% with D on follow-up.
Fenton & McGlashan (1989)	SPD, BPD	Follow-up interview	Of 105 subjects, 18 developed S on follow-up. Features of SPD but not of BPD were predictive of S.

Note. For explanation of abbreviations, see footnote to Table 7.1.

A number of issues were addressed in these studies. Those most frequently examined were the stability of the BPD diagnosis over time and the functional outcome of subjects with BPD as compared to other diagnoses. The question of which symptoms, if any, can predict the presence or absence of depression was not specifically addressed, and should be the subject of further study.

There appears to be a general finding that the diagnosis of BPD remains stable over time (Pope et al., 1983; McGlashan, 1983, 1987; Barasch, Frances, Hurt, Clarkin, & Cohen, 1985). This observation does not answer the question of the nosological status of BPD (i.e., a form of depression, a separate diagnosis); however, it does suggest that whatever BPD may be, it can be reliably identified in such a way that the diagnosis does not change. Second, a majority of studies found that depression frequently occurred in these patients. We (Pope et al., 1983) specifically compared outcome in patients who displayed BPD with and without a major affective disorder at index assessment, and found that those patients with a concomitant major affective disorder at index displayed a more frequent family history of affective disorders, a better response to medications, and better long-term outcome than patients with "pure" BPD. Of interest in the Pope et al. (1983) study was that three subjects were symptom-free at follow-up. All of these had BPD and a major affective disorder on index evaluation. This finding suggests that many, if not all, of these patients' "borderline symptoms" at the start of the study might have been attributable to depression, consistent with our discussion above.

No follow-up study supports a relationship between schizophrenia and BPD. One study (Fenton & McGlashan, 1989) noted that 18 of 105 subjects with schizotypal personality disorder or BPD were diagnosed as schizophrenic on follow-up. However, only features of schizotypal personality disorder and not BPD were predictive of this risk. In terms of outcome, most studies find that subjects with BPD do better than those with schizophrenia. Outcome of BPD compared to that of affective disorders was variable.

The studies in Table 7.3 generally do not address the issue of overlap between BPD and other Axis II diagnoses, although this is also an unresolved problem. However, it is worth noting that Barasch et al. (1985) found that depression developed as frequently among subjects with other personality disorders as among subjects with BPD. This, along with our findings (Pope et al., 1983), suggests that BPD and major affective disorders are distinct entities that frequently overlap.

In sum, outcome studies suggest that the diagnosis of BPD is stable over time. There is little evidence to support a relationship of BPD to schizophrenia, and much evidence against this relationship. Many but not all individuals with BPD will develop affective symptoms over time, if they do not already present with such symptoms. However, the latter findings may be true of other personality disorders as well.

THEORETICAL AND CLINICAL IMPLICATIONS

At this juncture, the weight of empirical evidence supports the diagnostic validity of BPD. There is perhaps a relationship between BPD and affective disorders, though its exact nature is uncertain. There appears to be no relationship between BPD and schizophrenia.

In the setting of an affective diagnosis, there is no proven means at present to distinguish BPD reliably from depression on presentation. Even structured interviews, as noted above, may not be reliable. Thus, when a patient with depression or another affective disorder presents, the clinician cannot reliably diagnose an Axis II disorder. It is particularly important, in a patient with possible major depression and BPD, that the clinician not dismiss the former diagnosis in favor of the latter. In such cases, potentially useful treatments for depression, such as cognitive therapy or thymoleptic medication, may be wrongfully withheld. From a research standpoint, more work is needed to see whether such traits as splitting, manipulation, and anger can be reliably identified and utilized as means of distinguishing BPD from affective disorders.

In the setting of BPD without an affective disorder, the data suggest that BPD is a stable diagnostic syndrome. However, its distinction from other Axis II disorders is imperfect at best. The clinician should be alert to the development of depression, however, since even subjects with "pure" BPD may develop affective symptoms.

The relationship of affective disorders and BPD has implications for pharmacological treatment in patients with BPD. There are a number of recent reviews of this topic (Gorton & Akhtar, 1990). We mention briefly several aspects of pharmacological treatment that relate to issues of Axis I comorbidity.

As we have discussed above, a large number of subjects with BPD will have affective symptoms. Given this, and the difficulty in separating BPD from affective disorders, we feel that affective symptoms should be actively treated in these patients, even if a clinician is skeptical that a patient truly has an Axis I disorder. The rationale for this statement is that failure to provide effective treatment for depression (especially pharmacological treatment) to a patient who may respond is a more serious tragedy than the reverse case, in which such treatment is administered to a patient who may not respond. Medication selection should be based upon target symptoms (e.g., antidepressants for depression or panic; lithium, carbamazepine, or valproate for affective instability or irritability) (Gardner & Cowdry, 1989). Given the difficulties with impulsivity and acting out that are described with these patients, it behooves the clinician to monitor serum levels to insure compliance. Anecdotally, many clinicians feel that in subjects with combined personality and affective disorders, therapeutic response may take longer to appear than usual. Thus, a minimum trial of antidepressants or lithium may last 4 or even 6 weeks at therapeutic levels.

The presence of an overt psychosis also may be suggestive of an affective diagnosis (Pope, Jonas, Hudson, Cohen, & Tohen, 1985), and the clinician should aggressively treat the affective disorder. However, many clinicians feel that subjects with BPD may have transient psychotic episodes and mild cognitive disturbances (e.g., paranoia, poor attention, illusions). For such cases, and sometimes as a general treatment, neuroleptics have been suggested (Soloff et al., 1989; Serban & Siegel, 1984). Because this is a nonapproved use of neuroleptics, the clinician should be sure to review with the patient all of the side effects of neuroleptics (including tardive dyskinesia) and to obtain informed consent.

CONCLUSIONS

The bulk of the available evidence suggests that BPD is a valid diagnostic entity, with a stable picture over time. The precise relationship of BPD and affective illness remains to be defined, and further work is still needed in the area of diagnosis, especially in distinguishing BPD from affective disorders. However, the presence of affective symptoms should move the clinician to caution in diagnosing BPD, and should motivate treatment for the affective disorder along with BPD.

REFERENCES

American Psychiatric Association. (1987). *Diagnostic and statistical manual of mental disorders* (3rd ed., rev.). Washington, DC: Author.

Andrulonis, P. A., & Vogel, N. G. (1984). Comparison of borderline personality subcategories to schizophrenic and affective disorders. *British Journal of Psychiatry*, *144*, 358–363.

Barasch, A., Frances, A., Hurt, S., Clarkin, J., & Cohen, S. (1985). Stability and distinctness of borderline personality disorder. *American Journal of Psychiatry*, *142*, 1484–1486.

Baxter, L., Edell, W., Gerner, R., Fairbanks, L., & Gwirtsman, H. (1984). Dexamethasone suppression test and Axis I diagnoses of inpatients with DSM-III borderline personality disorder. *Journal of Clinical Psychiatry*, *45*, 150–153.

Benjamin, J., Silk, K. R., Lohr, N. E., & Westen, D. (1989). The relationship between borderline personality disorder and anxiety disorders. *American Journal of Orthopsychiatry*, *59*, 461–467.

Davis, G. C., & Akiskal, H. S. (1986). Descriptive, biological, and theoretical aspects of borderline personality disorder. *Hospital and Community Psychiatry*, *37*, 685–692.

Fenton, W., & McGlashan, T. H. (1989). Risk of schizophrenia in character disordered patients. *American Journal of Psychiatry, 146*, 1280–1284.

Frances, A., Clarkin, J. F., Gilmore, M., Hurt, S. W., & Brown, R. (1984). Reliability of criteria for borderline personality disorder: A comparison of DSM-III and the Diagnostic Interview for Borderline Patients. *American Journal of Psychiatry, 141*, 1080–1084.

Fyer, M. R., Frances, A. J., Sullivan, T., Hurt, S. W., & Clarkin, J. (1988). Comorbidity of borderline personality disorder. *Archives of General Psychiatry, 45*, 348–352.

Gardner, D. L., & Cowdry, R. W. (1989). Anticonvulsant and personality disorders. In S. L. McElroy & H. G. Pope, Jr. (Eds.), *Anticonvulsants in psychiatry: Recent advances*. Clifton, NJ: Oxford Health Care.

Gorton, G., & Akhtar, S. (1990). The literature on personality disorders, 1985–1988: Trends, issues, and controversies. *Hospital and Community Psychiatry, 41*, 39–51.

Grunhaus, L., King, D., Greden, J. F., & Flegel, P. (1985). Depression and panic patients with borderline personality disorder. *Biological Psychiatry, 20*, 688–692.

Hirschfeld, R. M. A., Klerman, G. L., Clayton, P. J., Keller, M. B., McDonald-Scott, P., & Larkin, B. H. (1983). Assessing personality: Effects of the depressive state on trait measurement. *American Journal of Psychiatry, 140*, 695–699.

Jonas, J. M., & Pope, H. G. (1984). Psychosis in borderline personality disorder. *Psychiatric Developments, 4*, 295–308.

McGlashan, T. H. (1983). The borderline syndrome: II. Is it a variant of schizophrenia or affective disorder? *Archives of General Psychiatry, 40*, 1319–1323.

McGlashan, T. H. (1986). The Chestnut Lodge follow-up study: III. Long-term outcome of borderline personalities. *Archives of General Psychiatry, 43*, 20–30.

McGlashan, T. H. (1987). Borderline personality disorder and unipolar affective disorder: Long-term effect of comorbidity. *Journal of Nervous and Mental Disease, 175*, 467–473.

McManus, M., Lerner, H., Robbins, D., & Barbour, C. (1984). Assessment of borderline symptomatology in hospitalized adolescents. *Journal of the American Academy of Child Psychiatry, 23*, 685–694.

Perry, J. C. (1985). Depression in borderline personality disorder: Lifetime prevalence at interview and longitudinal course of symptoms. *American Journal of Psychiatry, 142*, 15–21.

Plakun, E. M., Burkhardt, P. E., & Muller, J. P. (1985). 14-year follow-up of borderline and schizotypal personality disorders. *Comprehensive Psychiatry, 26*, 448–455.

Pope, H. G., Frankenburg, F. R., Hudson, J. I., Jonas, J. M., & Yurgelun-Todd, D. (1987). Is bulimia associated with borderline personality disorder? A controlled study. *Journal of Clinical Psychiatry, 48*, 181–184.

Pope, H. G., Jonas, J. M., Hudson, H. I., Cohen, B. M., & Gunderson, J. G. (1983). The validity of DSM-III borderline personality disorder: A phenomenologic, family history, treatment response, and long-term follow-up study. *Archives of General Psychiatry, 40*, 23–30.

Pope, H. G., Jonas, J. M., Hudson, J. I., Cohen, B. M., & Tohen, M. (1985). An empirical study of psychosis in borderline personality disorder. *American Journal of Psychiatry, 142*, 1285–1290.

Rippetoe, P. A., Alarcon, R. D., & Walter-Ryan, W. G. (1986). Interactions between depression and borderline personality disorder: A pilot study. *Psychopathology*, *19*, 340–346.

Serban, G., & Siegel, S. (1984). Response of borderline and schizotypal patients to small doses of thiothixene and haloperidol. *American Journal of Psychiatry*, *141*, 1455–1458.

Snyder, S., Sajadi, C., Pitts, W. M., & Goodpaster, W. A. (1982). Identifying the depressive border of the borderline personality disorder. *American Journal of Psychiatry*, *139*, 814–817.

Soloff, P. (1981). A comparison of borderline with depressed and schizophrenic patients on a new diagnostic interview. *Comprehensive Psychiatry*, *22*, 291–300.

Soloff, P. (1987). Characterizing depression in borderline patients. *Journal of Clinical Psychiatry*, *48*, 155–157.

Soloff, P., George, A., Nathan, S., Schulz, P. M., Cornelius, J. R., Herring, J., & Perel, J. M. (1989). Amitriptyline versus haloperidol in borderlines: Final outcomes and predictors of response. *Journal of Clinical Psychopharmacology*, *9*, 238–246.

Tarnopolsky, A., & Berelowitz, M. (1987). Borderline personality: A review of recent research. *British Journal of Psychiatry*, *151*, 724–734.

Zanarini, M. C., Gunderson, J. G., & Frankenburg, F. R. (1989). Axis I phenomenology of borderline personality disorder. *Comprehensive Psychiatry*, *30*, 149–156.

Zimmerman, M., & Coryell, W. H. (1990). Diagnosing personality disorders in the community: A comparison of self-report and interview measures. *Archives of General Psychiatry*, *47*, 527–531.

CHAPTER 8

An Interpersonal Approach to the Diagnosis of Borderline Personality Disorder

LORNA SMITH BENJAMIN

PROBLEMS WITH THE DIAGNOSIS OF PERSONALITY DISORDER

The creators of the *Diagnostic and Statistical Manual of Mental Disorders*, third edition (DSM-III; American Psychiatric Association, 1980) discarded psychoanalytic theory and practice in favor of the Kraepelinian medical model (Blashfield, 1984). Their choice was intended to enhance the scientific status of the discipline of psychiatry, and the use of the medical model was inspired by the effectiveness of the newly developed neuroleptic, antidepressant, and anxiolytic drugs. Diagnosis is the centerpiece of the medical model, and the DSM-III advanced that model as it greatly improved agreement among independent diagnosticians. In the case of DSM-III Axis I diagnoses, kappas often reach the acceptable (Hartmann, 1977) level of .60 or more. However, Axis II, the domain of personality disorders, has not fared so well. Reliability for diagnoses made on Axis II in both the DSM-III and its revision, DSM-III-R (American Psychiatric Association, 1987), has been disappointing.

Two complications with Axis II labels for personality disorders are the coverage and the specificity problems. The coverage problem refers to the fact that a number of people who are personality-disordered according to the generic DSM-III definition do not fit into any of the Axis II categories. In other words, many individuals show inflexible maladaptive traits that interfere with functioning or cause subjective discomfort, but their patterns of interaction do not fit into any of the Axis II categories. The specificity problem marks the opposite dilemma: Some individuals fit into too many of the Axis II categories.

The coverage problem is easy to illustrate. Say a person is prickly with anger and consistently alienates his/her friends and colleagues. Everyone agrees that the person has a "personality problem." But he/she does not show the requisite four to six other symptoms needed to fit into one of the Axis II categories.

The specificity problem can be illustrated by considering the same symptom, anger, and noting that it characterizes several personality disorders. In slightly varying forms, the symptom of anger is a mark of each of the disorders in the dramatic, erratic cluster on Axis II: borderline personality disorder (BPD), antisocial personality disorder (ASP), histrionic personality disorder, and narcissistic personality disorder.[1] In addition to anger, these four diagnostic groups tend to share other symptoms, such as exploitativeness and various forms of self-centeredness. Because of confusing overlap in symptoms, practicing clinicians often express frustration and exasperation with the difficulty of choosing among several seemingly viable possibilities.

Widiger, Frances, Spitzer, and Williams (1988) offered a summary of the rationale for the changes from DSM-III, published in 1980, to DSM-III-R, published in 1987. To test the success of the changes, Morey (1988) analyzed a sample of 291 personality-disordered patients who had been seen at least 10 times by their treating therapists. Clinicians used a checklist to assess their patients for each of the 166 symptomatic descriptors on Axis II. Using a computer algorithm that implemented the rules of DSM-III and DSM-III-R exactly, Morey generated totally replicable diagnoses for the 291 individuals. He found that DSM-III-R yielded two or more diagnoses for 51.9% of the sample. Morey concluded that compared to DSM-III, the DSM-III-R had comparable internal consistency, and that it increased both coverage and overlap. In other words, the DSM-III-R left fewer people unlabeled, but its broader net worsened the overlap problem.

In an effort to resolve problems with diagnosing personality, many different structured or semistructured interviews and self-reports have evolved. Widiger and Frances (1985a) noted that some of the structured interviews show adequate reliability for some but not all the disorders. Klein (1988) found that agreement among the different structured interview and self-report methods was disappointingly low.

The self-report approach is especially plagued by the fact that many diagnostic signs for personality disorder are socially unacceptable. Moreover, information obtained directly from the patient may not be accurate. If the patient must directly acknowledge such undesirable traits as unreasonable anger, exploitativeness, and manipulativeness, and if the very nature of the disorder implies that the patient's information is untrustworthy, how can a

---

[1] Note that the acronym "BPD" is used in this chapter to refer either to "the diagnosis of borderline personality disorder" or to "a person diagnosed as having borderline personality disorder." The acronym "ASP" is used similarly.

questionnaire based on his/her reports be used to make the diagnosis? Should one expect a BPD to say that he/she is unstable, shows inappropriate anger, or has an identity disturbance? Should an ASP be counted upon to say that he/she has no regard for truth, is reckless regarding his/her own or others' personal safety, and lacks remorse? Finally, even if people would describe themselves in such negative terms, there remains the challenge of objectifying such concepts as "lack of remorse" or "instability."

CAN PERSONALITY DISORDERS BE CATEGORIZED?

Because of problems associated with reliability, coverage, specificity, validity, and definition of criteria, the very idea of thinking of personality disorders as diagnostic categories has been challenged. For example, Widiger and Frances (1985b) suggested that instead of classifying an individual in a category like BPD, it would be better to record how closely the person resembles a *prototype* for BPD. Prototypes can be drawn in terms of a set of underlying dimensions. These investigators proposed that the Axis II categories themselves could serve as the basic dimensions for personality disorder. Then, clinicians could "rate each patient on the extent to which he or she displays each set of maladaptive personality traits. Each patient would have a profile indicating the extent to which he or she is dependent, histrionic, schizotypic, paranoid, and so forth" (Frances & Widiger, 1986, p. 252). Their proposal would eliminate the overlap problem, because it builds overlap into the "diagnosis" itself.

Widiger, Trull, Hurt, Clarkin, and Frances (1987) added that still other definitions of underlying dimensionality could be used to describe prototypes. One alternative is Millon's (1981) three dimensions of self–other, activity–passivity, and pleasure–pain. Another is Eysenck's (1987) three dimensions of neuroticism, psychoticism, and introversion–extraversion. A third is the Interpersonal Circle (IPC; Leary, 1957), which arranges behaviors or traits in a circle constructed upon two axes. The IPC is the original of a group of models for personality, known as *circumplex models*, that are built on two axes (Guttman, 1966).

USE OF THE IPC TO DEFINE PERSONALITY DISORDERS

Leary's (1957) IPC specifies that one axis of the circumplex ranges from "hostility" (−4) through 0 to "friendliness" (+4). The other axis ranges from "dominance" (−4) through 0 to "submission" (−4). A given behavior is made up of these two underlying dimensions, and the more intense the behavior, the more pathological it is. For example, Leary (1957, p. 233) proposed that the "psychopathic, sadistic" personality would represent an intense version of an IPC category consisting of much hostility and some dominance.

Leary compared the psychiatric nomenclature of his time to the IPC. Since publication of the DSM-III, other IPC theorists have continued that practice by proposing that Axis II disorders be described by the IPC (e.g., Wiggins, 1982; Kiesler, 1986; Widiger & Frances, 1985b). Not everyone agrees that the IPC adequately characterizes all the Axis II disorders. BPD and ASP are two Axis II disorders that seem to have been particularly elusive.

For example, comparisons of the IPC to Axis II by Wiggins (1982) and by Widiger and Frances (1985b) did not include BPD at all. On the other hand, Kiesler (1986) did describe BPD in terms of the IPC. He suggested that the BPD DSM-III criteron 2—"a pattern of unstable and intense personal relationships, e.g., marked shifts of attitude, idealization, devaluation, manipulation" (American Psychiatric Association, 1980)—could be described by his IPC dimensions. Kiesler indicated that the dimensions "devoted" to "rancorous," "concurring" to "belligerent," and "flattering" to "disdainful" would describe criterion 2. Kiesler added that his "belligerent" would describe DSM-III criteron 3—"inappropriate, intense anger or lack of control of anger." Finally, DSM-III criterion 8—"chronic feelings of emptiness or boredom"—could be encompassed by Kiesler's IPC term "listless." Because the Kiesler analysis describes the BPD in terms of interpersonal conflict, it has promise. However, its descriptions of BPD in terms such as "listless," "belligerent," "rancorous," or "flattering" may seem incomplete to clinicians.

ASP was not included in Kiesler's analysis of Axis II because he concluded that the DSM-III descriptors for ASP are not interpesonal. He wrote: "Further, some disorders are defined almost exclusively by interpersonal descriptors (e.g., paranoid, histrionic), others provide a mix of interpersonal and other descriptors (e.g., passive–aggressive), while still others provide few, if any, interpersonal descriptors (e.g., antisocial)" (1986, p. 591).

The thought that ASP is not interpersonal is puzzling, since the ASP descriptors are widely regarded as being "behavioral," and many of the DSM-III-R items themselves certainly seem interpersonal. For example, the ASP attributes of defying social norms, fighting, defaulting, lying, and being reckless seem to involve interactions between one person and another. Widiger and Frances (1985b) have wondered whether the failure of the IPC to describe ASP might be due to shortcomings of the IPC itself:

> The antisocial personality disorder is also difficult to describe in IPC terms because the negative pole of the affiliation dimension is a mixture of hostile and detached behavior that does not adequately describe the criminal and guiltless exploitation of others. The antisocial person is neither hostile (aggressive) nor detached, but can in fact be superficially friendly although

disloyal, irresponsible, and exploitive. This difficulty in classifying the antisocial diagnosis may lend some support to those who argue for two circumplexes to define the interpersonal domain [reference to McLemore & Benjamin, 1979]. (p. 621)

Morey (1985) has tested some of the theoretical efforts to relate the IPC to Axis II disorders. He asked patients to rate themselves on the Inter-personal Check List (ICL), which measures traits in terms of Leary's IPC, and on the Millon Clinical Multiaxial Inventory (MCMI), a widely used self-report instrument that was constructed to correspond directly to Axis II of the DSM-III (Millon, 1981, 1982). Morey correlated the MCMI score for each personality disorder with the ICL affiliation and control scores. For example, each subject's BPD score from the MCMI was correlated with his/her ICL affiliation and control scores. The average of these two correlations was used to locate the BPD group on a two-dimensional (affiliation, control) graph. By this method, BPD was located in a "docile, dependent" position, with the next closest category being the "self-effacing, masochistic" position. Clinicians might feel that the characterization of BPD as "docile, dependent" is inadequate. Morey was critical of efforts to relate the IPC to Axis II disorders. He wrote: "The convergence of these two approaches to personality taxonomy is not as high as might be expected," and added, "it seems that the DSM-III personality disorders are not as differentiated with respect to affiliative needs as has been hypothesized" (p. 358).

Of course, Morey's challenge rests heavily on the assumption that the MCMI adequately describes the Axis II disorders, and this idea has itself been questioned (Widiger & Sanderson, 1987). Nonetheless, it should be noted that Millon was on the DSM-III task force and was very influential in the creation of Axis II. He, if anyone, is "the father of Axis II." Millon's 1981 book provides the most thorough available survey of the relevant literature on the disorders described by Axis II. His recent summary of his own view of personality disorders (Millon, 1990) is a very important, comprehensive theoretical contribution.

In sum, Leary's proposal that diagnosis be made in interpersonal terms is still being advocated for the Axis II personality disorders. However, an empirical test of the idea did not work as well as hoped. Even proponents of the IPC approach acknowledge that not every disorder is characterized adequately by the IPC.

The main theme of this chapter is that Structural Analysis of Social Behavior (SASB; Benjamin, 1974, 1984), a circumplex with three surfaces, does have the dimensionality needed to describe the personality disorders defined by Axis II. The arguments are presented in detail in an upcoming monograph (Benjamin, in press). The approach promises to improve both coverage and specificity of the DSM-III-R categories and has informed some of the revisions that will appear in the DSM-IV.[2] In accord with the goal of the present volume to emphasize empirical data that support interpretations of BPD, the balance of this chapter is restricted to discussion of data testing the validity of the SASB approach to BPD. For illustrative purposes, these data are compared to SASB data on ASP—a pattern that overlaps aspects of BPD, and one that also resists analysis by IPC. Normative data are added to provide a frame of reference for interpreting the findings on the two selected personality disorders.

ARE INTERPERSONAL TERMS ADEQUATE TO DESCRIBE AXIS II?

Before presenting the relation of the SASB model to BPD and ASP, it is important to consider arguments that interpersonal description may not be enough to describe these disorders. Focusing on BPD, Widiger and Frances (1985b) wrote that "these dimensions [of the IPC] might not be enough to account for the variance among personality disorders if the latter include more than interpersonal variables" (p. 621). Plutchik (1980) also argued that variables other than behavior may be crucial to the description of some personality disorders. He proposed that similar circumplexes can describe both the emotional and the interpersonal domains.

Plutchik and Conte (1985) developed the view that both emotions and behavior can be described by circumplexes, and both are necessary to describe personality disorder. These investigators asked psychiatrists to rate each Axis II disorder on semantic differential scales. Factor analysis of these clinicians' opinions yielded two factors to use as the basis of a circumplex (but not an IPC). Their empirical approach documented the overlap problem by placing BPD close to narcissistic personality disorder and ASP. Plutchik and Conte compared these results to other circumplex studies of emotion and personality traits. They concluded: "Personality traits represent mixtures of basic emotions that have frequently occurred together over time, and if personality disorder may be conceptualized as extremes or exaggeration of certain personality traits, then these personality disorders may be seen as derivatives of emotion" (1985, p. 11).

Elsewhere, I have also noted parallels between interpersonal behavior and emotion, and have added that parallel models for cognitive style could be developed (Benjamin, 1974, 1986). Together, the three corresponding models—interpersonal, emotional, cognitive—should provide definitive descriptions. If the three models (behavior, affect, cognition) move in parallel, they are redundant, and a useful description should therefore be possible

---

[2] First sent to the DSM-IV work force in December 1988.

with any one of them. Under the assumption that such parallel models can be developed, the present approach is restricted to the interpersonal model because it is the only version of SASB that has been well validated to date.

STRUCTURAL ANALYSIS OF SOCIAL BEHAVIOR: AN INTRODUCTION

Comparison of Features of the SASB and IPC Models

SASB (Benjamin, 1974, 1984) grew from Earl Schaefer's (1965) model of parenting behavior, and from the Leary (1957) IPC model, each of which has its own historical antecedents (reviewed in Benjamin, 1974). The SASB model and associated technology differ from the IPC approach in several significant ways:

1. There are three interpersonal surfaces in the SASB model. The dimension of focus (other, self, introject), which separates the surfaces, is not usually recognized within psychology or psychiatry, but awareness of focus is extremely useful to clinicians. BPDs, for example, consistently defy norms by focusing on the clinician rather than on themselves, as they are "supposed" to do in the patient role. Ability to identify this important dimension is very useful in the diagnosis and treatment of BPD.

2. Intrapsychic events as well as interpersonal events can be described by the SASB model, and there are explicit principles linking the interpersonal and the intrapsychic.

3. In contrast to the IPC, which holds "submission" to be the opposite of "dominance," the SASB model implements Schaefer's finding that "giving autonomy" is the opposite of "dominance." The SASB model posits that submission is the *complement*, not the *opposite*, of dominance. According to SASB, submission matches and goes with dominance; it does not oppose dominance.

4. Fifty percent of the space defined by the SASB model is devoted to describing various forms of differentiation, separation, or independence. By contrast, the IPC does not have an independence pole. This addition of the concept of separateness permits the SASB model to describe autonomous behaviors characteristic of ASP, avoidant personality disorder, and other personality disorders.

5. The IPC model defines pathology in terms of intensity, but the SASB model defines pathology qualitatively. SASB suggests that normal function is plotted in a different part of interpersonal space, and that normality and pathology are not on the same continuum.

6. The SASB method of identifying underlying dimensionality permits the detection of complex messages. It can, for example, easily describe the

"superficially friendly although disloyal, irresponsible, and exploitative" (Widiger & Frances, 1985b, p. 621) behavior of the person with ASP.[3]

Brief Description of the SASB Model

The SASB model has been well validated by factor analyses, dimensional analyses, and autocorrelational analyses. Individuals can be described by the SASB model on the basis of self-ratings (the INTREX Questionnaires), or on the basis of objective coding by observers (SASB coding).[4]

The SASB model is accompanied by a series of explicit predictive principles. These may be used to link specific early experiences with adult behaviors that may be characteristic of a given personality disorder. The SASB model may be used to describe interpersonal aspects of patient–therapist interactions, regardless of the therapist's theoretical orientation (Henry, Schacht, & Strupp, 1986; Hartley, 1991; Tress, Henry, Strupp, Reister, & Junkert, 1990; K. Grawe, personal communication, 1990). My personal preference for use of the SASB model in psychotherapy is a developmentally oriented social learning approach called "SASB-directed reconstructive learning" (SASB-RCL). Within that framework it is possible to develop and use the etiological theory to guide treatment interventions. Each therapy intervention can be defined as correct or incorrect in the light of the treatment plan.

The SASB model is introduced here by analyzing the anger in BPD, an attribute that is shared with ASP and other personality disorders. The goal of the analysis is to characterize BPD anger in interpersonal terms that distinguish it from ASP anger. If the symptom of anger is to be interpreted interpersonally, then one must consider *what sets off the anger*. The SASB therefore uses a psychosocial "stimulus–response" sequence analysis. The clinical method of interviewing, called "SASB-directed dynamic interviewing" (SASB-DI), requires that patient statements be expressed in interactional terms that are specific enough to be SASB-codable. Every interpersonal event should be understood in terms of (1) input, (2) response, and (3) the associated internalization of the event.

Inspection of clinical instances of anger in BPD suggests that its "input" usually is perceived abandonment or rejection. If the therapist is late, changes an appointment, cuts a phone call short, or takes a vacation, the BPD gives an angry response that starts a sequence that can end in internalized self-attack and mutilation (Benjamin, 1987a, in press). The SASB model is introduced by coding the BPD who is angry when the therapist is late.

---

[3] See Table 8.2, ASP baseline code: controlling, uninvolved affection (1-3 + 1-5 + 2-8).

[4] Low-cost software for personal computers (average per program is $10) is available for processing SASB data based on self-ratings and/or on coding of observed behaviors.

The input event for prototypical BPD anger is interactional (therapist in relation to BPD). The referents are therapist = X, and BPD = Y. SASB coding always is from the point of view of X. The first coding decision is directed by the three stick figures at the top of Figure 8.1. They represent transitive interpersonal focus on other (X to Y—focus is on what is happening to, for, or about Y), interpersonal focus on self (X to Y—focus is on what is happening to, for, or about X), and intrapsychic turning of transitive focus inward (X to X), respectively. The BPD's view of the therapist's lateness assumes the therapist is focused on the BPD. It does not occur to the BPD that the therapist might have concerns of his/her own that caused the lateness. The event is seen as transitive; that is, the therapist is seen as doing something to, for, or about the BPD.

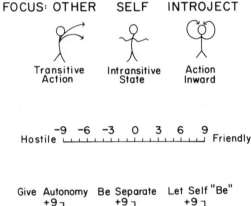

FOCUS: OTHER   SELF   INTROJECT

Transitive Action   Intransitive State   Action Inward

Hostile -9 -6 -3 0 3 6 9 Friendly

Give Autonomy   Be Separate   Let Self "Be"

Control   Submit   Self-Control

FIGURE 8.1. The three underlying dimensions of the SASB model. Interpersonal and intrapsychic events are evaluated in terms of focus (shown by the stick figures at the top), love versus hate (shown by the horizontal axis), and enmeshment versus differentiation (shown by the vertical axes). From "Adding Social and Intrapsychic Descriptors to Axis I of DSM-III" by L. S. Benjamin, 1986, in T. Millon and G. L. Klerman (Eds.), *Contemporary Directions in Psychopathology: Toward the DSM-IV.* Copyright 1986 by The Guilford Press. Reprinted by permission.

The second decision is shown by the horizontal axis in Figure 8.1. Like the IPC, this axis is anchored by hostility on the left and friendliness on the right. The prototypical BPD will see the therapist's lateness as quite hostile (say, about −6 on the horizontal scale).

The third decision is shown by the vertical axes in Figure 8.1. All three axes describe independence or differentiation at the top, and interdependence or enmeshment on the bottom. The specific anchor points for the three vertical axes differ for each type of focus. The therapist's lateness is transitive, so the vertical scale aligned underneath the transitive action figure in Figure 8.1 provides the anchor points for this dimension. It ranges from "control" to its opposite, "give autonomy." The therapist's lateness is seen as giving (unwanted) autonomy (say, about +3 on the vertical scale).

The SASB dimensional approach to the therapist's lateness suggests that the BPD sees lateness as transitive, hostile (−6), and autonomy-giving (+3). These three judgments alone yield a category[5] on the SASB model, which in full form has 108 categories. A simpler form of the SASB model, the cluster version, is shown in Figure 8.2 (Benjamin, 1987b).

The judgment that the therapist's lateness is seen as transitive locates the event on the top surface of the model. The second judgment, that the lateness is hostile, locates it 6 units in the negative direction (left) on the horizontal axis. The judgment that lateness gives autonomy locates the code 3 units in the positive direction (upwards) on the vertical axis. If a dot is drawn at the point (−6, +3) on the top surface of Figure 8.2, and a line is drawn from the origin to that dot, the classification can be made at the point where the vector (line drawn from the origin to the dot) intersects the boundaries of the model. Inspection of Figure 8.2 suggests that such a line would head for about 10 o'clock and would mark[6] the category 1-8, "igoring and neglecting." This is the SASB cluster model code for the BPD view of therapist lateness. In sum, therapist stimulus for BPD anger is SASB-coded 1-8, "ignoring and neglecting."

---

[5] The full model category is as follows: *123. Abandon, leave in lurch.* "Just when X is needed most, X abandons Y, leaves Y alone with trouble."

[6] If the dot falls inside the boundaries of the model, the behavior is less intense; if it falls outside the boundaries, it is more intense. Intensity does not define pathology. It is possible to have very intense normal behaviors, as when greeting a loved one after a long separation or becoming extremely aggressive if one's child is physically threatened.

FIGURE 8.2. The cluster version of the SASB model. The dimensions shown in Figure 8.1 can be combined to create the 24 categories shown here. From "Use of the SASB Dimensional Model to Develop Treatment Plans for Personality Disorders: I. Narcissism" by L. S. Benjamin, 1987b, *Journal of Personality Disorders, 1*, 43–70. Copyright 1987 by The Guilford Press. Reprinted by permission.

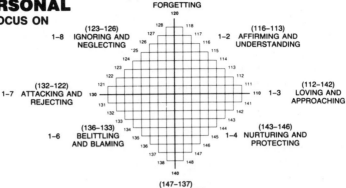

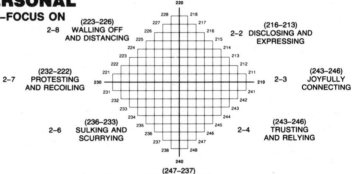

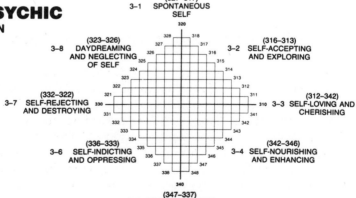

To understand subsequent data analyses and figures, the reader will need to know the logic of the number labels for the clusters on Figure 8.2. Each cluster number on the top, or transitive surface, begins with a 1. Cluster numbers on the middle surface begin with a 2, and those on the bottom surface begin with a 3. Within each surface, the second part of the number label ranges from 1 to 8, starting with 1 for the cluster located at the top (12 o'clock position), and proceeding in sequence in a clockwise direction. Cluster 1-8, "ignoring and neglecting," for example, is the eighth cluster on the top surface counting clockwise from the 12 o'clock position. Cluster 1-4, "nurturing and protecting" is the fourth one on the top surface. Inspection of Figure 8.2 shows that cluster 1-4, "nurturing" is opposite cluster 1-8, "neglecting."

SASB theory holds that anger has an interpersonal purpose, and the two most likely purposes are control and distance. Analyses of BPD patterns suggest that anger in response to cluster 1-8 is to control. Its purpose is to change the person who is seen as neglectful (1-8) into the opposite, a nurturer and protector (1-4).

The conclusion of the analysis is that the DSM-III-R description of anger in BPD should be modified to indicate that it is triggered by perceived abandonment (1-8). It has the interpersonal purpose of forcing the caregiver to deliver more and better caregiving (1-4).

A similar analysis of anger in the ASP will show that his/her anger is triggered by the wish to obtain something—dominance, money, sex, material goods—at the moment. An ASP will not care if the therapist or any other alleged caregiver is late, unless it humiliates or causes a loss of something material.

The SASB model dissects clinical events into the underlying dimensionality of focus (surfaces of the model), love−hate (horizontal axes), and enmeshment−differentiation (vertical axes). It also is associated with several predictive principles that are explained in context as needed to understand the data.

SASB-BASED DESCRIPTIONS OF BPD AND ASP

The preceding section illustrates how SASB codes can explicate the symptom of anger in BPD and in ASP. The complete SASB descriptions of all Axis II personality disorders were developed by (1) SASB-coding of the DSM descriptors in the way just illustrated; (2) SASB-coding the DSM-III and DSM-III-R casebook illustrations (Spitzer, Skodol, Gibbon, & Williams, 1981; Spitzer, Gibbon, Skodol, Williams, & First, 1989); (3) using the predictive principles of the SASB model to make inferences about social etiological factors and checking them against clinical material; and (4) using the principles of SASB-RCL to define appropriate and inappropriate interventions in psychotherapy.

Description of BPD

The "baseline" SASB codes of the DSM-III-R descriptors of BPD and the casebook illustrations are listed here, along with the INTREX Short Form items describing the cluster model points (Benjamin, 1988, pp. 14–16). In these statements, the BPD has the position of X.

> 1-5. *Watching and controlling.* INTREX Short Form item: To keep things in good order, X takes charge of everything and makes Y follow X's rules.
>
> 1-6. *Belittling and blaming.* INTREX Short Form item: X puts Y down, blames Y, punishes Y.
>
> 1-7. *Attacking and rejecting.* INTREX Short Form item: X fiercely attacks Y, very angrily rejects Y.
>
> 1-3. *Loving and approaching.* INTREX Short Form item: X happily, gently, very lovingly greets Y, and warmly invites Y to stay as close as possible.
>
> 2-4. *Trusting and relying.* INTREX Short Form item: X learns from Y, relies upon Y, accepts what Y offers.
>
> 3-7. *Self-rejecting and destroying.* INTREX Short Form item: X hatefully rejects and destroys himself/herself, uncaringly letting go of everything.
>
> 3-8. *Daydreaming and neglecting of self.* INTREX Short Form item: X is reckless and neglectful of himself/herself, sometimes "spacing out" altogether.
>
> 3-4. *Self-nourishing and enhancing.* INTREX Short Form item: X looks after, provides for, puts energy into developing himself/herself to the fullest.

To include goals (Allport, 1937, p. 48), the SASB codes of the underlying organizing wishes and fears are added to the description of BPD. If the clinician is aware of the organizing wishes and fears that maintain the patterns characteristic of the disorder, he/she is in a better position to choose effective treatment interventions. In the following descriptions of wishes and fears, BPD is the recipient, and has the position of Y:

> Wish: 1-4. *Nurturing and protecting.* INTREX Short Form item: With much kindness, X comforts, protects, and teaches Y.

Fear: 1-8. *Ignoring and neglecting.* INTREX Short Form item: X ignores, neglects, abandons Y.

Use of the SASB model to describe personality disorders clearly requires more than single-point descriptions. The SASB codes of the DSM-III-R descriptions of BPD can be summarized by text that integrates the codes into the usual context in which they are found:

> *Interpersonal summary of BPD:* There is a morbid fear of abandonment and a wish for protective nurturance, preferably by constant physical proximity to the rescuer (lover/caregiver). The baseline position is friendly dependency on a nurturer, which becomes hostile control if the caregiver/lover fails to deliver enough (and there is never enough). There is a belief that the provider secretly if not overtly likes dependency and neediness, and a vicious introject attacks the self if there are signs of happiness/success. (Benjamin, in press, Ch. 5).

The SASB coding of case histories in the DSM casebooks and in my own clinical practice generated a prototypical history for BPD. The typical BPD history is outlined on the left-hand side of Table 8.1. Briefly, the BPD

TABLE 8.1. Interpersonal Summary of BPD

History	Consequences of history
1. Chaotic, soap-opera lifestyle	1. Crises sought, created; no constancy
2. Traumatic abandonment (1-8 → 1-7) Incest prototype sets the patterns: Pain + love (2-7 + 2-3) Helplessness and omnipotence (2-5, 1-5) Modeled idealization (2-4) and devaluation (1-6)	2. Abandonment (1-8) sets off the "program" The structure of incest is repeated: Fuses pain and love (2-7 = 2-3) Helpless (2-5) and omnipotent (1-5) Idealizes (2-4) and devalues (1-6)
3. Self-definition (2-1), happiness (2-3) → attack (1-7)	3. Internalizes attack for doing well (2-1, 2-3 → 3-7)
4. Sickness (2-4) elicited nurturance (1-4)	4. Escalates sickness (2-4) to receive nurturance (1-4)

Note. From Benjamin (in press, Ch. 5).

Summary: There is a morbid fear of abandonment and a wish for protective nurturance, preferably by constant physical proximity to the rescuer (lover/caregiver). The baseline position is friendly dependency on a nurturer, which becomes hostile control if the caregiver/lover fails to deliver enough (and there is never enough). There is a belief that the provider secretly if not overtly likes dependency and neediness, and a vicious introject attacks the self if there are signs of happiness/success.

SASB baseline codes of BPD: Control (1-5), blame (1-6), attack (1-7), active loving (1-3), reliance on other (2-4), vicious self-attack (3-7), self-neglect (3-8), self-care (3-4). *Wishes:* To receive nurturance and protection (1-4). *Fears:* To be neglected, abandoned (1-8). *Necessary descriptors:* Transitive coercions to receive nurturance; happiness yields self-destruction. *Exclusionary descriptors:* Tolerance of aloneness on a long-term basis.

who shows all the criteria of DSM-III-R for this disorder has been raised in a chaotic environment and subjected to traumatic abandonment experiences. These confused pain with pleasure and helplessness with omnipotence, and they modeled idealization and devaluation. Self-definition and/or happiness were attacked, and sickness elicited nurturance. This pattern of experiences often is provided by painful incest with father or brothers. However, it is vital to note that the interpersonal dimensionality is what sets the pattern, not the category of experience. Painful incest often has the dimensionality that teaches the patterns of BPD, but incest does not *always* have that dimensionality, and it does not always create BPD. Experiences other than incest (e.g., cult abuse) can create the dimensionality needed for BPD, and therefore can set the pattern for BPD.

The consequences of the early BPD patterning are detailed in the right-hand column of Table 8.1. The connection between these SASB-based interpersonal descriptions of BPD and the DSM-III-R definitions of BPD are summarized by the following text from Benjamin (in press, Ch. 5):

> In a BPD who shows all the symptoms mentioned in DSM-III-R, the connections between the history and the symptoms would be as follows: The family abandonment (1-8) is internalized (3-8), so that the BPD is very reckless with himself/herself, as described by DSM-III-R criterion 2 (self-damaging impulsiveness). Internalization of neglect (1-8) and its association with boring aloneness and danger leads to unbearable feelings of emptiness, as described by DSM-III-R criterion 7. The fear of abandonment, described by DSM-III-R criterion 8, comes from its association with trauma and bad personhood (1-8 → 1-7, 1-6). The family devotion to chaos for high stakes accounts for the instability and intensity, described by DSM-III-R criteria 1 and 3. The famous anger of the BPD (1-6, 1-7), described by DSM-III-R criteron 4, is always set off by perceived abandonment and is always intended to coerce (1-5) the opposite of abandonment—namely, nurturance (1-4). The self-mutilation (3-7), described by DSM-III-R criterion 5, is a replay of the abuse and/or an effort to appease and/or reactivate an attacker. The identity disturbance (3-8, 3-7 → 3-4), described by DSM-III-R criterion 6, is a consequence of the internalization of objects who would attack (1-7, 1-6) if there were signs of differentiation or self-definition (2-1) and/or happiness (2-3). The thought disorder, soon to be reflected by DSM-IV criterion 9, may be the consequence of having reality testing negated: "What you think was hurt, was pleasure. What you think happened didn't happen."

The SASB approach has been used to construct a self-report inventory that captures the internal perspective of the individual with a personality disorder. This perspective accounts for the behaviors noted by the DSM-III-R. For example, the item for the highly controversial DSM-III-R BPD criterion 6 (describing identity disturbance) is worded: "I have a pattern of doing well in something important (school, job, relationship) and then suddenly dropping it altogether." The item describes the consequences of earlier attack directed at the BPD for signs of self-definition or happiness. It is far more concrete than the term "identity disturbance." Yet the item does address the BPD's noted inability to stay in school, in relationship, or in a job. These behaviors in turn assure that the BPD will not have a clear identity (other than as a failure at everything, a needy person). The BPD items are part of the Wisconsin Personality Inventory (WISPI). I constructed the original version of the WISPI, and it was carefully edited by M. Klein. Dr. Klein and her research team are now conducting extensive validation studies of the WISPI.[7] Because they were written from the internal perspective of raters with personality disorders, the WISPI items tend not to be ego-alien.

Description of ASP

The "baseline" SASB codes of ASP (the ASP is in the role of X), together with the appropriate INTREX Short Form items (Benjamin, 1988, pp. 14–16), are as follows:

Uncaring aggression, summarized by the following complex code:

1-7. Attacking and rejecting. INTREX Short Form item: X fiercely attacks Y, very angrily rejects Y.

2-8. Walling off and distancing. INTREX Short Form item: X walls himself/herself off from Y and doesn't react at all.

Uncaring control, summarized by the following complex code:

1-5. Watching and controlling. INTREX Short Form item: To keep things in good order, X takes charge of everything and makes Y follow X's rules.

2-8. Walling off and distancing.

Controlling, uninvolved affection, summarized by the following complex code:

1-3. Loving and approaching. INTREX Short Form item: X happily, gently, very lovingly greets Y, and warmly invites Y to stay as close as possible.

---

[7] For access to the WISPI, write Dr. Marjorie Klein, Department of Psychiatry, University Hospitals, 600 Highland Avenue, Madison, WI 53792.

1-5. *Watching and controlling.*
1-8. *Ignoring and neglecting.*

Self-indulgence without protective regard for the self, summarized by the following complex code:

3-4. *Self-nourishing and enhancing.* INTREX Short Form item: X looks after, provides for, puts energy into developing himself/herself to the fullest.
3-8. *Daydreaming and neglecting of self.* INTREX Short Form item: X is reckless and neglectful of himself/herself, sometimes "spacing out" altogether.

Self-indulgence without concern for others, summarized by the following complex code:

3-4. *Self-nourishing and enhancing.*
1-8. *Ignoring and neglecting.*

The prototypical ASP wishes to be in control and autonomous. The SASB codes for these wishes are as follows (the ASP has the role of X):

1-5. *Watching and controlling.*
2-1. *Asserting and separating.* INTREX Short Form item: X knows his/her own mind and "does his/her own thing" separately from Y. The ASP fears being controlled (i.e., being in the role of Y in cluster 1-5, above).

Here is a textual summary that integrates the SASB codes of ASP into their typical context:

> *Interpersonal summary of ASP*: A pattern of inappropriate and unmodulated desire to control others, implemented in a detached manner. There is a strong need to be independent, to resist being controlled by others, who are usually held in contempt. There is a willingness to use untamed aggression to back up the need for control and/or independence. The ASP usually presents in a friendly, sociable manner, but that friendliness is always accompanied by a baseline position of detachment—of not really caring about what happens to self or others. (Benjamin, in press, Ch. 8)

The left-hand side of Table 8.2 summarizes the hypotheses of how ASP is programmed; the right-hand side summarizes how those early experiences connect with the adult patterns characteristic of ASP. With ASP, as with all the Axis II disorders, it is possible to link the SASB codes back to each of the DSM-III-R descriptors (see Benjamin, in press, Ch. 8).

TABLE 8.2. Interpersonal Summary of ASP

History	Consequences of history
1. Harsh, neglectful parenting (1-8, 1-7)	1. Reckless self-destructiveness (3-8, 3-7), not bonded (2-7)
2. Sporadic, unmodulated parental control (1-5, 1-6), likely to be humiliating (1-6)	2. Fiercely protects autonomy (2-1, 2-8)
3. Inept parental caring (1-4 + 1-8)	3. Takes care of self in negligent ways, such as drug abuse, prostitution, crime (3-4 + 3-8)
4. Controlled family (1-5) due to parental dereliction of duty (1-8)	4. Control is an end in itself, implemented without bonding (1-5 + 1-8); exploitative

Note. From Benjamin (in press, Ch. 8).

Summary: A pattern of inappropriate and unmodulated desire to control others, implemented in a detached manner. There is a strong need to be independent, to resist being controlled by others, who are usually held in contempt. There is a willingness to use untamed aggression to back up the need for control and/ or independence. The ASP usually presents in a friendly, sociable manner, but that friendliness is always accompanied by a baseline position of detachment—of not really caring about what happens to self or others.

SASB baseline codes of ASP: Uncaring aggression (1-7 + 2-8); uncaring control (1-5 + 2-8); controlling, uninvolved affection (1-3 + 1-5 + 2-8); self-indulgence without protective regard for self (3-4 + 3-8) and/or any concern about others (3-4 + 1-8). *Wishes*: To be in control (1-5), to be independent (2-1). *Fears*: To be controlled (1-5). *Necessary descriptors*: Requires control of others and autonomy for self; utterly detached and without remorse. *Exclusionary descriptors*: Fear of abandonment; entitlement; dependency.

DATA DESCRIBING THE VIEWS OF BPD AND ASP

Research Methods

The data discussed in this section were gathered in a 4-year study of 194 psychiatric inpatients rating a large battery of tests, including the INTREX Long Form Questionnaires (Benjamin, 1984). Patients were diagnosed using information gathered by the Diagnostic Interview Schedule (Robins, Helzer, Croughan, & Ratcliff, 1981), by a scan of their charts using a formal checklist, and by a computer-driven series of decision rules (Greist et al., 1984). The results supported the proposal that there are statistically significant differences in the interpersonal perceptions of members of the various diagnostic groups (Benjamin, 1986). A subsample of the 31 individuals who were diagnosed as BPDs, and the 14 who were labeled as ASPs, provided the data to be discussed here. The BPDs came mostly from psychiatry units of three general hospitals, whereas the ASPs were all from a state hospital; most of the ASPs had been committed for murder, rape, or both.

SASB INTREX Short Form Questionnaire items allow raters to compare themselves and others to each of the points on the 24-point cluster model shown in Figure 8.2. The SASB INTREX Long Form Questionnaire is a more detailed and psychometrically sensitive version that conforms to the full 108-point SASB model (Benjamin 1974, 1984). Data from the Long Form can be reduced to conform to the simpler cluster form of Figure 8.2 by an averaging process.

Subjects used INTREX Questionnaires to rate different situations (relationships) and states (the "best" and the "worst"), including the following: the introject at best and worst; the relationship with a significant other person (SO) at best and worst; ratings of mother as remembered during the childhood ages 5–10, of father during childhood (5–10), and of the marital modeling seen during childhood (5–10). Patients rated each item on a scale ranging from 0 ("the item does not ever apply at all") to 100 ("the item applies always, perfectly").

To provide a frame of reference for any observed differences, data gathered independently on a normative sample of volunteer college students enrolled in psychology classes are also offered here. Because of differences in age and socioeconomic status and other circumstances, statistical tests did not include the normals. If they had, a large percentage of tests would have been significant; the ASPs and BPDs provided many ratings that differed from those of normals.

Results

The mean cluster scores for the BPD, ASP, and normal groups of raters are presented in Table 8.3. Simple *t* tests were performed on the cluster scores for BPD versus ASP. Multiple-comparison error need not be a major concern if an analysis is guided by highly specific theory, and if the patterns occur in a number of contexts. This requirement that results show logical and cross-situational consistency insures that an isolated finding cannot inappropriately be emphasized out of context.

The numbered lines in Table 8.3 describe different relationships: that with the rater's introject at best and worst (lines 1–2); that with the SO at best and worst (lines 3–10); the rater's remembered relationship with the mother during childhood (lines 4–14); and the rater's remembered relationship with father during childhood (lines 15–18).

Figure 8.3 presents a graph of the data shown in line 2 of Table 8.3. The cluster scores for the normal group followed an orderly pattern. There was relatively low endorsement of cluster 3-1, "spontaneous self" (shown at the 12 o'clock position on the introject surface in Figure 8.2). Endorsements increased to a high level for clusters 3-2, 3-3, and 3-4, and then progressively decreased to a minimum at cluster 3-7, "self-rejecting and destroying." This orderly progression resembles a cosine wave, and suggests that the introject scores conformed to circumplex ordering.

TABLE 8.3. Mean Cluster Scores for BPD, ASP, and Normal Groups

Focus	Relationship	BPDs ($n = 31$)							
		1	2	3	4	5	6	7	8
Inward	1. Introject—Best	40*	43	48	58	60	44	45	40
Inward	2. Introject—Worst	42	18†	13†	27	41	81†	74†	71
He/she	3. SO focuses—Best	45	66	53	59	35	18	13	19
He/she	4. SO reacts—Best	54	65	57	52	30	22	12*	21*
I	5. Focus on SO—Best	49	67	52	51	24*	17	13	15
I	6. React to SO—Best	47†	61	57*	55	35	27	15	25
He/she	7. SO focuses—Worst	44†	40	27*	31	41	37	28	40
He/she	8. SO reacts—Worst	53	37	29†	33	22	27	27	42
I	9. Focus on SO—Worst	49	38	24†	29†	28†	34	24	33
I	10. React to SO—Worst	41†	36	25†	37	40	41	37	44
She	11. Mother focused	31*	27*	32	40	62	48	34	46
She	12. Mother reacted	47	35	31	30	18†	24	35	42
I	13. Focused on mother	44†	46	32	34	22	27	21	21
I	14. Reacted to mother	38	37	37	52	56	50	39	43
He	15. Father focused	36	43	41	45	58	33	27	38
He	16. Father reacted	59	43	39	36	19	16†	21	37
I	17. Focused on father	52	53	36	38	19*	20	18*	20*
I	18. Reacted to father	39	42	42	56	54	43	31	33

* $p < .05$ by t test (BPDs vs. ASPs only).

† $p < .01$ by t test (BPDs vs. ASPs only).

The group averages suggest that even at their worst, normals were friendly to themselves, and engaged in relatively little self-attack or neglect. The profile for the BPD group is almost the inverse of that for the normal group: Rather than assigning maximal scores to items describing friendliness toward the self, the BPDs showed maximal endorsement in the region of self-attack. ASPs failed to show convincing circumplex order in their self description at worst: They were friendlier to themselves than were the BPDs, but not so friendly as normals. Self-attack was less in ASPs than in BPDs, but greater than in normals.

Line 2 of Table 8.3 shows that the BPDs' self-attack (clusters 6 and 7) was significantly greater than the ASPs' self-attack. BPDs' willingness to be nice to themselves was significantly lower than that of ASPs. BPDs had a significantly more destructive introjects than did ASPs, and the ASPs' self-concept was less favorable than that of normals.

ASPs ($n = 14$)								Normals ($n = 133$)							
1	2	3	4	5	6	7	8	1	2	3	4	5	6	7	8
52	53	57	56	53	48	39	46	27	70	71	74	52	17	9	15
54	41	39	38	48	57	57	62	27	70	71	74	52	17	9	15
52	70	57	48	40	32	22	26	48	82	75	72	23	9	4	9
57	61	58	56	37	30	24	34	57	82	81	69	20	13	5	12
56	72	58	58	42	33	18	25	48	84	77	73	20	7	3	5
59	67	71	59	43	36	29	30	57	84	84	72	24	15	5	11
62	49	42	37	42	41	33	38	45	60	48	49	31	20	13	22
59	51	48	37	34	39	33	41	55	54	51	52	21	22	16	28
55	50	44	44	46	45	31	41	43	63	51	49	29	20	12	17
57	45	51	42	40	44	36	48	52	56	53	54	27	27	16	27
44	46	45	50	64	40	27	43	32	68	64	73	55	17	6	11
54	45	47	34	36	35	36	43	50	64	60	51	17	12	10	13
64	52	45	33	27	30	26	27	52	68	48	51	14	14	9	11
42	44	49	63	54	58	46	45	45	64	62	76	48	38	15	17
36	41	40	47	66	42	35	41	37	64	55	66	51	17	9	17
62	42	36	33	27	34	31	47	56	61	58	53	46	13	10	8
56	45	33	40	30	37	36	37	55	66	42	44	12	11	8	12
46	44	46	52	48	53	45	42	49	57	56	73	45	37	16	19

The SASB principle of "introjection" is a codification of Sullivan's (1953) idea that self-concept comes from treating the self as important others have done. Introject theory suggests that a BPD's self-attack should correspond to treatment received at the hands of primary caregivers—namely, the mother and father. If, for example, a given BPD's mother consistently engaged in 1-6, "belittling and blaming" of the BPD, the resulting introject would include 3-6, "self-indicting and oppressing." Both these clusters are located at the 8 o'clock position on the SASB model shown in Figure 8.2.

To test the introject theory, Figure 8.4 presents the data from lines 11 (mother focused on the rater) and 15 (father focused on the rater) of Table 8.3. Within the normal group, the patterns of parental focus compared almost exactly to the pattern of their introject: Mothers and fathers focused on the raters with warmth and control, and the internalized patterns showed both self-love and self-control.

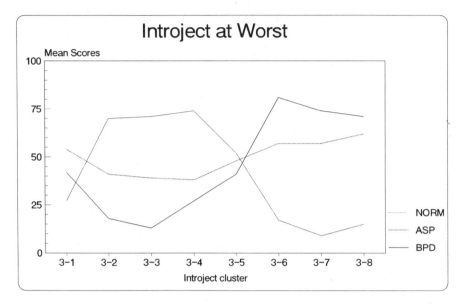

FIGURE 8.3. Mean cluster scores for "rater's introject at worst" for the BPD, ASP, and normal groups. Numbers on the abscissa mark clusters on the "introjection" surface of Figure 8.2. Normals show circumplex order oriented around friendliness toward self, while BPDs show circumplex order oriented around self-attack. ASPs do not show well-articulated circumplex order in their introject.

Figure 8.4 suggests that parenting patterns for BPDs and ASPs were different from those of normals. Both ASPs and BPDs reported that parental focus peaked on control (rather than on warmth), and both described parental hostility substantially above normal levels. Line 11 of Table 8.3 shows that friendly maternal affirmation of the typical BPD as a separate person (1-2, "affirming and understanding") was significantly less than that received by the typical ASP. Finally, mothers of ASPs gave significantly more autonomy (1-1, "freeing and forgetting") than did mothers of BPDs.

These analyses suggest that ASPs and BPDs had introjects that were more hostile than normal, and, as predicted by introject theory, that their perceived parenting was more hostile than that of normals. The ASPs were given more autonomy, and they showed significantly more "letting go of self" (3-1, "spontaneous self") than did BPDs. BPDs were given significantly less affirmation, and they showed significantly less self-acceptance (3-2, "self-accepting and exploring") than ASP.

Despite these important correspondences, the nearly exact parallel between patterns for parental input and patterns for the introject shown in the normal group did not obtain for BPDs or for ASPs. Better parallels are seen for

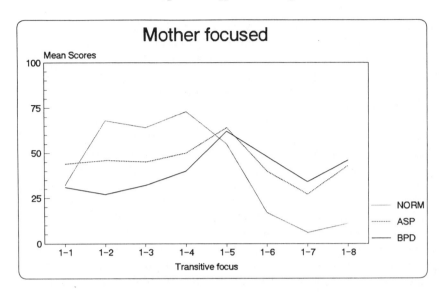

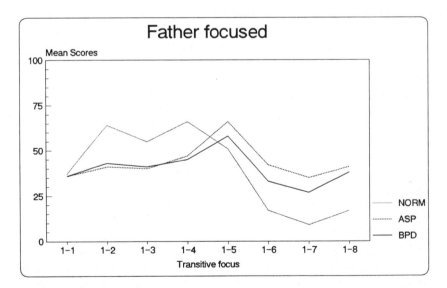

FIGURE 8.4. Mean cluster scores for "mother focused on the rater" (top) and "father focused on the rater" (bottom) for the BPD, ASP, and normal groups. Numbers on the abscissa mark clusters on the "focus on other" surface of Figure 8.2. Parents of normals were seen as friendly and nurturant, whereas parents of BPDs and ASPs centered on control and were noticeably more attacking than parents of normals.

them if the parental focus (line 11) is compared to the introject at best (line 1) instead of to the introject at worst. The question of how experience with important caregivers is internalized to form the self-concept is so central to the understanding of personality disorder that a more detailed analysis of the relation between remembered parental input (lines 11 and 15) and self-concept is warranted.

The top part of Figure 8.5 shows the product—moment r between BPD mothers' friendly (transitive) focus, and the BPDs' internalizations in the worst state. The bottom part of Figure 8.5 shows correlations between the mothers' hostile focus and the BPDs' internalizations. The correlations suggest that friendly initiations from mother were associated with friendly internalizations (top part of the figure), and hostile initiations from mothers (lower part of the figure) were associated with hostile internalizations. However, correlations for autonomy giving (1-1) and control (1-5) did not show the predicted relations. Maternal 1-1, "freeing and forgetting," was associated as predicted by introject theory with 3-1, "spontaneous self," but maternal autonomy giving also was associated with degrading the self (3-6, "self-indicting and oppressing"). This deviation from introject theory supports a minor hypothesis based on clinical observations that autonomy giving in families of BPDs is associated with blame (Benjamin, in press, Ch. 5). Not only is the prototypical BPD subject to traumatic abandonment experiences, but often there is the implication in the family that the BPD was left alone *because* he/she was a bad person. If a BPD learned to equate maternal 1-1, "freeing and forgetting," with 1-6, "belittling and blaming," the large correlation with 3-6, "self indicting and oppressing," would make sense.

Figure 8.6 presents for ASPs the same product—moment correlations shown for BPDs in Figure 8.5. Unlike Figure 8.5, Figure 8.6 shows little sensible ordering. The only nearly consistent pattern is that unequivocal maternal hostility (1-7) and neglect (1-8) were associated with self-attack (3-7 and 3-6), and, strangely, with self-affirmation (3-2).

Speculation on the meaning of the patterns, or lack of them, in figure 8.6 is beyond the scope of the present chapter. For the moment, the conclusions based on Figures 8.5 and 8.6 are as follows: (1) The very self-destructive BPD introjects showed orderly correspondence to perceived maternal attack, with the added twist that maternal autonomy giving also was associated with self-attack. (2) By contrast, the ASP self-concept was not well articulated according to circumplex order, and it did not directly relate to perceived maternal focus. The BPDs had taken in maternal hostility, and the ASPs had not taken in much at all from their mothers.

The lack of order in Figure 8.6 is neither an artifact of the small sample size for ASPs nor the result of a general lack of interpersonal consistency for ASPs. Figure 8.7 shows that this relatively small sample of ASPs did exhibit orderly *interpersonal* complementarity to their remembered maternal focus.

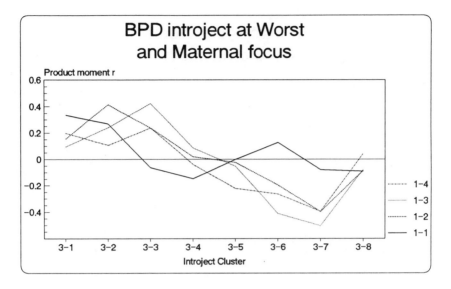

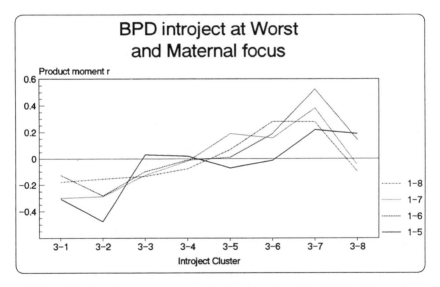

FIGURE 8.5. Product–moment correlations between "rater's introject at worst" and "mother focused on the rater" for BPD subjects. Friendly maternal focus is shown at top; hostile maternal focus is shown at bottom. The patterns of the correlations show that the hostile BPD introject of Figure 8.3 is directly associated with the perceived maternal attack profiled in Figure 8.4.

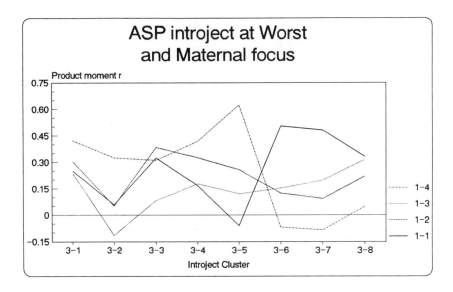

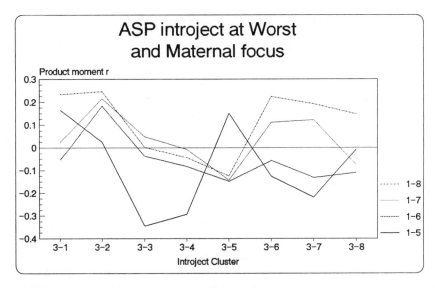

FIGURE 8.6. Product–moment correlations between "rater's introject at worst" and "mother focused on the rater" for ASP subjects. Friendly maternal focus is shown at the top; hostile maternal focus is shown at bottom. For the ASP group, there is little discernible correspondence between maternal input and self-concept.

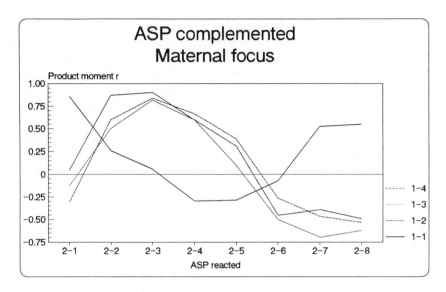

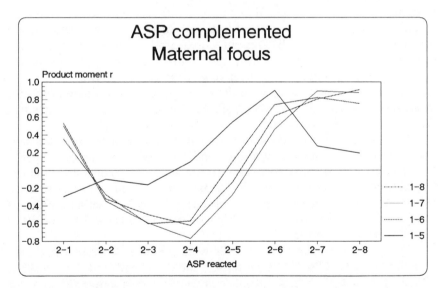

FIGURE 8.7. Product–moment correlations between "rater's reaction to mother" and "mother focused on the rater" for ASP subjects. Friendly maternal focus is shown at top; hostile maternal focus is shown at bottom. The strong circumplex order shown in this figure provides support for the SASB principle of complementarity, and shows that the lack of order in the ASP data in Figure 8.6 is not a simple artifact of the smaller sample size.

The SASB principle of "complementarity" holds that behavior at any given point on an interpersonal surface will be matched by behavior marked at that same topological location on the other interpersonal surface. For example, if the mother affirmed the child with 1-2, "affirming and understanding," the child would be likely to respond with friendly self-definition (2-2, "disclosing and expressing"). SASB complementarity theory (unlike IPC complementarity theory, discussed by Orford, 1986) has been confirmed in a variety of contexts. It held in the present normal sample, in the BPD sample, *and in the ASP sample*. Together, Figures 8.7 and 8.8 establish that although interpersonal relations between ASPs and their mothers were complementary, something went wrong with the internalization process in the ASP group.

The examination of lines 2, 11, 14, 15, and 18 of Table 8.3 has shown how the SASB ratings can create a profile for each relationship, and how profiles can be compared using mean scores and product–moment r. Space limitations preclude examination of all possible relations among all lines of the table. The balance of this review is restricted to the highlights suggested by lines in the table that yielded a significant difference between ASP and BPD.

The differential diagnostic comparisons of BPDs and ASPs were made by means of the t test. When BPD and ASP differed significantly from each other, these variables are compared to the normative data offered for frame of reference. If an ASP or BPD mean score on the variable was within one-half of one standard deviation from the normal mean, the clinical group is declared "within normal range" by a very conservative margin.

Line 1. ASPs showed significantly more letting go of self than did BPDs (3-1, "spontaneous self"). Neither ASPs nor BPDs were within normal range ($SD = 13.8$) on this variable.

Line 2. Compared to ASPs, BPDs at worst showed significantly less self-love (3-2, "self accepting and exploring," and 3-3, "self loving and cherishing"). Neither group was within normal range (both SD's = 19.9) on these variables. In addition, compared to ASPs, BPDs at worst showed significantly more self-attack (3-6, "self-indicating and oppressing," and 3-7, "self-rejecting and destroying"). Neither group was within normal range (SD's = 23.3 and 19.7, respectively) on these variables.

Line 4. At best, the SOs of ASPs were significantly more withdrawn than the SOs of BPDs (2-7, "protesting and recoiling," and 2-8, "walling off and distancing"). Neither group was within normal range (SD's = 7.5 and 12.9, respectively) on these variables.

Line 5. At best, ASPs exerted significantly more control over their SOs than did BPDs (1-5, "watching and controlling"). BPDs were within normal range ($SD = 14.4$) for this variable.

Line 6. At best, BPDs were significantly less autonomous and loving in relation to their SOs than were ASPs (2-1, "asserting and separating," and

2-3, "joyfully connecting"). ASPs were within normal range (*SD* = 12.6) for the assertion.

Line 7. At worst, the SOs of ASPs gave significantly more autonomy than did the SOs of BPDs (1-1, "freeing and forgetting"). BPDs were within normal range (*SD* = 14.8) on this variable. Also, at worst, the SOs of BPDs were significantly less loving than were the SOs of ASPs (1-3, "loving and approaching"). ASPs were within normal range (*SD* = 23.8) on this variable.

Line 8. At worst, the SOs of BPDs were significantly less loving than were the SOs of ASPs (2-3, "joyfully connecting"). ASPs were within normal range (*SD* = 24.0) on this variable.

Line 9. At worst, ASPs were significantly more controlling of their SOs than were BPDs (1-5, "watching and controlling"). BPDs were within normal range (*SD* = 19.0) on this variable. In addition, at worst, BPDs were significantly less loving and nurturant of their SOs than were ASPs (1-3, "loving and approaching," and 1-4, "nurturing and protecting"). ASPs were within normal range (*SD*'s = 24.5 and 20.7, respectively) on these variables.

Line 10. At worst, BPDs were significantly less autonomous and loving with their SOs than were ASPs (2-1, "asserting and separating," and 2-3, "joyfully connecting"). ASPs were within normal range (*SD*'s = 15.8 and 24.6, respectively) on these variables.

Line 11. Mothers of ASPs were seen as giving significantly more autonomy than mothers of BPDs (1-1, "freeing and forgetting"). BPDs were within normal range (*SD* = 15.1) on this variable. In addition, mothers of BPDs gave significantly less friendly affirmation of their children's separate identities than did mothers of ASPs (1-2, "affirming and understanding"). Neither group was within the normal range (*SD* = 25.1) for this variable.

Line 12. Mothers of ASPs were far more submissive than were mothers of BPDs (2-5, "deferring and submitting"). BPDs were within normal range (*SD* = 12.6) on this variable.

Line 13. BPDs gave their mothers significantly less autonomy than did ASPs (1-1, "freeing and forgetting"). Neither group was within normal range on this variable. The direction of differences suggests that BPDs showed less autonomy than did normals, whereas the ASPs showed more than normals did.

Line 16. Fathers of ASPs showed significantly more resentful submission than did fathers of BPDs (2-6, "sulking and scurrying"). BPDs were within the normal range (*SD* = 14.2) on this variable.

Line 17. APSs directed significantly more control, blaming and overt attack toward their fathers than did BPDs (1-5, "watching and controlling," 1-6, "belittling and blaming," and 1-7, "attacking and rejecting"). BPDs were within normal range (*SD* = 12.8) for controlling their fathers, but not for blaming (*SD* = 11.6) or attacking (*SD* = 13.3) them.

DIFFERENTIAL DIAGNOSTIC IMPLICATIONS

According to the data in Table 8.3, ASPs and BPDs shared some attributes that were not within the normal range. Compared to normals, both groups were more self-critical and self-attacking (line 2), and more likely to let themselves go unrestrained (line 1). Both were less self-accepting or self-loving than normals (line 2). Members of each group were more alienated from their SOs at their best (line 4), and both reported less than normal affirmation from their mothers (line 11). These findings suggest that both groups were generally more alienated from themselves and others than were the people who provided the normative data.

Many of these attributes are expected of people with personality disorders. The significant differences between the two diagnostic groups are more informative. Compared to ASP, BPDs were less self-loving, more self-attacking (line 2), less autonomous (lines 6, 10, 11, 13), and in less loving relationships (lines 7, 8, 9, 10). Compared to BPDs, ASPs were more autonomous (lines 1, 7, 11), more controlling (lines 5, 9, 12, 16, 17), and had more alienated SOs (lines 4).

The BPDs' tendencies to self-attack, their underdeveloped autonomy, and their perception that they do not receive enough love were predicted. The ASPs' tendencies to be hostile, autonomous, and controlling also were predicted.

On the othe hand, some of the predictions in Tables 8.1 and 8.2 were not confirmed. Data did not confirm the prediction that both groups would engage in more self-care (3-4, "self-nourishing and enhancing") than normals. Perhaps the failure occurred because "self-care" in the ASP and BPD groups theoretically is embedded (complex-coded) in self-destructive activity such as drug and alcohol abuse or crime. Another predictive failure was that the BPDs would show more enmeshment in general and dependency in particular, which they did not.

Not all the hypotheses in Tables 8.1 and 8.2 can be tested by the present data set. For example, the data do not lend themselves to a direct test of the idea that painful incest often programs the BPD prototype. That theory would suggest that BPDs would be more likely to endorse items describing overt sexual advances and explicit attack from a parental figure. The INTREX Long Form includes two such explicit items:

110. *Tender sexuality.* With gentle loving tenderness, X connects sexually if Y seems to want it.
130. *Annihilating attack.* X murders, kills, destroys, and leaves Y as a useless heap.

Ratings of father as both sexual and murderous (items given a score of 50 or more) were given by two of 31 BPDs, no ASPs, and no normals. One more BPD and one ASP[8] reported this pattern with mother. The addition of ratings of mother brought the total for BPDs to 3 of 31, nearly 10%. This extremely "unlikely" procedure of asking for straightforward endorsement of highly ego-alien material in relation to only two of many possible incest perpetrators does provide suggestive support for the hypothesis.

In sum, the SASB measures did confirm important predictions for BPD and ASP. The clinician needing to make the differential diagnosis between BPD and ASP could look for greater control and autonomy in the ASP, and for greater self-attack along with a sense of not receiving enough love in the BPD.

The IPC, which does not distinguish assertion (intransitive, differentiated focus on the self) from dominance (transitive, enmeshed focus on others), is theoretically unable to make these distinctions between ASP and BPD. The autonomy pole of the SASB model and the introject surface were especially important in making the differential diagnosis between these disorders. The present data bank did include measures on a well-validated version of the ICL (Wiggins, 1982), and t tests of the octant scores yielded only one difference. ASPs rated themselves as more "aloof−introverted" than did BPDs ($p < .053$).

TREATMENT IMPLICATIONS

Kiesler (1986) has used his version of the IPC to generate treatment suggestions for personality disorders: "Finally, we can predict that in later sessions the therapist can exert greatest pressure for positive change in the Compulsive by offering therapeutic responses anticomplementary on the [IPC] Circle to the patient's maladaptive style" (p. 595). The "anticomplementarity" principle (Kiesler, 1983) is similar to the SASB principles of "antithesis" (Benjamin, 1974). The latter specifies that the best chance of changing a patient's behavior to its opposite is for the changer (e.g., the therapist) to show the complement of the desired opposite. The principle of antithesis would predict that if a BPD is too dependent (2-4), the opposite behavior of walling off and distancing (2-8) would be more likely if the therapist were "not to pay attention" (1-8). However, any therapist who has tried this (fatal) bit of folk wisdom

---

[8] The fact that this same pattern was seen in one ASP, in a group of individuals committed for murder or rape, serves as a reminder that "one pattern does not a diagnosis make." A painful incestual experience can result in patterns other than BPD, depending on the dimensionality and the context of the experience.

(codified by the antithesis principle) with a BPD will have discovered that it does not work. In fact, "not paying attention" is likely to escalate BPD dependency rather than to reduce it as predicted. Unfortunately, the patterns of personality disorder are ingrained and complicated enough that it is not possible to specify simple algorithms using antitheses to specify corrective therapist positions, disorder by disorder.

Nonetheless, the SASB does provide guidelines for treatment planning, albeit not simple ones. Briefly, the thesis is that the major tasks in therapy are for the patient to learn what his/her patterns are, where they came from, and what they are for, and then to decide whether or not they are "worth it." If the patient decides that they are not, then therapy becomes a matter of learning new patterns. Usually, the most problematic stage of therapy involves the decision to give up the (often unconscious) wishes and fears that organize the patterns. The prototypical BPD must recognize that the desperate dependency on the therapist represents a re-enactment of a tumultuous love—abuse relationship, while that same relationship also is supposed to represent safe haven from such dangers. Once the BPD decides to give up the wish to merge with the therapist and to work instead on differentiation, usual and customary therapy techniques work well. Before that decision is made, therapy with BPD can be a frustrating whirlwind of love and hate, intimacy and alienation, control and helplessness for both the patient and the therapist.

If therapy is defined in terms of learning about patterns, a therapist's intervention is correct if it falls into one of five categories:

1. Facilitate the alliance between the therapist and the patient against "it"—the maladaptive patterns.
2. Help the patient learn to recognize his/her patterns and where they came from.
3. Block maladaptive patterns.
4. Help the patient mobilize the will to give up the underlying wishes, challenge the fears.
5. Help the patient learn new more adaptive patterns.

The therapist can reflect the BPD's patterns clearly so that he/she can recognize them and accomplish the five tasks just outlined. A summary of the SASB-RCL approach to therapy appears in Benjamin (1991), and an extended discussion of specific treatment interventions helpful in BPD is found in Benjamin (in press, Ch. 5). Some aspects of the recommended approach to BPD are supported by the present data set. The analysis clearly marked some of the key patterns: BPDs' self-attack, weakness in autonomy taking, and perceived lack of affirmation and affection from important others. One implication is that the BPD will be unable to express his/her own view if it differs from that of another, *while at the same time remaining friendly.* Being differentiated, having a separate identity of one's own, is "not OK" to the mind of the BPD. A major therapy task is to change this idea.

Concentration on understanding of interpersonal patterns and their purposes can help the therapist avoid costly errors. For example, a therapist who uses the cathartic model might think it wise to facilitate expression of anger when a BPD is complaining about his/her lover. If, however, the anger is for the interpersonal purpose of coercing nurturance, the therapist's endorsement of it would reinforce a presenting problem (see Benjamin, 1989). Similarly, if the therapist unilaterally decides to discourage dependency by reducing the number of sessions per week, BPD programming is likely to lead to a reactive self-destructive act (Benjamin, 1987a). Therapist understanding of the structure of BPD phenomenology should lead the therapist to approach the dependency problem more constructively and effectively.

SUMMARY AND DIRECTIONS FOR FUTURE WORK

It is my belief (1) that the dimensionality of the SASB Model (Benjamin, 1974, 1984) permits faithful capturing of key interpersonal features of all of the Axis II disorders; (2) that the use of the SASB model to study the dimensional structure of DSM-III-R yields interpersonal descriptors for the Axis II categories that can greatly reduce the overlap problem; and (3) that the SASB analysis of Axis II has clear psychosocial, etiological, and treatment implications. In sum, the SASB model helps define personality disorders as categories that have etiological and treatment implications. Careful development of the arguments and results for each disorder on Axis II are available in Benjamin (in press).

Highlights of the present data analyses suggested that both BPDs and ASPs were generally more alienated from themselves and others than were the people who provided the normative data. There were important differences between the clinical groups in self-concept. BPDs had an introject organized around self-attack, which was related directly to perceived maternal attack. Although interpersonal relations between ASPs and their mothers were complementary, something went wrong with the internalization process in the ASP group. They did not have well-articulated self-concepts. The BPDs also differed from the ASPs interpersonally. BPDs felt they received less affirmation and affection from important others, and they had a weak sense of their own autonomy. ASPs, on the other hand, had a very strong sense of autonomy and saw themselves as having control over others, including their parents during childhood. The SASB model was better able than the IPC to characterize and differentiate BPD from ASP.

The SASB-DI method (Benjamin, in press, Ch. 2) will provide better tests of the theory (Tables 8.1 and 8.2). Recorded interviews with patients will be SASB-coded for input, response, and internalization of perceptions of early and current important relationships. There will be cross-sectional comparisons such as those illustrated by Table 8.3. Predictions also will be tested in the complex contexts specified by theory, but not tested by the present cross-sectional survey methods. If results of the proposed interview study are promising, then a longitudinal study of parent–child interactions might be justified.

It is important to note that studies showing connections between patient perceptions of family life and psychopathology should be used to help rather than to blame families. Although the present data suggest that experiences in the family may shape temperament, they do not establish that ASP and BPD are "the family's fault." The role of temperament and other genetically based factors in the emergence of psychopathology must not be forgotten. In addition, I have become increasingly convinced that the role of the patient's *will* (wishes and fears) is central to the appearance and the disappearance of many mental disorders. Probably the most difficult and elusive aspect of psychotherapy is the challenge of how to mobilize the will to change. In any case, understanding and insight should enable constructive change in both the patient and the family rather than engender defeat.

ACKNOWLEDGMENT

The study described in this chapter was supported by National Institute of Mental Health Grant No. MH-33604, by the Wisconsin Alumni Research Fund, and by the University of Wisconsin Department of Psychiatry Research and Development Fund.

REFERENCES

Allport, G. W. (1937). *Personality: A psychological interpretation*. New York: Henry Holt.

American Psychiatric Association. (1980). *Diagnostic and statistical manual of mental disorders* (3rd ed.). Washington, DC: Author.

American Psychiatric Association. (1987). *Diagnostic and statistical manual of mental disorders* (3rd ed., rev.). Washington, DC: Author.

Benjamin, L. S. (1974). Structural Analysis of Social Behavior. *Psychological Review*, *81*, 392–425.

Benjamin, L. S. (1984). Principles of prediction using Structural Analysis of Social Behavior. In R. A. Zucker, J. Aronoff, & A. J. Rabin (Eds.), *Personality and the prediction of behavior*. New York: Academic Press.

Benjamin, L. S. (1986). Adding social and intrapsychic descriptors to Axis I of DSM-III. In T. Millon & G. L. Klerman (Eds.), *Contemporary directions in psychopathology: Toward the DSM-IV*. New York: Guilford Press.

Benjamin, L. S. (1987a). Commentary on the inner experience of the borderline self mutilator. *Journal of Personality Disorders*, *1*, 334–339.

Benjamin, L. S. (1987b). Use of the SASB dimensional model to develop treatment plans for personality disorders: I. Narcissism. *Journal of Personality Disorders*, *1*, 43–70.

Benjamin, L. S. (1988). *Short Form INTREX Users' Manual*. Madison, WI: INTREX Interpersonal Institute.

Benjamin, L. S. (1989). Interpersonal Analysis of the cathartic model. In R. Plutchik & H. Kellerman (Eds.), *Emotion: Research and experience* (Vol. 5). New York: Academic Press.

Benjamin, L. S. (1991). Brief SASB-directed reconstructive learning therapy. In P. Crits-Christoph & J. Barber (Eds.), *Handbook of short-term dynamic therapy*. New York: Basic Books.

Benjamin, L. S. (in press). *Diagnosis and treatment of personality disorders: A structural approach*. New York: Guilford Press.

Blashfield, R. K. (1984). *The classification of psychopathology: Neo-Kraepelinian and quantitative approaches*. New York: Plenum Press.

Eysenck, H. J. (1987). The definition of personality disorders and the criteria appropriate for their description. *Journal of Personality Disorders*, *1*, 211–219.

Frances, A. J., & Widiger, T. (1986). The classification of personality disorders: An overview of problems and solutions. In A. J. Frances & R. E. Hales (Eds.), *Review of psychiatry* (Vol. 5). Washington, DC: American Psychiatric Press.

Greist, J. H., Mathiesen, K. S., Klein, M. H., Benjamin, L. S., Erdman, H. P., & Evans, F. J. (1984). Psychiatric diagnosis: What role for the computer? *Hospital and Community Psychiatry*, *35*, 1089–1090.

Guttman, L. (1966). Order analysis of correlation matrixes. In R. B. Cattell (Ed.), *Handbook of multivariate experimental psychology*. Chicago: Rand McNally.

Hartley, D. (1991). Assessing interpersonal behavior patterns using Structural Analysis of Social Behavior (SASB). In M. Horowitz (Ed.), *Person schemas and maladaptive interpersonal patterns*. Chicago: University of Chicago Press.

Hartmann, D. P. (1977). Considerations in the choice of interobserver reliability estimates. *Journal of Applied Behavior Analysis*, *10*, 103–116.

Henry, W., Schacht, T., & Strupp, H. H. (1986). Structural analysis of social behavior: Application to a study of interpersonal process in differential psychotherapeutic outcome. *Journal of Consulting and Clinical Psychology*, *54*, 27–31.

Kiesler, D. J. (1983). The 1982 interpersonal circle: A taxonomy for complementarity in human transactions. *Psychological Review*, *90*, 185–214.

Kiesler, D. J. (1986). The 1982 Interpersonal Circle: An analysis of DSM-III personality disorders. In T. Millon & G. Klerman (Eds.), *Contemporary directions in psychopathology: Toward the DSM-IV*. New York: Guilford Press.

Klein, M. H. (1988). [Report at an NIMH meeting on personality disorders], Bethesda, MD.

Leary, T. (1957). *Interpersonal diagnosis of personality: A functional theory and methodology for personality evaluation*. New York: Ronald Press.

McLemore, C. W., & Benjamin, L. S. (1979). Whatever happened to interpersonal diagnosis? *American Psychologist, 34,* 17–34.

Millon, T. (1981). *Disorders of personality: DSM-III, Axis II.* New York: Wiley–Interscience.

Millon, T. (1982). *Millon Clinical Multiaxial Inventory Manual* (2nd ed.). Minneapolis: National Computer Systems.

Millon, T. (1990). *Toward a new personology: An evolutionary model.* New York: Wiley.

Morey, L. C. (1985). An empirical comparison of interpersonal and DSM-III approaches to classification of personality disorders. *Psychiatry, 48,* 358–364.

Morey, L. C. (1988). Personality disorders in DSM-III and DSM-III-R: Convergence, coverage, and internal consistency (1988). *American Journal of Psychiatry, 145,* 573–577.

Orford, J. (1986). The rules of interpersonal complementarity: Does hostility beget hostility and dominance, submission? *Psychological Review, 93,* 365–377.

Plutchik, R. (1980). *Emotion: A psychoevolutionary synthesis.* New York: Harper & Row.

Plutchik, R., & Conte, H. R. (1985). Quantitative assessment of personality disorders. In R. Michels, J. O. Cavenar, Jr., & H. K. H. Brodie (Eds.), *Psychiatry* (Vol. 1). Philadelphia: J. B. Lippincott.

Robins, L. H., Helzer, J. E., Croughan, J. L., & Ratcliff, K. S. (1981). National Institute of Mental Health Diagnostic Interview Schedule: Its history, characteristics and validity. *Archives of General Psychiatry, 38,* 381–389.

Schaefer, E. S. (1965). Configurational analysis of children's reports of parent behavior. *Journal of Consulting Psychology, 29,* 552–557.

Spitzer, R. L., Gibbon, M., Skodol, A. E., Williams, J. B. W., & First, M. B. (1989). *DSM-III-R casebook.* Washington, DC: American Psychiatric Press.

Spitzer, R. L., Skodol, A. E., Gibbon, M., & Williams, J. B. W. (1981). *DSM-III casebook.* Washington, D.C.: American Psychiatric Association.

Sullivan, H. S. (1953). *The interpersonal theory of psychiatry.* New York: Norton.

Tress, V. W., Henry, W. P., Strupp, H. H., Reister, G., & Junkert, B. (1990). Die strukturale Analyse sozialen Verhaltens (SASB) in Ausbildung und Forschung. *Zeitschrift für Psychosomatische Medizin und Psychoanalyse, 36,* 240–257.

Widiger, T. A., & Frances, A. (1985a). Axis II personality disorders: Diagnostic and treatment issues. *Hospital and Community Psychiatry, 36,* 619–627.

Widiger, T. A., & Frances, A. (1985b). The DSM-III personality disorders. *Archives of General Psychiatry, 42,* 615–623.

Widiger, T. A., Frances, A., Spitzer, R. L., & Williams, J. B. W. (1988). The DSM-III-R personality disorders: An overview. *American Journal of Psychiatry, 145,* 786–795.

Widiger, T. A., Trull, T. J., Hurt, S. W., Clarkin, J., & Frances, A. (1987). A multidimensional scaling of the DSM-III personality disorders. *Archives of General Psychiatry, 44,* 557–563.

Widiger, T., & Sanderson, C. (1987). Convergent and discriminant validity of the MCMI as a measure of the DSM-III personality disorders. *Journal of Personality Assessment, 51,* 228–241.

Wiggins, J. S. (1982). Circumplex models of interpersonal behavior in clinical psychology. In P. C. Kendall & J. N. Butcher (Eds.), *Handbook of research methods in clinical psychology.* New York: Wiley.

PART FOUR

TREATMENT

CHAPTER 9

Borderline Behavioral Clusters and Different Treatment Approaches

STEPHEN W. HURT
JOHN F. CLARKIN
HEATHER MUNROE-BLUM
ELSA MARZIALI

Effective treatment planning begins with a clear description of a patient's focal areas of difficulty and associated problems. However, such a description in itself is not sufficient for focused and efficient intervention. For the latter, one needs to go beyond the phenomenological description and develop a model of the behaviors that is based upon the covariation of behaviors and hypotheses about the proximate and distal causes of the dysfunctional behaviors. With the improvements in the reliability and specificity of psychiatric diagnoses embodied in the *Diagnostic and Statistical Manual of Mental Disorders*, third edition (DSM-III) and its revision, DSM-III-R, models (at various stages of development) for some disorders have been sufficiently well articulated for investigators to propose specific treatment strategies and techniques. Schizophrenia (Falloon, Boyd, & McGill, 1984; Anderson, Reiss, & Hogarty, 1986), anxiety disorders (Barlow, 1988), and major depression (Beck, Rush, Shaw, & Emery, 1979; Klerman, Weissman, Rounsaville, & Chevron, 1984) are among the disorders that have received this sort of attention. These disorders are defined as Axis I disorders in DSM-III-R; the development of treatment manuals for Axis I disorders has been more rapid, since these symptom complexes have generated the most research and specific pharmacological interventions are widely available.

Attempts to develop systematic treatment strategies and techniques directed at Axis II disorders have lagged behind. Luborsky (1984) and Strupp and Binder (1984) have developed psychodynamic treatment strategies for individuals with chronic, repetitive interpersonal difficulties—a set of difficulties commonly experienced by individuals with personality disorders as well as others. Efforts to develop specific treatment strategies and techniques for the Axis II disorders have been hindered by the lack of models for these disorders that would help to guide their treatment. This difficulty besets attempts to develop not only psychotherapies for Axis II disorders, but pharmacotherapies as well (Cowdry, 1987).

In this chapter, we consider recent data on borderline personality disorder (BPD) in the context of ongoing research efforts to develop treatment strategies for behaviors characteristic of BPD individuals. Psychotherapy outcome studies, at least those that compare two different treatment approaches, have been very disappointing to date. Few data useful to the clinician have come from these studies. The treatments are usually found to be equally effective and are more effective than a placebo treatment. This finding has been repeated so often that we wonder whether the comparative design, adopted from double-blind pharmacological treatment studies, should be abandoned. We argue here that with a model of the disorder, one can more effectively design a comparative treatment study that will yield information useful for differential treatment planning. The field does not need a simple, comparative study of the behavioral, psychodynamic, and relational treatments for BPD considered here.

BPD AS A SYNDROME

Development of a general treatment strategy for Axis II disorders such as BPD might begin with the identification of common or core problems manifested by individuals with the disorder. The diagnostic criteria of DSM-III and DSM-III-R represent an effort to provide phenomenological criteria for the diagnosis of BPD, and, as such, can be considered a working definition of common difficulties presented by individuals with the diagnosis. However, the criteria vary widely in their sensitivity, specificity, and predictive powers with respect to the diagnosis (Clarkin, Widiger, Frances, Hurt, & Gilmore, 1983). In general, very few of the individuals classified as having the disorder manifest all the criteria. Because BPD, like most DSM-III and DSM-III-R disorders, is polythetic (i.e., a fixed number of criteria— fewer than the total number of possible criteria—are minimally required to make the diagnosis), it is inevitable that individuals with the disorder will be quite heterogeneous with regard to the criteria and the problem areas they represent.

This heterogeneity among individuals with the disorder makes it difficult to develop a unified treatment strategy. Designing treatment strategies for each of the individual criteria themselves or for the many possible combinations of criteria seems overly detailed. On the other hand, a treatment strategy designed to address the entire complex of criteria would fail to address the modal individual with the diagnosis who has fewer than the complete set.

Equally daunting are the difficulties imposed by the presence of concurrent disorders. Insofar as DSM-III and DSM-III-R encourage multiple diagnoses, it is likely that studies of Axis II disorders will be carried out in populations with different concurrent Axis I and Axis II disorders. Fyer, Frances, Sullivan, Hurt, and Clarkin (1988), in studying the comorbidity of BPD and other Axis II disorders with Axis I disorders, reported no significant relationships between a BPD diagnosis and Axis I diagnoses. The patterns of occurrence of various Axis I diagnoses in conjunction with BPD were similar to those found in conjunction with other personality disorders (taken as a group) and with the absence of an Axis II disorder. In reviewing several previous studies, Fyer et al. (1988) noted that the likelihood of finding BPD in conjunction with any specific Axis I diagnosis appeared to depend principally on the prevalence of the Axis I diagnosis in the populations studied. A similar influence of the base rates of the various Axis II diagnoses in the populations studied might parsimoniously account for the often-reported finding that BPD and schizotypal diagnoses are commonly found in combination.

The common co-occurrence of various Axis I and Axis II conditions with BPD can be seen as consistent with either of two equally plausible propositions. First, BPD might be considered an independent diagnostic entity that is commonly encountered, and so can be found in conjunction with a wide variety of other Axis II and Axis I conditions. Second, it may be that BPD represents no specific syndrome per se, but is rather a point on more general dimensions of impulsivity, affective turbulence, and inconsistent self-representations that can be attained through a wide variety of means.

BPD Criteria and Their Relationships

Borderline personality disorder (BPD) represents a heterogeneous group of individuals with important differences between them, considering both the criteria used to assign the BPD diagnosis and accompanying Axis I and Axis II diagnoses. We argue that considerations of these conjoint relationships should inform the development of treatment strategies for this disorder.

Recently reported data (Hurt et al., 1990) relate to one part of this problem. Combining data from four separate studies of BPD in patients with a primary personality disorder diagnosis, Hurt et al. explored the relationships among the criteria used in making the diagnosis to develop homogeneous clusters of criteria. They then identified those cluster combinations that were related to the BPD diagnosis more often than would be expected by the simple mathematical permutations of the criteria involved. The joint associational structure of the criteria indicated that three relatively distinct subsets of criteria could be extracted from the eight DSM-III criteria. One cluster, referred to as the Identity cluster, consisted of the criteria of chronic feelings of emptiness or boredom, identity disturbance, and intolerance of being alone. This cluster reflects commonly described borderline features such as a need for involvement with others and a reliance on external support for self-definition. A second cluster, referred to as the Affect cluster, consisted of the criteria of intense, inappropriate anger, instability of affect, and unstable interpersonal relationships. These criteria capture the frequently stormy, often dramatic, and intense affective qualities of interpersonal relations described in the clinical literature. The third cluster, referred to as the Impulse cluster, consisted of self-damaging acts and impulsive behaviors. This cluster taps the behavioral inconsistency and proneness to engage in self-destructive behaviors; it represents the more dramatic life- and treatment-threatening qualities of BPD patients frequently discussed in the treatment literature.

At a descriptive level, these three clusters of criteria constitute relatively homogeneous collections of behaviors that identify three core problems presented by individuals with BPD. Hurt et al. (1990, Fig. 1, p. 125) also used these combinations to explore the taxonomy of the disorder. Using cluster combinations allows a more parsimonious consideration of subtypes than is possible with the eight criteria considered individually. In this mixed group of inpatient and outpatient samples, subtypes with criteria combinations involving the Affect and Impulse clusters occurred 2.5 times more often than would be expected by chance alone, whereas subtypes involving the Identity and Impulse clusters occurred only one-half as often as expected by chance.

More recently, this cluster solution was partially replicated (Clarkin, Hurt, & Hull, 1991) in data from borderline patients uniformly assessed for the DSM-III-R criteria for BPD with the Structured Clinical Interview for DSM-III-R Personality Disorders (SCID-II). The Impulse cluster readily emerged from the data. The Identity cluster was replicated in large part, with identity diffusion and feelings of emptiness/boredom forming the core of the cluster. Anger and unstable interpersonal relations again combined, replicating the central features of the Affect cluster. The remaining two criteria of frantic efforts to avoid being alone and instability of affect failed to show their previous associations.

We believe that the treatment of these groups of patients would be quite different and would demand different treatment foci, different treatment strategies, and different ways of accommodating to and forming a therapeutic alliance.

These three clusters of criteria might be referred to as "core problems," in that the individual criteria in a cluster might be construed as reflecting dispositional markers for a more general psychological construct. For example, the criteria of self-damaging acts and impulsive behaviors (which form the Impulse cluster) might reflect a general disposition to engage in high-risk activities for the sake of excitement, accompanied by a disregard for the deleterious consequences of such behaviors. Individuals with BPD for whom these criteria are prominent might be expected, at the more pathological extreme, also to manifest problems with substance abuse to a sufficient degree to warrant a concurrent Axis I diagnosis. BPD individuals with less prominent difficulties in these areas might still engage in high-risk activities that are more socially acceptable—for example, gambling as a hobby. The dispositions reflected in these clusters are not, in themselves, pathological; as an example, risk taking is present to some degree in many human activities. Attempts to develop behavioral or attitudinal descriptions that indicate a pathological degree of such an underlying construct should lead to the development of criteria which potentially fulfill one of the DSM-III-R's general requirements for personality disorder criteria: behaviors or traits that cause either significant impairment in social or occupational functioning or subjective distress.

The interrelationships among the clusters themselves might be equally informative. Making use of these relationships might allow us to develop parsimonious therapeutic strategies and to anticipate broader consequences from our interventions. For example, given the observed relationship between the Affect and Impulse clusters, we would anticipate that interventions directed at one would predictably influence the other. Exploring conditions under which impulsive behaviors are expressed would produce an understanding of the characteristic affects with which they are associated. In turn, an exploration of this relationship might suggest more appropriate self-management strategies, as well as additional therapeutic interventions. Greater understanding of these interrelationships might possibly be theoretically informative, although this is not necessary for treatment planning. For example, the behavioral association of these dispositions might be fundamentally influenced by specific biological substrates. Cloninger (1986) and Siever, Klar, and Coccaro (1985) have postulated that Axis II disorders may, in part, be causally related to an underlying biological system; they offer the specific suggestion that the impulsive behaviors of BPD are related to serotonergic functioning.

Treatment Strategies and Behavioral Clusters

These three clusters of the DSM-III and DSM-III-R criteria for BPD and their observed relationships to one another form a basis for the development of treatment strategies for BPD. Efforts to develop an effective program of specified treatment strategies—as, for example, in a treatment manual—must address several issues, including the following:

1. Specification of treatment strategies and techniques for the three clusters of behaviors noted in the above-described analyses.
2. Particular emphasis on impulsive behaviors, because of their episodic nature and life- and treatment-threatening implications.

3. Some indication of the sequence of addressing each of the clusters in the treatment.
4. Incorporation of appropriate shifts in strategy, given the likelihood and array of comorbid conditions on both Axis I and Axis II.

These issues develop naturally from a consideration of DSM-III-R's schema and the criteria for BPD. Other relevant issues can be perceived outside the domain of DSM-III-R. For example, the general approach to the development of treatment manuals has often originated in theoretical or metapsychological considerations relevant to psychological disorders generally, or certain aspects of human psychology thought to underlie the development of a particular disorder. Although the issue of the relative merits of a phenomenological strategy based on DSM-III-R (such as the one we present here) and a more theoretical strategy developed from other foci is certainly arguable, we choose in what follows to compare three treatment strategies in the context of their relationship to the DSM-III-R criteria for BPD. In doing so, we hope to highlight the relationships between these strategies and the clusters described, rather than to focus on their relative theoretical merits. We prefer to await outcome studies based on these approaches before attempting to decide on their relative merits.

The three treatment approaches chosen are those developed by Kernberg, Selzer, Koenigsberg, Carr, and Appelbaum (1989); Linehan (1984, 1987); and the McMaster University group (Dawson, 1988; Marziali, Newman, Munroe-Blum, & Dawson, 1989). Kernberg's model represents an attempt to develop treatment strategies within the context of psychodynamic theory; Linehan's model is developed from a cognitive–behavioral orientation; the McMaster University group's model is based on an object relations approach.

The treatment strategy of Kernberg et al. (1989) relies principally on the psychodynamic techniques of clarification, confrontation, and interpretation within the evolving transference relationship between the patient and the therapist. Clarifying the roles of both the therapist and the patient, particularly with regard to self-destructive behaviors outside of and within the treatment hour, is the chief focus of the initial consultations. As treatment proceeds, these efforts are supplemented with confronting the disparate aspects of the patient's self—efforts that challenge the fragmented sense of identity allowing the expression of self-destructive tendencies. In Kernberg et al.'s view, these split-off aspects of the patient's identity are repositories of seemingly inconsistent emotional polarities. Shifts in affect emerge as these identity facets are brought to the fore; interpreting these shifts and understanding their relationship to the evolving transference relationship between the patient and the therapist become the central work of the therapy. Thus, by turns, these techniques are applied to the core problems of Impulse, Affect, and Identity through the medium of the transference. The format for the treatment is individual psychotherapy.

Linehan's (1984, 1987) treatment strategy relies principally on the cognitive and behavioral techniques of support, education, contingency management, and construction of alternatives. Patients are asked to make a commitment to diminishing self-destructive behaviors and are supported in their efforts to do so. They are educated about the maladaptive nature of such behaviors, which are framed as habits and, as such, are difficult to control. Through a format of both individual and group psychotherapy, they are provided with alternative means of tolerating and expressing distressful affects, and are encouraged to engage actively in problem solving around these historically difficult emotional constellations. Furthermore, the therapists use all available contingencies to reinforce adaptive responses and discourage maladaptive ones. The relationship between the individual therapist and the patient is viewed as the primary vehicle for this contingency management.

The treatment strategy of the McMaster University group is focused on observing and processing the meanings of the contextual features of the patient–therapist interactions—a strategy referred to as "relationship management psychotherapy" (RMP; Dawson, 1988). According to this perspective, the borderline patient's self-system contains conflicting attributes that have not been resolved. This results in a state of instability and ambiguity, which the patient seeks to resolve in the context of interpersonal relationships, including the therapeutic relationship. As in other relationships, the borderline patient externalizes his/her conflict in the therapeutic dialogue. If the therapist takes up one side of the dialogue by being supportive and optimistic, the patient will assume the other side by being argumentative and pessimistic. As long as the therapist and patient replicate the self-system conflict, no resolution takes place. Since the patient has little knowledge of how internal conflict is externalized in the therapeutic interaction, it is the therapist who must behave in a manner that will alter the dialogue and disconfirm the patient's distorted expectations. In psychodynamic psychotherapy, the self-system conflict is addressed when the therapist explores and interprets the nature of the conflict, its developmental antecedents, and its manifestations in the treatment relationship. The McMaster University group (Dawson, 1988; Marziali et al., 1989) argues that these dynamic therapeutic strategies perpetuate the conflict because they reinforce the patient's "helpless, hopeless" role and maintain the therapist in the "healthy, responsible" role. In RMP, the therapist avoids the patient's projected expectations (i.e., that the therapist will rescue, protect, admire, control, humiliate, and devalue) by attending to the process rather than the content of the interaction. It requires of the therapist a bland, neutral stance, in which the patient's propositions are acknowledged, reflected, and affirmed. These therapist responses are provided in the context of an unwavering interest in the patient's dialogue. RMP emphasizes that it is the patient who has control and it is the therapist who communicates uncertainty and confusion while maintaining a "working" therapeutic stance.

RMP reflects a therapeutic approach that Settlage (1977) proposed as a method for addressing the borderline patient's developmental conflicts with separation–individuation. The format for the treatment is exclusively a time-limited, group psychotherapy. The patient's control over the therapist serves the developing task of self-regulation. Settlage proposes that control by the patient avoids the liability of intruding into the patient's psychic functioning. The repetition of this experience in the therapeutic interaction allows the patient to gain control over internal confusion; the patient identifies with the therapist's tolerance for ambiguity, and with the therapist's thoughtful exploration of the patient's confused representations of self and other.

APPLICATIONS OF THE THREE TREATMENT APPROACHES

To consider the application of these treatment approaches to the treatment of BPD, we consider the treatment of a patient with BPD whose diagnostic phenomenology is characterized by core problems involving the Affect and Impulse clusters. This is the most typical type of patient in our samples, and we expect that it is the kind of patient who gives the clinician the most difficulty. Such a patient is typically female, in her 20s or early 30s; she is single, and holds a job with difficulty if she is working at all. She is also angry, has a history of intense relationships marked by alternating feelings of love and hate, engages impulsively in sex or perhaps goes on eating binges, often abuses alcohol or drugs, may burn or cut herself, or may have threatened or tried several times to kill herself. The most immediate treatment goal with such an individual is to initiate and maintain a pattern in which she comes to treatment on a regular basis.

Reaching even this limited, preliminary goal can be quite difficult, as many BPD individuals seek treatment during periods of crisis that often arise from episodic, impulsive behaviors. The potential disruptiveness of such behaviors makes it difficult to induce appropriate treatment role behaviors, and their episodic nature makes it difficult to sustain motivation for treatment once the crisis has passed. Consequently, early in the treatment the therapist must manage the anger that the patient is likely to focus on the therapist and the treatment being offered, and must organize an effective strategy for the most seriously destructive of these behaviors.

In our view, these immediate treatment goals will be present whether the conceptual framework for approaching such problems is cognitive–behavioral, psychodynamic, or relational. However, because different theoretical orientations conceptualize these behaviors differently, different strategies are employed in meeting these early treatment goals. The immediate treatment goals and the strategies employed within each of the three treatment approaches are discussed below.

Reduction and Control of Impulse Cluster Behaviors

Impulsive and self-destructive behaviors are of immediate concern to the therapist for several reasons. First, the self-destructive behavior is often quite serious and even life-threatening, especially when the patient first comes to treatment. Its potentially lethal consequences often demand immediate attention. Consequently, it is crucial that these difficulties be managed successfully from the outset of treatment. If these difficulties are not met directly and early with appropriate interventions, little if any therapeutic gain with regard to the other difficulties will be manifested on the remaining behavioral clusters. A final reason for our emphasis on impulsivity is its prevalence in the data discussed earlier (Hurt et al., 1990). We confine our discussion here to the management of potentially suicidal behavior as it occurs in the context of chronic, repetitive patterns of self-destructive behavior. Intermittent suicidal impulses, particularly those that occur in response to intercurrent episodes of depression, should be managed differently.

Kernberg et al. (1989) and Linehan (1984, 1987) focus the initial treatment consultations on the establishment and negotiation of a treatment contract consistent with the therapeutic framework underpinning each of the treatment approaches. The presentation and development of a treatment contract addresses, at the outset of treatment, several issues pertinent to the management of impulsive behavior. Although these two approaches overlap to some degree, they also offer different perspectives and emphases.

Kernberg et al.'s approach to the development of a treatment contract emphasizes (1) clarifying the role of the therapist, (2) clarifying the role of the patient, and (3) developing a structure for the treatment as a framework for subsequent interpretations of any deviations from the structure. In clarifying the role of the therapist, the goals of the therapy are stated and the activities of the therapist are outlined. The therapist emphasizes a commitment to understanding feelings, thoughts, and behavior, and their relationships to one another. The patient is not expected to refrain from self-destructive behaviors or to make a commitment to do so. Rather, the patient is expected to work at understanding these behaviors, since these behaviors have undermined past efforts to benefit from therapeutic encounters. The therapist is instructed to specify the limits of his/her involvement with the patient's self-destructive behavior as it occurs outside of the therapy hour. Rather than intervening repeatedly to prevent the patient's possible death, the therapist suggests alternative means of seeking help at these times, such as going to hospital emergency rooms. Thus, right from the beginning of treatment, the therapist acts to limit the patient's power over the treatment by being able to force a choice between continuing treatment or ending life. Open acknowledgment of the difficulty of this task for the patient and the possibility of failure, as well as genuine acceptance of this possibility on the part of the therapist, is necessary. Accepting the possibility of failure requires the therapist to convey to the patient that although the patient's death would sadden the therapist, the therapist's life would not be altered significantly by the patient's death. If appropriate, this attitude and these feelings are also conveyed to the patient's family.

The role of the patient is to bring to therapy all thoughts and feelings related to self-destructive impulses, so that the material can be explored and understood. The importance of the patient's role as organizer, recorder, and presenter of personal experiences is emphasized for its value in providing material for and structure to the treatment situation. Thus, the shared re-sponsibility for the therapeutic work provides a framework for the patient—therapist interactions. For Kernberg and colleagues, the provision of such a framework and adherence to its demands by both parties provides a structure for the patient that helps her to achieve the goal of self-restraint, and provides the setting for the material that forms the substance of the therapeutic work.

Deviations from the role assigned to the patient provide the therapist with opportunities for clarifying and understanding the vicissitudes of the patient's self-destructive wishes. By focusing the work on this aspect of the patient's experience, the therapist reaffirms the original commitment of helping the patient to explore and understand. In doing so, the therapist honors his/her own commitment to the treatment and invites the patient to re-engage in the therapeutic work.

Linehan's approach to the development of a treatment contract includes many of the same components. In the initial sessions, the therapist provides information about the treatment program and focuses on both the role of the patient and the role of the therapist. The program is contractual; although these contracts are time-limited, they are renewable if progress has been made. The program also has within it a large educational component. There is a much more explicit focus on the underlying theory of parasuicidal behavior, and a greater emphasis on bibliographic materials as aids to understanding.

Linehan also emphasizes the role of the therapist in helping the patient to gain insight into the reasons for her suicidal behavior in the context of the theory of parasuicidal behavior. In addition, the therapist is expected to help the patient learn new skills for coping with suicidal impulses. The patient is informed of the therapist's rights to assess the potential risk involved in a patient's behavior, and to insist on hospitalization or other unwanted inter-ventions if the patient convinces the therapist that death by suicide is imminent. The therapist's acting as a monitor and triage consultant to the patient thus adds a further dimension to the therapist's role. The therapist also informs the patient that urges to continue suicidal behavior are expected, since such behavior is a maladaptive, habitual response to stress, and such habits are difficult to curtail.

The role of the patient requires a general commitment to the specific goal of reducing the frequency of suicidal behavior. Because of the multimodal nature of the treatment strategy, the patient must also make a number of interrelated, specific commitments. Individual and group psychotherapy are conducted concurrently, and attendance at all psychotherapy sessions is expected. Missing four sessions (group or individual) in a row will result in termination of treatment. The terms of the treatment contract impose a clear structure on the roles and relationships as they involve impulsive, self-destructive behavior. The first topic of any psychotherapy session is the occurrence of any parasuicidal behavior since the last session. The purpose of the structure is to remove any impediments to the completion of the time-limited course of therapy. Disruptions of the therapeutic framework that derive from impulsive, self-destructive behaviors of the patient do not immediately result in termination of the therapy unless the previously identified thresholds for such behavior are crossed.

The RMP approach (Dawson, 1988; Marziali et al., 1989) places little emphasis on the development of a treatment contract. RMP does not focus on parasuicidal behaviors or any other patient actions or threats that Linehan and Kernberg et al. view as potentially disruptive to therapy. The patient is invited to join a treatment group that will meet weekly for 30 sessions. The decision to attend the group is left up to the patient. Each patient is given the opportunity to meet individually with the cotherapists the week prior to the first group session. This is not a group induction session, however. Rather, the patient decides whether or not to attend the session, and may use the time to inquire about group treatment or to share doubts about attending the group. Of importance is the fact that the therapists do not attempt to structure these pregroup sessions, and the patient has full control over how she wishes to use the session.

The objectives of the initial group sessions are similar to those established for any psychotherapy group: engagement, testing the group parameters, developing connections, and forming some commitment to group membership. The therapists are actively involved in the process, but their interventions are largely exploratory, open-ended questions that are phrased tentatively. Questions that require specific answers and interpretations are avoided. When challenged, the therapists acknowledge and affirm the patients' doubts about the ultimate benefits that might be gained from participating in the group. Similarly, patients' frustrations with the futility of previous treatment experiences are affirmed.

There is no explicit discussion of a treatment contract in RMP. Instead, from the outset, the therapist attempts to establish an atmosphere of interest and respect for the patient's own thoughts, feelings, and decisions. Behaviors that could disrupt the treatment process are not explained or interpreted. Attendance at group is voluntary, participation is voluntary, and silences are accepted. In RMP, the primary therapeutic task is deducing, from the group's interactions, the "core message" intended for the therapists. Regardless of which patient is speaking, or to whom a patient is speaking, a message is communicated that polarizes the patients' status vis-à-vis the therapists. From these observations, the therapists generate and test hypotheses about the intent of the "core message." For example, if the polarization reflects "incompetent patients and competent therapists," the therapists' interventions communicate doubt, not knowing, and confusion. If the patients' interactions begin to shift to competent attempts to solve problems, the therapists' hypothesis has been confirmed, and therapeutic error has been aborted. It is the repetition of this cycle of patient–therapist interactions that validates the patients' importance, feeling states, abilities, and skills. The therapists demonstrate repeatedly that the patients' wishes, frustrations, doubts, and errors can be tolerated, managed, and contained.

Managing Anger toward the Therapist and the Therapy

One of the major tasks in beginning the treatment is to set a framework in which the patient's anger toward the therapist and the treatment can be managed and absorbed, while still allowing the therapist to proceed with the work of the therapy. Kernberg et al. (1989) and Linehan (1984, 1987) both do this through a careful explication, at the beginning of the treatment, of how self-destructive behaviors will be handled. They both acknowledge (at least implicitly) that the patient will probably continue such behaviors and that the plan for their management, however well articulated, is likely to contain some inconsistencies that will be noted by the patient. As a consequence, both approaches emphasize a need to make every attempt to be explicit in describing how such behaviors will be managed, and emphasize the need for the therapist to be consistent in the implementation of these plans.

RMP (Dawson, 1988; Marziali et al., 1989) does not attempt to explain or interpret the patient's anger or potentially self-destructive behaviors. No attempt is made to help the patient gain insight into what motivates maladaptive and self-destructive behaviors. The therapist does not educate or attempt to exert control over the patient through therapeutic management of behaviors that threaten disruption of the therapy. If a patient reports engaging in potentially life-threatening behaviors, the therapist responds by empathically stating that he/she does not want the patient to harm herself, but realizes that he/she cannot do anything to stop the patient; the therapist also reiterates that help is always available at a hospital emergency service. This approach is the antithesis of Linehan's approach to the management of self-destructive behaviors, but parallels Kernberg et al.'s approach to some extent. However, in the RMP approach, the implications and meanings of such behaviors are not explored or interpreted.

Angry, self-destructive patients frequently engender feelings of anger and helplessness in therapists, and these feelings are probably a major obstacle to treating these patients. It has been suggested, for example, that when medications are used with such patients, it has much to do with feelings of anger and/or helplessness on the part of the therapist (Nurnberg & Suh, 1978; Silver, Book, Hamilton, Sadavoy, & Slonim, 1983; Silver, Cardish, & Glassman, 1987). Of major importance in helping to redirect and diffuse such feelings is the consistent application of the specific techniques recommended in these treatment strategies. Although Kernberg and colleagues, Linehan, and the McMaster group take different approaches to managing this important stage of treatment (and these are discussed in some detail below), we note here that Kernberg et al. and Linehan recommend a consistent attempt on the part of the therapist to manage self-destructive behaviors as initially outlined to the patient, and to make every effort to engage the patient in a collaborative treatment relationship as initially outlined. Since RMP is not concerned with controlling the patient's potentially self-destructive behaviors, the initial therapeutic phase parallels the beginning of any psychotherapy group. The therapists attend carefully to group member interactions that reflect polarizations in which the therapists are viewed as directing the group and having answers, and the patients are viewed as having no control, having no answers, and being at risk of humiliation. When the therapists effect a shift in this polarization by being interested but nondirective, and by taking the nonexpert role, the patients begin to assume responsibility for developing a collaborative working environment in the group. They often begin to exert control over each other's potentially destructive behaviors. Whereas a group of neurotic patients may take four to six sessions to gain commitment to treatment, a borderline group may require twice as long to test out anxieties and doubts about commitment to the therapeutic process.

It is commonly assumed that cognitive–behavioral treatments such as those offered by Linehan are more supportive than those such as Kernberg et al.'s psychodynamic treatment, with its requisite posture of therapeutic neutrality. Comparing the different publications makes it possible to explore the similarities and differences with regard to the actual therapist behaviors each approach prescribes. This helps to reduce any vagueness regarding the nature of a supportive versus an exploratory treatment. Linehan (1984, 1987) recommends the active use of information and the giving of this information to the patient as a supportive activity. The patient is explicitly asked to contract to try to reduce suicidal behavior and is told that the therapist assumes that such behavior *will not immediately subside*. Such concrete information is not directly transmitted to the patient involved in a psychodynamic treatment.

The approaches also differ with regard to the degree of prescribed contact between patient and therapist. Linehan recommends that during an emergency (a condition defined by the patient), the patient be told how to achieve telephone contact with the therapist between sessions. Emergency consultations are permitted with the express purpose of involving the therapist in helping the patient to actively solve an immediate problem, in order to prevent hospitalization or medical treatment. Kernberg et al. (1989) explicitly forbid any contact between sessions, and instead recommend that the therapist discuss, within the consultation hour, the requirement that the patient utilize such emergency services as needed without involving the therapist in such consultations. RMP (Marziali et al., 1989) neither prescribes nor prohibits between-session contacts with the therapists.

In Linehan's view, the extra contact serves to increase the strength of the relationship by providing concrete opportunities for the patient to employ newer coping strategies with the support and guidance of the therapist. In Kernberg et al.'s view, such contact is disallowed because it must, by definition, occur at times when the therapist must forgo the original treatment contract of helping the patient to understand, and instead must assume an active posture that is incompatible with the primary task of therapy. Within the parameters of RMP, between-session contacts are not discussed during sessions unless the issue is raised by one of the patients. The therapists tell the patients that they can call if they wish, but that this might result in frustration because they often will not be able to reach a therapist immediately. If the concern is with suicidal risk, the patients are told that hospital emergency departments are available to them.

Insofar as all three positions are clearly articulated as consistent with the long-range goals of treatment, as originally defined, adherence to the framework of the treatment contract helps the therapist to manage the patient's inevitable anger at the therapist and disappointment in the initial outcome of the therapy.

Another major difference among the three treatment approaches is Linehan's use of both individual and group modalities. The use of the combined treatment format allows the patient contact with a number of people, and may help to diffuse anger toward the individual therapist, as well as providing additional time and support for developing more adaptive coping strategies. In contrast, Kernberg et al. recommend meeting twice a week with the patient for individual psychotherapy only. This creates a situation in which the therapist becomes a major figure in the patient's life—one onto which many transferential feelings are projected. The promotion of the early development of such feelings provides an enriched treatment opportunity by helping to focus these feelings for the patient and the therapist, so that they can be more quickly understood. RMP uses a group approach and is time-limited. The group meets weekly for 1½ hours. Although the group therapists scan the group interactions in order to infer the "core message" intended for the therapists, they avoid becoming the focus of the exchange by not interpreting the transference.

Establishing Regular Appointments

BPD patients are notorious for premature ending of therapy (Gunderson, 1984), and this makes it difficult both to treat them and to investigate their treatment. It is most often assumed that aspects of borderline psychology (i.e., angry, intense relationships combined with self-destructive behaviors) are directly related to this treatment-aborting behavior. Such a view simply blames the disorder for the failure of the treatment, without suggesting how the treatment might be made more congenial for those with the disorder. In contrast, two of the treatment manuals, those of Kernberg et al. (1989) and Linehan (1984), begin with a recognition of the likelihood of this very phenomenon and so place a heavy emphasis on the careful induction of the patient into treatment. Both manuals outline specific efforts and strategies for describing in detail the roles of the patient and the therapist, so that a more productive, working relationship may be established. Linehan teaches these behaviors explicitly by providing information about the cognitive–behavioral conceptualization of self-destructive behavior. Kernberg et al.'s teaching efforts are embedded in exploratory interpretations involving idiographic hypotheses relating these behaviors to feelings about the treatment situation. Both manuals also have in common an implicit statement to the patient that the therapist believes that a regular, scheduled, and sustained treatment relationship is the only arrangement that will be workable.

In contrast, the RMP manual (Marziali et al., 1989) provides no instruction for inducting the patients into either a treatment contract or into the group. When group treatment is offered to the patient, she is told about the structure of the group, including its time boundaries and the frequency, time, and place of the meetings. In addition, as noted earlier, each patient is offered the opportunity to meet with the group therapists individually prior to the first group meeting. Each patient is free either to take up or to ignore this option. Furthermore, the way in which the pregroup session is used by each patient who selects the option is left entirely up to the patient. In taking this stance at the onset of the treatment encounter, RMP affirms the patient's control over whether or not to accept treatment.

Dealing with Identity Cluster Issues

Whereas the other clusters involve overt behaviors that are more easily observed and measured, the Identity cluster involves inner states that are quite dependent upon the reporting of the subject and therefore less accessible to observation and careful measurement. This does not mean that they are less important, but their relative importance may be more difficult to assess.

The dynamic formulation of BPD puts theoretical weight on identity diffusion and considers it one of the core features of the entire borderline personality organization. The behavioral formulation gives it less prominence. This relative degree of prominence is also reflected in the treatment strategies focused upon identity cluster issues.

Kernberg et al. (1989) are constantly attentive to how the patient manifests disparate and contradictory aspects of the self as they are played out in the immediate relationship with the therapist. The therapeutic strategy of confrontation—that is, identifying the contradictory nature of the patient's experience and/or behavior in the here and now—is utilized in order to provide an opportunity for the BPD patient to integrate these split-off features.

Linehan (1985) seems to approach some of the issues that Kernberg et al. would refer to as primitive defenses of "splitting" and "identity diffusion" in other terms. She speaks of the "black-and-white" cognitive style of the patient, and utilizes dialectical techniques to assist the patient in overcoming this all-or-none thinking and approach to life's situations.

The RMP therapist (Marziali et al., 1989) searches for manifestations of identity diffusion in a manner similar to Kernberg et al.; that is, the therapist observes the interactions between patients, and between patients and therapists, during the group process. Patients dichotomize versions of the self by playing out interpersonal paradigms in which self and other are polarized. The RMP therapist does not interpret, clarify, or explain the patient's discrepant or contradictory behaviors; instead, the therapist avoids enacting any of the projected, polarized positions. For example, the angry patient who expects either punishment or rejection receives a therapeutic response that affirms the anger and that acknowledges aspects of the confusion associated with the anger. When the therapist actively identifies with and tolerates the patient's confusion and anger without enacting any of the polarized projections, the patient has the opportunity to reclaim and process in a different manner the split-off aspects of the self.

DISCUSSION

We have attempted to illustrate how data from diagnostic studies might be utilized to focus on and compare treatment strategies, even those that arise from conceptualizations as disparate-seeming as the cognitive–behavioral and the psychodynamic. This approach has been empirical, in that it extracts core problems that serve to define a disorder of interest, and compares treatment strategies that are directed at these problems and their relationships to one another. This approach helps to illustrate the treatment strategies to be employed and the goals of the treatment. With these clearly in mind, attempts to assess the relative merits of one therapeutic approach in relation to another are easier to realize. Although none of the three treatment approaches discussed here has as yet generated sufficient data to warrant a comparison regarding outcomes, they nevertheless have been sufficiently well developed to form the basis for a clear discussion of their approaches to the core problems represented by patients with BPD.

The Focus of Treatment

In contrast to the McMaster group, neither Linehan nor Kernberg et al. developed their manuals to focus directly on the DSM-III or DSM-III-R criteria for BPD. Linehan's (1984) manual is focused on the treatment of parasuicidal women, many of whom meet the DSM-III-R criteria for BPD. Kernberg et al.'s (1989) efforts are focused on theoretical considerations stemming from Kernberg's conceptualization of borderline personality organization, a diagnostic construct that is broader in scope that the BPD of DSM-III-R. Although BPD is not the sole consideration in either case, the groups for whom these treatments have been developed overlap with the DSM-III-R BPD group to a significant degree. The RMP manual (Marziali et al., 1989) was developed to respond specifically to the symptoms and behavioral manifestations of BPD as specified in DSM-III.

The most interesting point of similarity between the Kernberg et al. and Linehan approaches is their emphasis on a clear and explicit treatment contract as the first therapeutic task. The need for such a contract stems directly from the life- and treatment-threatening behaviors frequently displayed by the BPD patient. It is thought that if these episodic behaviors were allowed to rule the therapeutic relationship, then little of therapeutic value would be accomplished. In emphasizing the therapeutic work, the patient is expected to establish a commitment to refrain from engaging in such behavior to the degree that it undermines the potentially therapeutic nature of the relationship. Both Linehan and Kernberg et al. clearly specify that this means accepting the fact that treatment may fail; in fact, all other things being equal, that is the most likely possibility. Such a presentation runs the risk of engendering a dangerous amount of stultifying pessimism, were it not for the fact that for those engaged in a chronic, repetitive pattern of potentially self-destructive behavior, this very outcome is a virtual certainty. What can be offered genuinely, having accepted that the treatment will most likely fail, is a consistent effort to address the difficulty by the best means available to the therapist, and a clear commitment not to deviate from this effort in spite of a limited chance of success. In RMP, a treatment contract is implied but never specifically articulated. That is, patients are never asked to commit themselves to the time-limited group. Thus, avoidant behaviors, including potentially self-destructive behaviors, are not addressed in the context of their implications for continuing treatment. In contrast to the approaches of Kernberg et al. and Linehan, it is hypothesized in RMP that the act of focusing on these behaviors allows the intensified concern for the behaviors to rule and possibly to derail the therapeutic encounter. RMP is based on the assumption that only responding to potentially self-destructive behaviors in a truly neutral fashion will cause them to diminish in influence.

The Kernberg et al. and Linehan approaches have in common a clear commitment to the treatment as the central issue for both patient and therapist. It is thought that specifying what is required and expected of both parties establishes a framework of expectations and shared experiences that can be called upon to help contain impulsive, self-destructive modes of expression. Both approaches offer an opportunity for expression, management, and understanding of the sources of the self-destructive behavior, and focus their attention on the therapeutic advantages of such an endeavor, rather than allowing the interaction to be driven by the impulsive behavior itself.

By focusing, at the outset, on the life- and treatment-threatening behaviors, both approaches deal directly with a significant core problem and do so in an organized and structured therapeutic context. Although this is the preliminary step in the overall treatment strategy, its concretization provides an important setting in which to develop and improve the tactical advantages of each approach. Developments in the science of differential therapeutics clearly depend on being better able to specify what treatment approaches yield the greatest advantages to which kinds of patients under what sort of circumstances. Our ability to make effective treatment choices is enhanced by our efforts to arrive at answers to these questions. We believe that empirical study of the relationships between criterion-based diagnoses such as those of DSM-III-R, and treatment strategies such as those of Kernberg et al., Linehan, and the McMaster group, can provide us with answers to these questions.

In the context of process-oriented psychotherapy studies, these three treatment approaches invite comparisons. The Kernberg et al. and Linehan approaches both directly address impulsive behaviors at their outset, whereas RMP only indirectly addresses these. Thus, tracking the incidence of such behaviors over time would be one method of studying the impact of these treatments. A more elegant approach might be to consider the impact of these treatments on the Affect and Identity clusters in relation to changes in the Impulse cluster. Although all three treatments directly or indirectly respond to the problem of impulsive behaviors at the outset of treatment, we believe that they do so for somewhat different reasons. Kernberg et al. emphasize these behaviors initially in order to make clear the limits of the therapist's responsibility, and thereby to undermine the power of these behaviors to nullify the therapy. Linehan, on the other hand, emphasizes these behaviors in order to make clear the patient's commitment to reducing them. The McMaster group takes no active role in relation to these problems, leaving them to the responsibility of the individual patients. It should be noted that patients generally perceive this as an active stance of neutrality on the part of the therapists.

Emphasizing the potentially conflictual, cooperative, or neutral aspects of the treatment relationship, respectively, sets the stage for the subsequent treatment strategies proposed. These emphases also imply different models of the therapeutic relationship. Process-oriented investigations of these treatments might profitably focus on the relationships between different constellations of the three core problems and the success or failure of the treatment at various stages.

How the Changes Are Made

Bringing suicidal behavior (and other impulsive behavior) under control is a goal of all three treatments, but *how* this is done differs in the three models. What are the accompanying changes that we would expect from the three models? In the Linehan model, we would expect that the patients would learn to utilize the skills and tactics they have been taught to exert increasing self-control over their self-destructive feelings. In contrast, we would expect patients treated under the Kernberg et al. model to exhibit a greater understanding of their self-destructive wishes and to acknowledge the manner in which this aspect of the self operates to their own detriment. These patients should have a heightened awareness of their self-destructive behaviors and how they operate in intense interpersonal relationships, including the one with the therapist. In the McMaster model, we might expect that patients would show a diminished interest or awareness of their self-destructive behaviors as they gradually gain greater confidence in their own decisions.

An obvious question is how the various approaches might be combined so as to utilize the most efficient and effective approach. One might think that Kernberg et al. would resist any attempt to intermingle behavioral and dynamic strategies, particularly in light of their belief that supportive and dynamic methods cannot be mixed. The stance of therapeutic neutrality—essential, in their view, to the dynamic method—is in some respects consistent with RMP, but it overtly excludes supportive and behavioral methods. On the other hand, we might suggest that Kernberg and colleagues are mixing psychodynamic and behavioral interventions, the latter not identified as such, in their own manual. Certainly the focus of the initial consultations on arriving at a treatment contract approaches the behaviorists' notion of contingency contracting. This approach is explicitly disavowed by the McMaster group, which adopts a dialectical stance toward the resolution of conflicting self-representations.

As Linehan has suggested, there may be a staged approach to combining different models. BPD patients with extensive histories of impulsive and self-destructive behaviors and no fruitful work experience may need the structure, support, and direction of the behavioral approach to begin to get the impulsive behaviors under control. Once this is accomplished, the dynamic approach may add depth to the patient's changes and understanding of the self. It may also be argued that with such understanding in hand, the opportunity to test and validate newer self-representations is directly offered by the RMP approach.

Future research could add useful information regarding the optimal match of patient profile and treatment strategy associated with the effects of these three approaches to treating the BPD subgroups represented in the Impulse, Affect, and Identity clusters.

REFERENCES

Anderson, C. M., Reiss, D. J., & Hogarty, G. E. (1986). *Schizophrenia and the family*. New York: Guilford Press.

Barlow, D. H. (1988). *Anxiety and its disorders: The nature and treatment of anxiety and panic*. New York: Guilford Press.

Beck, A. T., Rush, A., Shaw, B. F., & Emery, G. (1979). *Cognitive therapy of depression*. New York: Guilford Press.

Clarkin, J. F., Hurt, S. W., & Hull, J. W. (1991). *Subclassification of borderline personality disorder: A cluster solution*. Unpublished manuscript, New York Hospital–Cornell Medical Center, Westchester Division, White Plains, NY.

Clarkin, J. F., Widiger, T. A., Frances, A., Hurt, S. W., & Gilmore, M. (1983). Prototypic typology and the borderline personality disorder. *Journal of Abnormal Psychology, 92*, 263–275.

Cloninger, R. C. (1986). A systematic method for clinical description and classification of personality variants: A proposal. *Archives of General Psychiatry, 44*, 573–588.

Cowdry, R. W. (1987). Psychopharmacology of borderline personality disorder: A review. *Journal of Clinical Psychiatry, 48*, 15–22.

Dawson, D. (1988). Treatment of the borderline patient: Relationship management. *Canadian Journal of Psychiatry, 33*, 370–374.

Falloon, I. R. H., Boyd, J. L., & McGill, C. W. (1984). *Family care of schizophrenia*. New York: Guilford Press.

Fyer, M. R., Frances, A. F., Sullivan, T., Hurt, S. W., & Clarkin, J. F. (1988). Comorbidity of borderline personality disorder. *Archives of General Psychiatry, 45*, 348–352.

Gunderson, J. G. (1984). *Borderline personality disorder*. Washington, DC: American Psychiatric Press.

Hurt, S. W., Clarkin, J. F., Widiger, T. A., Fyer, M. R., Sullivan, T., Stone, M. H., & Frances, A. (1990). Evaluation of DSM-III decision rules for case detection using joint conditional probability structures. *Journal of Personality Disorders, 4,* 121–130.

Kernberg, O., Selzer, M., Koenigsberg, H., Carr, A., & Appelbaum, A. (1989). *Psychodynamic psychotherapy of borderline patients.* New York: Basic Books.

Klerman, G. L., Weissman, M. M., Rounsaville, B. J., & Chevron, E. S. (1984). *Interpersonal psychotherapy of depression.* New York: Basic Books.

Linehan, M. M. (1984). *Dialectical behavior therapy for treatment of parasuicidal women: Treatment manual.* Unpublished manuscript, University of Washington.

Linehan, M. M. (1987). Dialectical behavioral therapy: A cognitive behavioral approach to parasuicide. *Journal of Personality Disorders, 1,* 328–333.

Luborsky, L. (1984). *Principles of psychoanalytic psychotherapy: A manual for supportive–expressive treatment.* New York: Basic Books.

Marziali, E., Newman, T., Munroe-Blum, H., & Dawson, D. (1989). *Manual and training materials for relationship management psychotherapy.* Unpublished manuscript.

Nurnberg, H. G., & Suh, R. (1978). Time-limited treatment of hospitalized borderline patients: Considerations. *Comprehensive Psychiatry, 19,* 419–431.

Settlage, C. F. (1977). The psychoanalytic understanding of narcissistic and borderline personality disorders: Advances in developmental theory. *Journal of the American Psychoanalytic Association, 25,* 805–833.

Siever, L. F., Klar, H., & Coccaro, E. (1985). Psychobiologic substrates of personality. In H. Klar & L. J. Siever (Eds.), *Biologic response styles: Clinical implications.* Washington, DC: American Psychiatric Press.

Silver, D., Book, H., Hamilton, J., Sadovoy, J., & Slonim, R. (1983). The characterologically difficult patient: A hospital treatment model. *Canadian Journal of Psychiatry, 28,* 91–96.

Silver, D., Cardish, R., & Glassman, E. (1987). Intensive treatment of characterologically difficult patients. *Psychiatric Clinics of North America, 10,* 219–245.

Strupp, H. H., & Binder, L. L. (1984). *Psychotherapy in a new key.* New York: Basic Books.

CHAPTER 10

The Therapeutic Alliances of Borderline Patients

ARLENE F. FRANK

The role of the doctor–patient relationship in facilitating recovery from illness has long been recognized by the medical establishment. Though significant in all clinical specialties, this relationship is most important in the practice of psychotherapy. Psychotherapy is, after all, a uniquely interpersonal endeavor that gains its meaning largely from the emergent interactions of the individuals involved (Docherty, 1985; Butler & Strupp, 1986). Even those who maintain that change derives primarily from the skillful selection and use of specific therapeutic techniques acknowledge that the successful application of those techniques depends upon a certain degree of openness, trust, understanding, and mutuality between patient and therapist. This constellation of relationship factors has been known variously as a "therapeutic" (Zetzel, 1956), "working" (Greenson, 1965; Bordin, 1979), or "helping" (Luborsky, 1976) alliance.

Since Freud introduced the concept, much has been written about the alliance. The most extensive discussions can be found in the psychoanalytic literature. However, the subject has been of interest to practitioners and theorists of all orientations. In fact, at least some concept of alliance can be found in every corner of the psychotherapy literature; and, increasingly, the concept has been incorporated into discussions of pharmacotherapy (Gutheil, 1978, 1982; Bowers & Greenfeld, 1980; Adelman, 1985; Docherty & Fiester, 1985; Book, 1987; Smith, 1989; Waldinger & Frank, 1989a, 1989b).

The alliance has captured the interest of researchers as well as clinicians. The result has been a burgeoning empirical literature on this subject. The emerging consensus from this literature is that the alliance is a highly significant prognostic indicator, with considerable power for predicting compliance with disposition plans (Eisenthal, Emery, Lazare, & Udin, 1979) and medication regimens (Docherty & Fiester, 1985; Waldinger & Frank, 1989b; Frank & Gunderson, 1990); the tenure of psychotherapy (Howard et al., 1970; Feister

& Rudestam, 1975; Saltzman, Leutgert, Roth, Creaser, & Howard, 1976; Tracy, 1977; Kolb, Beutler, Davis, Crago, & Shanfield, 1985; Tracey, 1986; Eaton, Abeles, & Gutfreund, 1988; Gunderson et al., 1989; Frank & Gunderson, 1990); and treatment outcome (Horwitz, 1974; Saltzman et al., 1976; Gomes-Schwartz, 1978; Marziali, Marmar, & Krupnick, 1981; Morgan, Luborsky, Crits-Christoph, Curtis, & Solomon, 1982; Moras & Strupp, 1982; Luborsky, Crits-Christoph, Alexander, Margolis, & Cohen, 1983; Luborsky, Crits-Christoph, Mintz, & Auerbach, 1988; O'Malley, Suh, & Strupp, 1983; Horowitz, Marmar, Weiss, DeWitt, & Rosenbaum, 1984; Marziali, 1984; Allen, Tarnoff, & Coyne, 1985; Allen, Deering, Buskirk, & Coyne, 1988; Kolb et al., 1985; Marmar, Horowitz, Weiss, & Marziali, 1986; Marmar, Gaston, Gallagher, & Thompson, 1989; Horvath & Greenberg, 1986; Alexander & Luborsky, 1986; Clarkin, Hurt, & Crilly, 1987; Eaton et al., 1988, Budman et al., 1989; Gerstley et al., 1989; Saunders, Howard, & Orlinsky, 1989; Frank & Gunderson, 1990).

Although the alliance–outcome relationship is probably not simple or direct, it seems to hold across diverse patient populations and treatment modalities (Horvath & Symonds, 1990). This has provided incentive and justification for careful scrutiny of the nature of the alliance, as well as systematic delineation of the factors in the patient, therapist, and treatment process that contribute to its development and maintenance.

For those who treat borderline patients, this information would prove especially useful. Although there is disagreement about the therapeutic interventions that are most effective with borderline patients, there is widespread agreement that securing an alliance is crucial—and difficult to achieve. The nature and severity of the borderline patient's impairments in ego functioning and interpersonal relations are precisely what impede the formation of the kind of open, trusting, collaborative therapeutic relationship that generally is considered the hallmark of an alliance. Yet these same impairments make the development of an alliance a goal of paramount importance (Masterson, 1978). It has been argued that with borderline patients, in contrast to healthier patients, the development of an alliance is more a consequence of successful treatment than a prerequisite for it (Adler, 1979; Frieswyk et al., 1986).

BARRIERS TO EMPIRICAL RESEARCH

Although the alliance probably plays a key role in the treatment of borderline patients, little empirical research has been devoted specifically to this subject. This lack of research can be related to at least six factors: time-limited treatment, diagnostic controversies, conceptual ambiguities, measurement problems, high patient dropout rates, and therapist resistance.

Time-Limited Treatment

Most alliance studies have dealt with short-term (10- to 20-session) treatments. It has become something of a clinical truism that in selecting patients for such treatments, evidence of a capacity to rapidly form and sustain an alliance is essential; moreover, lack thereof is considered reasonable grounds for rejecting as "unsuitable" the prospective therapy candidate (Rush, 1985)—in this case, the borderline patient. Although the use of such selection/suitability criteria has recently been challenged, even by proponents of short-term psychotherapy (Binder, Henry, & Strupp, 1987), it remains the basis for many treatment and research decisions.

Diagnostic Controversies

In the last decade, there has been a virtual explosion of research aimed at isolating the defining features of borderline patients and establishing reliable and valid methods for diagnosing borderline personality disorder (BPD). This research has provided considerable support for the existence of BPD as a distinct diagnostic entity. Nonetheless, the diagnosis remains controversial; questions about the nature, etiology, and boundaries of the disorder continue to occupy center stage in current research efforts. As Greene, Rosenkrantz, and Muth (1986) have pointed out, this disproportionate focus on diagnosis-oriented research has precluded to some extent treatment-oriented research on borderline patients, including studies of the alliance.

Conceptual Ambiguities

A problem not specific to the study of BPD is the lack of consensus regarding how best to conceptualize and operationalize the alliance. The term "alliance" continues to be used in confusing, inconsistent, and sometimes idiosyncratic ways to describe a variety of phenomena (see Gutheil & Havens, 1979; Frieswyk, Colson, & Allen, 1984; Gaston, 1990). For example, some have asserted that the alliance is best conceptualized narrowly, in unidimensional terms, as the patient's active collaboration with the therapist in an effort to solve a problem (Frieswyk et al., 1984, 1986). Others have advocated a broader, multidimensional conceptualization—one that also includes the affective bond of trust and attachment that the patient forms with the therapist (Luborsky, 1976; Bordin, 1979), as well as the contractual agreement that the patient reaches with the therapist regarding treatment goals and methods (Bordin, 1979). Except for one published study (Tichenor & Hill, 1989), these competing conceptualizations have not been directly compared. This has led to difficulties in determining which is most accurate and under what circumstances (e.g., with what kinds of patients, in what stages of their illness or treatment).

It has also been difficult to distinguish the alliance from the transference. As a number of authors have observed, it is misleading to think that an alliance can be founded solely on the "real" (nontransferential) aspects of the patient−therapist relationship. Invariably, the fantasies, expectations, and wishes derived from earlier experiences with significant others will intrude upon and shape that relationship (Gill & Hoffman, 1982; Horowitz & Marmar, 1985; Frieswyk et al., 1986; Gabbard et al., 1988).

Separating core features of the alliance from other factors that contribute to its development and maintenance is a related problem. For example, it is unclear in many studies to what extent the alliance has predictive power in its own right, or derives its predictive power from its association with other change measures or other good prognostic indicators present at the start of treatment. Also unclear is whether the development of an alliance reflects the skillful application of specific therapeutic interventions, or is simply a product of the fortuitous pairing of a particular patient and therapist. Especially problematic has been the linking of the alliance to the use of supportive treatment techniques (Zetzel, 1956, 1971). Despite recommendations to maintain a distinction between the alliance and those therapist activities that influence it, investigators have tended to blur these boundaries, adding to the confusion surrounding the concept.

Measurement Problems

The diversity and lack of clarity in conceptualizations of the alliance have been mirrored in the instruments used to assess it. Since Barrett-Lennard's (1962) pioneering work with the Relationship Inventory, no fewer than seven different instruments have been developed specifically for the purpose of measuring the alliance. These include the Quality of Alliance Scale (Ryan & Cicchetti, 1985); the Penn Helping Alliance Scales (HAcs, HAr, HAq; Luborsky, 1976; Morgan et al., 1982; Luborsky et al., 1983; Alexander & Luborsky, 1986); the Vanderbilt Therapeutic Alliance Scale (Hartley & Strupp, 1983); the Working Alliance Inventory (WAI; Horvath & Greenberg, 1986, 1989; Tracey & Kokotovic, 1988); the Menninger Therapeutic Alliance Scales (Newsom, Gabbard, & Coyne, 1984, 1988; Frieswyk et al., 1984); and the Therapeutic Alliance Rating System (TARS; Marziali et al., 1981; Marziali, 1984; Horowitz et al., 1984; Marmar et al., 1986) and its successors, the California Psychotherapy Alliance Scales (Marmar et al., 1986; Marmar, Gaston, et al., 1989; Marmar, Weiss, & Gaston, 1989).

In addition, at least five other instruments were not developed specifically for the purpose of measuring the alliance, but have been used to yield information about it. These include the Therapy Session Report (Orlinsky & Howard, 1975; Saunders et al., 1989), the Vanderbilt Psychotherapy Process Scales (Gomes-Schwartz, 1978; O'Malley et al., 1983; Suh, Strupp, & O'Malley, 1986), the Vanderbilt Negative Indicators Scale (Sachs, 1983; Suh et al., 1986), the Psychotherapy Status Report (Stanton et al., 1984; Frank & Gunderson, 1990), and the Motivation for Psychotherapy Scales (Rosenbaum & Horowitz, 1983).

Since most of the available assessment instruments were developed for and have been used with relatively healthy outpatients receiving short-term psychotherapy exclusively, the possibility remains that they may not be entirely adequate for use with borderline patients. This hypothesis is consistent with an observation first made by Bordin (1979) and subsequently echoed by Gaston, Marmar, Thompson, and Gallagher (1988)—namely, that alliances may vary considerably, depending upon the demands of the treatment being provided and the characteristics of the patient being treated. Clinical experience supports the notion that the alliances formed by borderline patients are apt to differ both qualitatively (in type or pattern of development) and quantitatively (in strength, stability, or rate of development) from those formed by other patients (Frank, 1985). Without measurement methodologies that take such differences into account, clinically relevant research on the alliances of borderline patients will continue to lag.

High Dropout Rates

Another explanation for the paucity of studies in this area stems from the nature of the treatment itself. To say that the psychotherapy of BPD is complex, arduous, and fraught with difficulties is an understatement. Accumulating evidence suggests that even when treatment is conducted by experts, outright successes are rare (Waldinger & Gunderson, 1984, 1987), and premature terminations are more often the rule than the exception (Skodol, Buckley, & Charles, 1983; Waldinger & Gunderson, 1984; Gunderson et al., 1989).

The fact that so many borderline patients drop out of treatment, and do so early, has hindered the conduct of those studies that would be of greatest clinical interest. These include studies of how good alliances are developed and maintained with borderline patients, as well as how their alliances affect and are affected by other changes that occur during treatment. Even descriptive research efforts to identify early manifestations or antecedents of an alliance have foundered in the face of the difficulties and costs of obtaining sufficiently large and representative samples of borderline patients for study.

No wholly adequate solution to this problem has yet been found. However, progress has been made in developing new methods for dealing with high attrition rates (see Howard, Krause, & Orlinsky, 1986; Flick, 1988). The field also has witnessed the development of new methods for tracking the complex and shifting events that characterize the interactions of individual patients and therapists (see Rice & Greenberg, 1984; Benjamin, 1982, 1987). The advent of these discovery-oriented approaches to psychotherapy research is especially welcome, since they partially obviate the need for recruiting large samples of patients.

Therapist Resistance

Recruitment problems extend to therapists as well. Introducing research into the matrix of a treatment that from the outset is problematic and easily subject to disruption is more than many therapists are willing to risk, despite the potential benefits. Compounding the problem is the well-known capacity of borderline patients to evoke in their treaters intense countertransference reactions and doubts about the treaters' own sense of control, competence, and self-worth. It therefore is not surprising that therapists of borderline patients are somewhat reluctant to open up their work for scrutiny, especially if the subject of investigation is the patient–therapist relationship itself.

Summary

Obviously, there are many barriers to research on the alliances of borderline patients. Nonetheless, interest in this subject remains high, and empirical studies are appearing with increased frequency. These are mostly exploratory, naturalistic studies, subject to the methodological limitations inherent in such work. The available studies also deal largely with hospitalized patients receiving intensive, dynamically oriented, individual psychotherapy. Moreover, though all yield data relevant to borderline patients, not all focus exclusively on them. Yet these studies provide a useful starting point for understanding the role of the alliance in the treatment of BPD. They also set the stage for more definitive studies in the future. The remainder of this chapter is devoted to a critical review of the studies done to date, their methodological strengths and weaknesses, and their implications for both research and clinical practice.

EXISTING EMPIRICAL STUDIES

Most of the studies that have been done have drawn their inspiration from the Menninger Foundation's Psychotherapy Research Project (PRP), a study conceived in the mid-1950s and carried out over a span of nearly 20 years (Wallerstein, 1989). The PRP was a prospective, naturalistic study of 42 severely disturbed but nonpsychotic patients, many of whom would be considered borderline by current standards. The patients were treated over a long period of time by experienced therapists, either in psychoanalysis or in some form of psychoanalytic psychotherapy. Most treatment was conducted on an outpatient basis, but a number of the patients required hospitalization at some point during the study. Comprehensive and multifaceted assessments of the patients were done at the start and termination of treatment and at 2–3 years posttreatment. A variety of procedures were used to analyze a large array of patient, therapist/treatment, and situational measures. Results were based on a combination of traditional statistical and nonmetric analyses (see Kernberg et al., 1972), more qualitative patient prediction studies (see Horwitz, 1974), and in-depth clinical case studies (see Wallerstein, 1986).

The prediction studies are the ones most relevant to this discussion; from them, Horwitz (1974) drew a number of important conclusions. First, for borderline patients, the development and internalization of a therapeutic alliance is a major vehicle of change. Second, this internalization process is a slow, evolutionary one, in some cases taking months or even years. Third, good alliances do not develop by accident or with time alone. They require a certain disposition on the part of the patient to perceive the therapist as a good object; this disposition has to be cultivated and reinforced by the therapist, through a variety of need-gratifying actions and occasionally through hospital containment. A fourth conclusion that can be inferred from Horwitz's other comments is that the alliance is not a simple construct, and that assessments of it must capture its complexity of forms and development.

Today, these conclusions might seem intuitively obvious. However, this was not the case at the time the prediction studies were done. Despite research design limitations, Horwitz's observations have withstood the tests of time and of further research. His work has had several other useful consequences. It underscored the importance of adopting a multivariate approach to the study of the alliance. It showed that patient dispositional variables and process variables (e.g., therapist actions) can interact in subtle and sometimes unpredictable ways to affect the alliance and its relation to outcome. This has since been confirmed by others (see Horowitz et al., 1984; Alexander & Luborsky, 1986; Suh et al., 1986). Horwitz's work also demonstrated that the prediction-failure-by-inspection methodology is a viable alternative to traditional group comparison designs and linear statistical models, which not only require large samples but can obscure interesting and important changes in the alliance and associated measures. Variations on this methodology have now been used effectively in several studies of the alliance (Foreman & Marmar, 1985; Suh et al., 1986; Gabbard et al., 1988).

Most important, Horwitz's work helped to crystallize what have become the major questions that require empirically based answers:

1. What types of alliances are formed by borderline patients, and how can they best be characterized?
2. What specific factors in the patient, therapist, and/or treatment situation facilitate (or inhibit) the development and maintenance of a good alliance with a borderline patient?
3. To what extent and in what ways do the alliances formed by borderline patients change over time?
4. How precisely does the development of an alliance (or lack thereof) affect the borderline patient's subsequent clinical course and outcome?

To a greater or lesser extent, all of the studies that have been done since the PRP address these questions, and should be evaluated with them in mind. These studies have come primarily from two ongoing research projects, both initiated in the early 1980s: the Menninger Treatment Interventions Project, directed by L. Horwitz,[1] and the McLean Borderline Psychotherapy Engagement Project, directed by J. Gunderson.[2] Relevant results from each are reviewed in turn.

The Menninger Treatment Interventions Project

There seemed little doubt from the PRP that a more precise assessment of the alliances of borderline patients would be useful. To this end, investigators at the Menninger Foundation developed a number of alliance scales. Initially, their measurement scheme, like their conceptualization of the alliance, was fairly broad. It included assessments of the patient's trust in the therapist, sense of acceptance by the therapist, optimism about the likely outcome of therapy, tolerance for and expression of affect in the treatment relationship, and mutual collaboration in the work of therapy.

In a pilot study, Horwitz and Frieswyk (1980) tested these measures with an outpatient described as having a borderline personality organization. Independent judges rated five tape-recorded therapy sessions selected to represent the early, middle, and end phases of what was a 1½-year treatment. Measures of the therapy process also were obtained, using a modified version of Gill and Hoffman's (1982) rating procedure. The alliance measures were evaluated in terms of their reliability, stability, and relation to the process measures.

As expected, some shifts in the alliance, first downward and then upward, occurred over the course of treatment. These were accompanied by parallel

---

[1] In collaboration with J. Allen, D. Colson, L. Coyne, S. Frieswyk, G. Gabbard, G. Newsom, and the staff of the Menninger Memorial Hospital and Outpatient Clinics.

[2] In collaboration with myself, E. Ronningstam, S. Wachter, S. Brody, R. Waldinger, and the staff of the McLean Hospital Psychosocial Research Program.

shifts in the therapy process, notably in the occurrence of both direct and indirect references to the therapeutic relationship made by both patient and therapist. However, the reliability of the alliance ratings was rather low (r's below .64), casting some doubt on the validity of the shifts in those ratings across therapy sessions. There also was some question as to the representativeness of the case and the five sessions chosen for study. In addition, the process evaluations, like the diagnosis, were based more on qualitative than on quantitative data. Nonetheless, the authors' methodology and alliance scales showed sufficient promise to warrant further development and application. This was done in two subsequent studies.

The first was devoted to a revision of the original alliance scales (Allen et al., 1984). In an effort to achieve greater conceptual clarity and reliability of measurement, the alliance was defined more narrowly as the patient's active collaboration in the treatment process. The measures of trust, acceptance, optimism, and affect tolerance/expression were retained, but were now viewed as mediating variables in the alliance formation process, separate from collaboration. Both sets of refined measures then were applied to typescripts of 16 therapy sessions (held with 15 different patients).

Interrater reliability improved markedly for the collaboration scale ($r =$ .79) and its eight component subscales (r's ranged from .63 to .83), as well as for all of the mediating-variables scales except the measure of affect tolerance/ expression, largely because little affect toward the therapist was evident in the sessions sampled. Unfortunately, the two sets of measures did not emerge as independent (r's ranged from .66 to .91), raising questions now about the authors' narrow conceptualization of the alliance. Despite this, Allen et al. (1984) maintained that assessments of collaboration should be kept separate from other relationship measures. As they correctly pointed out, patients can show variations in their level of collaboration, depending upon their level of trust, acceptance, optimism, or affect tolerance/expression. In fact, one of their stated research goals was to discover what therapist interventions might enhance patient collaboration when an affective bond with the therapist was weak or lacking.

This issue was addressed more directly in a second, single-case study of a borderline patient who was seen three times per week in analytically oriented psychotherapy for several years (Gabbard et al., 1988). The aim of the study was to track *within-session* shifts in the alliance and to link those shifts to specific therapist interventions. Using the refined alliance measure, independent judges rated transcribed segments of six therapy sessions spanning the entire treatment. They recorded instances in which there was an observable increase, decrease, or lack of change in collaboration. Other judges independently rated therapist interventions, using Gill and Hoffman's (1982) process coding categories. The two rating groups then met to determine how a given intervention may have influenced a subsequent shift in collaboration.

Although no standard reliability statistics were presented, the authors reported that it was fairly easy for judges to identify and agree about when shifts in collaboration occurred. Such shifts were apparent in all sessions studied. There also was good agreement regarding the therapist's contribution to those shifts. Consistent with the earlier findings (Horwitz & Frieswyk, 1980) and those of Foreman and Marmar (1985), 10 of 11 shifts toward increased collaboration were preceded by relationship-focused interventions (e.g., transference interpretations). However, both of the observed shifts toward decreased collaboration also followed transference interpretations. Further examination of the process material suggested that in the latter instances, the interpretations were laden with countertransference anger, which aroused fears in the patient that could not be assimilated at that point.

This last observation fits with earlier suggestions that borderline patients' difficulties in managing affect may be a limiting factor in the development of an alliance. It also underscores one of the most interesting, but heretofore neglected, aspects of the Allen et al. (1984) study—namely, the inclusion in their measurement scheme of a scale that dealt not simply with the valence or intensity of emotions directed toward the therapist, but with the range of emotions expressed and the patient's ability to modulate and reflect upon them. In most other alliance schemes, the focus has been exclusively on the former. The more positive affect (and the less negative affect) expressed by the patient toward the therapist, the stronger the bond between the two is assumed to be, and hence the better the alliance. This has made for easier assessment. However, it has put research on the alliance somewhat at odds with clinical reality, and with the work that has been done by social and developmental psychologists on interpersonal attraction and attachment. This work suggests that the strongest and most durable alliances will permit and be characterized by the balanced expression of both positive and negative affects.

Achieving such a balance is something that borderline patients have particular difficulty with. Fluctuating ego states and frequent shifts from idealization to devaluation of significant others are hallmarks of BPD. A rating system that takes these affective shifts or imbalances into account is a significant contribution indeed. So too is Gabbard et al.'s (1988) demonstration of the feasibility and utility of bringing empirical methods to bear on the complex clinical problems presented by individual borderline patients. Both this study and its predecessor (Horwitz & Frieswyk, 1980) showed how it is possible to capture some of the instability that clinicians know is so characteristic of the alliances formed by borderline patients, but that researchers have rarely documented.

At the same time, these studies show how limited our understanding of the alliance formation process still is. Needed are studies that establish more direct causal connections between the alliance and a range of specific interventions, applied at various times and in various ways. As Gabbard et al. (1988) pointed out, characterizing therapist interventions solely by type (e.g., transference-related vs. non-transference-related) is inadequate, since many interventions derive their power from the tone, timing, appropriateness, and skill with which they are made. Finally, it is useful to remember that the alliance may affect and be affected by factors outside of, as well as within, the therapy. This is especially likely with borderline patients, who often receive a variety of treatments in addition to individual psychotherapy.

Many borderline patients require hospitalization at one time or another. Colson and Coyne (1978) studied the conceptual frameworks used by hospital staff members and found that the alliance occupied a prominent place in the thinking of all disciplines. But few systematic assessments of the role of the alliance in hospital treatment have been done. Three studies have attempted to address this issue (Allen et al., 1985, 1988; Clarkin et al., 1987). None of these dealt exclusively with borderline patients. Moreover, all employed correlational designs, precluding inferences about the specific effects of the alliance on hospital treatment or vice versa. In addition, the methods and measures used in these studies differed somewhat from each other and from those used in studies of individual psychotherapy. Yet together they attest to the importance and complexities of assessing the alliance in the variety of settings in which borderline patients are seen.

The first study (Allen et al., 1985) was a prospective examination of 37 inpatients, 25 of whom had a personality disorder as their primary diagnosis. To assess the alliance, the investigators used a modified version of the collaboration scale they had developed previously (Allen et al., 1984). On admission and again at discharge (an average of 10.6 months later), ratings on this scale were made independently by members of what were multidisciplinary treatment teams. These subsequently were averaged after it was determined that there was a high degree of concordance in ratings made by different staff members. A similar procedure was used to assess outcome. In addition to rating overall improvement and global psychopathology, staff members rated patients on a number of measures of ego functioning and on potential for violent or self-destructive behavior. These ratings also were made on admission and at discharge.

Several noteworthy findings emerged from this study. One was that even after an extended period of intensive hospital treatment, good alliances remained rare and collaboration was limited. Which patients were more (and less) likely to form a good alliance by discharge was not predictable from their level of alliance on admission. Nor was outcome predictable from admission alliance ratings. Outcome was, however, related to changes in the alliance from admission to discharge (r's above .66, $p < .001$). Improvement in one went hand in hand with improvement in the other, and with longer hospital stays.

In an effort to understand why some patients showed a consistent level of alliance over the course of treatment while others showed a shift in their collaborative involvement, Allen et al. (1985) performed some additional clinical analyses. They found that two groups of patients whose alliances decreased—those with histories of psychosis and those with severe character pathology—had a distinctive clinical course. Both groups initially appeared motivated for treatment and willing to participate in the hospital program, albeit in a somewhat passive and compliant manner. But this "honeymoon" did not last. When the patients were faced with the demands of treatment and deepening treatment relationships, their vulnerability and ambivalence, respectively, increased; their ability and willingness to collaborate decreased; and they often left treatment prematurely.

Although the samples were small, these findings suggest that alliances do not change in linear fashion—a point made previously by Hartley and Strupp (1983). They also show how a particular pattern of change may depend upon the characteristics of the patient involved. The key task, according to Allen et al. (1985), is to identify which patient characteristics and which other factors are associated with which patterns.

This view was echoed by Clarkin et al. (1987) in a study done with 96 hospitalized patients. Of these, 19 had a *Diagnostic and Statistical Manual of Mental Disorders*, third edition (DSM-III) Axis II diagnosis in the "dramatic" cluster (which includes BPD), and 33 had other personality disorder diagnoses. Like Allen et al. (1985), Clarkin et al. used an alliance scale that focused on the patient's active involvement in the hospital treatment program, and they were similarly interested in the alliance–outcome relationship. However, they also were interested in those pretreatment patient characteristics that contributed to that relationship, and their alliance measure consisted of a single rating of the patient's level of collaboration *throughout* hospitalization. All data for the study, including admission and discharge Global Assessment Scale (GAS) scores, were obtained or derived from the patients' medical records.

As Allen et al. (1985) had done, Clarkin et al. (1987) found a significant (though more modest) relationship between alliance level and outcome, as measured by discharge GAS scores ($r = .39$, $p < .001$). They also found that a number of patients achieved a good outcome despite having a poor alliance, and a number had a poor outcome even though their alliance was judged to be quite good. The interaction of Axis I and Axis II pathology accounted for some of this variance in outcome, and significant differences in alliance levels were found for patients with different Axis I diagnoses. But there were no differences in the alliance as a function of the presence or type of Axis II pathology alone. Nor were any other pretreatment patient characteristics related to the alliance.

Although the findings of these studies are of interest, they have their limitations. For example, in both studies, some staff members made both alliance and outcome ratings. This raises the possibility that halo effects contributed to the correlation between the ratings. Questions also can be raised about the meaning of the term "alliance" as used in the context of hospital treatment. Unlike individual psychotherapy, hospital treatment permits and even encourages patients to become involved in a variety of potentially therapeutic activities and relationships. It also affords ample opportunity for patients who are so inclined (e.g., borderline patients) to engage in "splitting." Under these circumstances, it is somewhat misleading to measure an alliance with a hospital treatment program in the same way that one measures an alliance with an individual therapist. A third limitation derives from the fact that both studies looked at the alliance–outcome relationship only from the perspective of the clinicians. Patients may have viewed the alliance, and their progress, quite differently.

To address the limitations of the previous studies, Allen et al. (1988) conducted a study in which they examined the alliance from the perspective of the patients as well as various hospital staff members, using scales better suited to the complexities of inpatient treatment. Their sample consisted of 107 long-term inpatients and 90 hospital staff members representing all professional disciplines. Most (78%) of the patients had a DSM-III diagnosis of either BPD ($n = 41$) or another personality disorder ($n = 42$). In addition to assessments of patient progress, two measures of alliance were used: a 12-item, patient-rated collaboration scale adapted from the clinician-rated scale used previously (Allen et al., 1985), and a single scale on the working relationship, which was rated by both patients and staff. The latter reflected Luborsky's (1976) conceptualization of the alliance as involving a feeling of being helped/helpful and of working together toward treatment goals. The time frame for all ratings was the preceding month.

In contrast to their previous study, Allen et al. found little concordance in this study among staff members from different disciplines in the quality of the working relationships they formed with patients. Patients likewise judged their working relationships with various staff members to be different. The investigators also found evidence that "splitting" did occur, but that it was not uniquely associated with borderline patients. Nor did it extend to staff members. In fact, there was little agreement between patients and staff members in either their views of working relationships or their judgments of patient progress. This underscores the importance of considering the alliance from many vantage points.

Expanding existing conceptions of the alliance also may be necessary. A principal-components factor analysis of the patients' 12 collaboration ratings indicated that collaboration had three dimensions: (1) goal orientation, (2) affective involvement and communication, and (3) adherence to and use of treatment structures. Scores on all three factors, especially the goal orientation factor, were positively and significantly correlated with patients' ratings of their progress and the quality of their working relationships with staff members. However, only goal orientation scores were significantly correlated with staff ratings of patient progress.

This study has a number of implications for both research and clinical practice. First, it suggests that an accurate and complete picture of the alliance and its relation to treatment course and outcome will probably not be obtained from assessments made by either clinicians or patients alone. Second, different treatment interventions may have an impact on different aspects of the alliance, and thus may be more (or less) useful under various circumstances. For example, relationship-oriented interventions may enhance collaboration by virtue of their effect on the affective involvement/communication dimension of the alliance, and they may be especially useful with more withdrawn or depressed patients. Those same interventions may have less effect on the alliance dimension dealing with goal orientation, or on more disorganized patients. That dimension and those patients may be affected more by the clinician's active efforts to set clear and realistic treatment goals. It follows that among severely disturbed, hospitalized patients, the alliance may take different forms. In fact, there may be multiple alliances comprised of multiple dimensions, which may change alone or in concert over the course of treatment. To determine whether this is the case, more longitudinal studies will be needed.

Allen et al. (1988) came to essentially the same conclusions. However, they felt that their results were limited to situations in which patients have contact with multiple treaters. They maintained that "in the context of [in-dividual] psychotherapy, one can justifiably speak of *an* alliance . . . most clearly manifested in the patient's collaboration" (p. 298). Recent work done at McLean Hospital suggests that even this may be an oversimplification.

The McLean Borderline Psychotherapy Engagement Project

The point has often been made that establishing guidelines for the use of psychotherapy with borderline patients has been complicated by the relative absence of controlled outcome studies. Such studies are made difficult by the fact that so many borderline patients drop out of psychotherapy before its effects can be ascertained. Even those who remain often fail to become actively engaged in the therapy process. To understand why this occurs and how therapists can combat the problem, it is necessary to understand the nature of the early engagement process. The McLean Borderline Psychotherapy Engagement Project was designed to address this issue.

Unlike the studies done at the Menninger Foundation, the McLean project focused only on the first 3–6 months of treatment. Subjects were drawn from consecutive hospital admissions over a period of several years. To be included, patients had to meet current clinical (DSM-III or DSM-III-R) and research (Diagnostic Interview for Borderlines, or DIB; Gunderson, Kolb, & Austin, 1981) criteria for BPD. Prior to starting what typically was a three-times-per-week psychotherapy, patients received a comprehensive social and psychiatric evaluation. At 3 and 6 months after baseline, the patients were re-evaluated. If and when the psychotherapy was discontinued, patients and therapists were asked to complete a questionnaire describing their respective reasons for the termination and their reactions to it. A series of studies employed this data base.

One of the first of these studies dealt with the hypothesized relationship between the development of an alliance and continuance in psychotherapy (Gunderson et al., 1989). As expected, there was a high rate of attrition from psychotherapy. Of the first 60 patients studied, 36 (60%) discontinued their therapy within 6 months, and 26 of these (43% of the total) unilaterally dropped out for reasons directly related to the clinical situation. Efforts to identify patient characteristics that were associated with dropping out proved disappointing, prompting a more in-depth examination of the clinical records of the dropouts and the termination questionnaires. These evaluations indicated that a majority of the clinical dropouts (77%) had what might be construed as problems in forming or sustaining an alliance.

One subgroup of 5 patients displayed a consistent lack of motivation for treatment and a superficial involvement in it from the outset. All attempts to engage these patients proved unsuccessful. A second, larger subgroup of 15 patients showed a pattern virtually identical to that seen by Allen et al. (1985). Initially, they appeared motivated for treatment, involved in the process, and positively disposed toward the therapist—until their therapists confronted their denial regarding the extent or severity of their problems. According to both the patients and therapists, this led to open conflict over treatment goals and methods, and the feeling on the part of the patients that the therapist was not understanding; was critical and judgmental; or was cold, distant, and uncaring. All these feelings are negative indicators of an alliance, or what Safran, Crocker, McMain, and Murray (1990) have termed "alliance rupture markers." In anger, the patients left treatment.

These findings are of interest for several reasons. First, they extend to borderline patients previous observations regarding the alliance–continuance relationship. Second, they suggest that within a carefully diagnosed and presumably homogeneous sample of borderline patients, it is possible to identify subgroups of patients on the basis of the alliances they form. Of course, these conclusions must remain tentative, given the study's limitations. To begin with, no quantitative measures of the alliance were included, and the assessments that were made were retrospective. Neither were any formal process measures obtained, precluding definitive judgments about the therapists' role in the alliance formation process. Finally, only the alliances of dropouts were investigated. Obviously, the patients who remained in treatment did not complete a termination questionnaire. It thus could not be determined what alliance formation problems they experienced (if any), and whether or how they resolved those problems.

To address these design weaknesses, the sample was expanded (to an *n* of 75); the follow-up period was extended (to 1 year); and a more systematic examination of the alliance formation process was undertaken. This was done using data that were being collected prospectively on all cases, not just dropouts. Included were measures of the alliance obtained from both patients and therapists after 1, 3, and 6 months of treatment, using one or more established, self-report alliance questionnaires (i.e., the TARS, WAI, and HAq). Additional alliance measures were obtained from therapists and independent judges, using a new instrument designed specifically for this project (i.e., the Therapeutic Alliance Interview Schedule, or TAIS; Frank, 1985).

Although similar in content to other instruments, the TAIS differs from them in scope and method of administration. It is a semistructured interview in which a trained clinician queries a patient about his/her relationship and work with a therapist during the previous month. A parallel version of the instrument was designed for completion by the therapist. The questions are quite specific, but the scope of the TAIS is intentionally broad, covering four alliance dimensions. The first, termed the "behavioral" dimension, deals with the degree to which the patient is meeting basic treatment obligations and adhering to the parameters of the treatment. This dimension was included because of its particular relevance to borderline patients who are inclined to express themselves via acting out, often in regard to the treatment framework. The frequency with which they do so, and the ways in which they respond to limits set on this behavior, are sometimes the primary (even the only) clues to the state of their alliance. The second dimension, termed the "contractual" dimension, was derived from Bordin's (1979) conceptualization of the alliance. It refers to the degree to which the patient has reached a consensus or formed a contract with the therapist regarding treatment goals, methods, roles, and responsibilities. The third, called the "affective" dimension, reflects Luborsky's (1976) and Allen et al.'s (1984) thinking about the alliance. It refers to the degree to which the patient has formed a bond of trust and attachment with the therapist and feels secure enough in the relationship to express a full range of feelings, both positive and negative. For this reason, it is further subdivided into separate positive and negative dimensions. The last dimension, termed the "cognitive–motivational" dimension, is most like the one used by investigators at the Menninger Foundation. It refers to the degree to which the patient is actively collaborating with the therapist in an effort to solve problems. Each dimension can be considered in its own right or in relation to the others; this makes it possible to study alliance profiles and derive information about the form as well as the strength of the alliance.

As part of the instrument development process, the TAIS was administered to a subsample of the borderline patients who were participating in the main project. The interviews were tape-recorded and scored independently by a second, trained rater. Analyses of these ratings (Frank & Brody, 1987) showed that the TAIS as a whole, as well as its component scales, had good interrater reliability (r's ranged from .71 to .93) and internal consistency (Cronbach's alphas ranged from .50 to .72). Except for the contractual and cognitive–motivational scales, which were correlated .75, the scales were also relatively independent of each other (all r's below .66). Evidence of the instrument's discriminant/convergent validity was obtained from analyses showing that TAIS ratings were not correlated with type or severity of patient symptomatology at baseline (as measured by the Symptom Checklist—90 [SCL-90] and GAS), but were correlated with similar measures of the alliance taken from the TARS, WAI, and HAq, and with TAIS ratings made by therapists (all r's above .58).

On the basis of these initial findings, the TAIS was administered to the entire sample. This was done (1) to substantiate earlier impressions regarding the developmental course of the alliance with borderline patients and its stability over the first 6 months of treatment, and (2) to examine more systematically the relationship of the alliance to premature termination of psychotherapy and short-term outcome in this patient population.

As expected, the development of an alliance in all its facets proved to be a difficult task, requiring considerable time. After 1 month of treatment, only 60% of the patients were consistently meeting even their minimum treatment obligations—to attend therapy regularly, stay for the entire session, and talk. Only one-third had reached a consensus with their therapists regarding treatment methods and goals. Even fewer (25%) were actively and regularly collaborating with their therapists in pursuit of those goals. Strong expressions of both positive and negative feelings for the therapists were likewise rare, with fewer than 20% of the patients showing a full range of emotions in therapy.

Even after 6 months of treatment, good alliances were the exception rather than the rule. Nearly half of the patients still were violating the treatment framework. Two-thirds still were having difficulty forming a viable and mutually acceptable therapeutic contract. However, the affective bond between patients and therapists was considerably stronger (McNemar's $\chi^2 = 4.90$, $df = 1$, $p < .05$), and more direct expressions of both positive and negative feelings for the therapist were evident. More patients (one-third) also were making a sustained, active effort to collaborate in the work of therapy, but the gains in this area were not statistically significant. These findings, all based on TAIS scores, were mirrored in both patient and therapist TARS, WAI, and HAq ratings.

It should be noted that the relative consistency in alliance ratings observed for the sample as a whole belied the considerable variability in ratings of individual cases over the first 6 months of treatment. The weak correlation between the 1- and 6-month TAIS ratings (r's ranging from $-.02$ to .42) confirmed this and indicated that initial alliance levels were not particularly good harbingers of later levels. However, they were predictive of continuance in psychotherapy. This is important because of the observation that borderline patients are not likely to receive the putative optimal benefits of psychotherapy until they have been in it for an extended period of time (Waldinger & Gunderson, 1987). In this study, the higher the patients' scores on the TAIS at 1 month, especially on the cognitive–motivational scale and the two affective scales, the more likely they were to remain in therapy for a year or more. This finding held even when statistical adjustments were made for time spent in the hospital ($R = .65$, $p < .001$), a factor shown previously to affect continuance (Gunderson et al., 1989).

Interestingly, 1-month TAIS ratings, especially those made by independent judges, were better predictors of premature termination than were any of the other alliance measures used. However, they were not better predictors of short-term outcome. For that matter, none of the alliance measures had a strong or consistent relationship to outcome, as measured by change over the first 6 months in symptoms, ego functions, suicidal behavior, major role performance, and interpersonal relations. Most correlations ranged only from .35 to .45 ($p < .05$), and rarely did alliance ratings account for more than 25% of the variance in outcome ratings. This may have been due to measurement error, progressive sample attrition over time, and the fact that different patients were administered different combinations of alliance instruments. Another possibility is that in the early phase of treatment with borderline patients, factors other than the alliance (e.g., therapist interventions) are more important determinants of change.

Although no formal process measures were included in this project, indirect support for the role of therapist actions was obtained from the 30 patients and therapists who were administered the TARS. Unlike the other alliance instruments used in the study, the TARS contains items that deal specifically with the therapist's contribution to the alliance, both positive and negative. Analyses of those items revealed an interesting and unexpected *positive* correlation between therapists' ratings of their own negative contribution to the alliance in the first month of treatment and patients' ratings of symptomatic improvement over the first 6 months, including reductions in paranoid ideation, psychotic thinking, and identity diffusion (r's ranged from .44 to .67, $p < .01$).

Marziali (1984) found a similar relationship between negative therapist contributions to the alliance and symptomatic improvement in a study of 42 "neurotic" outpatients who were receiving brief psychotherapy. But she dismissed this finding as spurious. It may have been spurious in this study as well, since a relatively large number of analyses were done, and the sample used for those analyses was relatively small and possibly not representative. However, it makes sense, considering which TARS items accounted for the observed relationship in this study: the therapist's being overly active and directive; exclusively pursuing his/her own agenda in the sessions; being critical of the patient; displaying intolerance of the patient's need to perpetuate problems; and conveying disappointment, annoyance, or frustration because the patient was not making sufficient progress. For some patients, these actions may indeed impede the formation of a good alliance and have a negative impact on outcome. For hospitalized borderline patients, these same interventions may be just what is needed to limit regressions, anchor the patients in reality, make maladaptive behaviors ungratifying, and otherwise enable a solid alliance to evolve and structural change to occur.

If these findings are borne out in subsequent studies, they would have implications for the treatment of borderline patients and for future research on their alliances. In particular, they suggest that existing alliance scales may not be as well suited for, or have the same meaning when used with, hospitalized borderline patients as for and with other patients. Further support for this was obtained from a principal-components factor analysis of the TARS ratings made by patients and therapists in this study. That analysis yielded somewhat different alliance dimensions from those that have been found in previous studies using relatively healthy outpatients (Marziali et al., 1981; Marmar et al., 1986; Marmar, Gaston, et al., 1989; Marmar, Weiss, & Gaston, 1989). The small n's and the lack of independent corroboration of therapists' reports of their actions preclude any definitive conclusions about either the factor structure of the TARS when applied to borderline patients or the therapists' contribution to their alliances. Yet the findings are intriguing.

Also noteworthy was this study's lack of success in demonstrating the unique contribution of the alliance to outcome. This suggests that conventional methods of data analysis may be inadequate for capturing the complexity and variability in the process of alliance formation and change. For this reason, the data were reanalyzed, using an approach adopted by Suh et al. (1986). Instead of seeking an overall statistical relationship between measures of the alliance and treatment outcome for the entire sample, an effort was made to identify clinically meaningful subgroups of patients on the basis of their *profiles* of 1-month TAIS scores. The groups then were compared on a variety of other measures. Although the classification initially was done by inspection, it was largely confirmed by a cluster analysis. The result was seven subgroups, ranging in size from 7 to 14 patients. Each was characterized by what was considered to be a different type of alliance, and each had what proved to be distinctive clinical presentation and early course.

One group of patients ($n = 9$) was judged to have an "ideal" alliance, in the sense that they scored high on all of the TAIS scales. They were not the healthiest patients in the sample, but they did have the best early course. Their hospital stays were the shortest, and they had the lowest incidence of premature termination from psychotherapy. Most (88%) remained in treatment for a year or more, sustained their "ideal" alliances, and showed significant symptomatic improvement.

At the other extreme was a group ($n = 11$) deemed "distant–uninvolved" by virtue of their low scores on all of the TAIS scales. That this group kept themselves at arm's length was not surprising, since they were the most symptomatic patients in the sample, scoring higher than all others on the SCL-90 scales measuring interpersonal sensitivity, paranoid ideation, and psychotic thinking. They also had the clearest history of resistance to treatment in the past. Their response to the current treatment episode was equally poor. The majority (82%) dropped out of therapy within the first 6 months, showing minimal evidence of improvement in any area prior to leaving.

Although differing in their clinical presentation, both groups had alliances that were fixed in the first month of treatment and were relatively resistant to change thereafter. This is consistent with findings from studies of healthier outpatients (Gomes-Schwartz, 1978; Marziali et al., 1981; Morgan et al., 1982; Luborsky et al., 1983; Eaton et al., 1988; Tichenor & Hill, 1989). It suggests that some patients come to treatment with a predisposition to form, or not to form, an alliance. Their experiences in treatment do little to alter this predisposition or the patients' early course, which proceeds in a fairly predictable fashion consistent with their overall level of alliance. However, this is not true for all patients, as shown by this study and others (see Hartley & Strupp, 1983; Horowitz et al., 1984; Marziali, 1984; Allen et al., 1985; Foreman & Marmar, 1985; Marmar et al., 1986; Marmar, Weiss, & Gaston, 1989; Frank & Gunderson, 1990; Klee, Abeles, & Muller, 1990).

A good example was provided by those patients ($n = 7$) who formed what was termed a "negative–oppositional" alliance. At the start of treatment they scored high on the negative affective scale of the TAIS, but low on all others. Yet they were hardly uninvolved in the treatment. Quite the contrary: They were highly engaged with their therapists, but by means of a struggle over everything from the treatment framework (which they violated persistently) to the treatment goals and methods (which they overtly disagreed with) to the therapist's collaborative overtures (which they actively resisted).

This group typifies the borderline patients often seen in inpatient settings. They were chronically self-destructive and tended to act out impulsively, usually by cutting themselves. They also were quite depressed, but otherwise asymptomatic. Surprisingly, the majority of them (57%) stayed in therapy 9 months or more, and eventually made good use of treatment. Over time, they became less devaluing of their therapists and more allied in all other respects. Their self-destructive behavior decreased accordingly, though they remained fairly depressed. From their case records, it appeared that this group had the most unflappable therapists, who communicated in words and actions that they could survive the patients' rage. This and the fact that they had ongoing institutional support for therapy (i.e., a lengthy index hospitalization) seemed to be important factors in their better-than-expected early course.

These findings suggest that the predominance of negative affects within treatment sessions does not invariably signify a poor alliance, so long as these affects are directly expressed and dealt with early on. Further support for the idea that it is easier to engage an overtly angry borderline patient than a covertly or passively resistant one was obtained from a comparison between the "negative–oppositional" patients and those who were equally negativistic, but not explicitly oppositional. The latter group ($n = 11$) had many narcissistic features and a fairly high level of denial regarding their problems and their need for treatment. The alliances they formed in the first month could best be termed "negative–compliant." Like the previous group, they expressed many negative feelings for their therapists, but they generally adhered to the treatment framework. Disagreements over treatment goals and methods occurred, but they were muted. Moreover, some degree of collaboration was evident, though it was limited.

This group did not have nearly as good an early course. They never developed a positive affective bond with their therapists or much in the way of a collaborative working relationship; over time, they showed progressively less adherence to the treatment framework. Their case records indicated that at some point during the first 6 months, their therapists confronted them about this behavior and about their defensive use of denial or grandiosity. Apparently this proved too much for these narcissistically vulnerable patients. Most (82%) simply fled treatment, without having made many gains in any area. What was interesting about this group was their similarity to a group of borderline patients hypothesized by Horwitz and Frieswyk (1980) to need a more supportive, noninterpretive approach throughout treatment. By all indications, this was something they did not receive.

A group of patients who did receive a less interpretive and less confrontational approach were those who formed a type of alliance termed "positive–compliant" ($n = 8$). Initially they too adhered to the treatment framework, but they did not collaborate much with their therapists in either the development or implementation of a treatment plan. Mostly they did what they were told, largely out of enormous positive regard for the therapists. They were a very interpersonally connected, even dependent group of patients, who sought and received a lot of support from their therapists. Yet their behavior was deceptive. It seduced therapists into believing that all was well when in fact it was not. This became evident in the first few months. As their treatment unfolded, the patients regressed and revealed considerable underlying disorganization. By the 6-month follow-up, all but one (88%) had either been in seclusion for a prolonged period, been transferred to a state hospital, or left treatment against medical advice.

These findings again point to the important contribution that therapists can make to the alliance formation process. They also show how a failure to attend to all aspects of the alliance can cause problems in the treatment of borderline patients. In this case, it was the presence of a strong, positively toned affective bond that was misleading. A high-level collaboration can be equally misleading.

Evidence of this was obtained from another group of patients ($n = 14$) who displayed what many dynamically oriented therapists would consider to be a very good alliance. From the outset, they adhered to the treatment framework, negotiated a solid therapeutic contract, and were highly collaborative. But they scored relatively low on both affective scales of the TAIS, indicating a weak emotional connection to their therapists. Hence their alliances were termed "controlled–collaborative." At baseline, these were the most depressed patients in the sample. On the surface they were socially appropriate and cooperative, though rather withdrawn. They denied all anger and consistently tried to remain unemotional. But there was an ominous, controlled quality to their interactions. A review of their histories confirmed their explosive potential. Three of the patients had been assaultive, and seven had made carefully planned and potentially lethal suicide attempts.

Their treatment course was a study in contrasts as well. Over time, all of the patients became much more affectively connected to their therapists, but somewhat less collaborative. They remained quite depressed, and although they showed evidence of greater impulse control, they showed a continued preoccupation with self-destructive thoughts. Within 6 months, half of the group dropped out of treatment. Again, the therapists' approach seemed to be a determining factor: Those patients who dropped out were treated more supportively, whereas those who stayed were treated more interpretively, but with little early interpretation of negative transference material.

Of course, it would be a mistake to attach too much significance to these differences, given that the treatments were not administered in a controlled manner. Moreover, conclusions regarding therapist actions were based largely on clinical impressions and case records, which varied in quality and completeness. It likewise would be unwarranted to infer any causal connections among the use of specific therapeutic interventions, the development of an alliance, and early treatment course or outcome. As the more traditional, statistical analyses of these data showed, it was difficult to separate changes in the alliance from changes in patient functioning. It was equally difficult to know whether a given therapist intervention was a determinant of or a response to these changes. And although the total sample was large, the subgroups were relatively small, and comprised only of inpatients who were studied for a fraction of what was intended to be long-term psychotherapy. Whether the same subgroups would emerge in outpatient settings, in other forms of psychotherapy, or in the later stages of treatment is unknown.

Also unknown is the role that ancillary treatments may have played in this study. Most (80%) of the patients received medications at some point during their hospitalization. A retrospective survey of therapists—many of whom participated in this study—indicated that the use of medications strengthens the alliances of borderline patients (Waldinger & Frank, 1989b). Yet the precise role of medications, as well as of milieu treatment, in the alliance formation process remains unclear.

SUMMARY AND CONCLUSIONS

As this discussion suggests, much has been learned about the alliances of borderline patients, but much still is not known. The existing empirical studies indicate that in both form and course of development, the alliances of borderlines are highly variable. Those patients who do form good alliances do so gradually, over a prolonged period of time, and with the assistance of therapists who are attuned to potential derailments of the process. How therapists deal with these alliance ruptures can markedly influence the patients' subsequent clinical course. Yet the complex ways in which specific therapist interventions and patient characteristics interact to affect both the alliance and outcome are far from understood. Also not well understood is the alliance–outcome relationship in this patient population. Clarification of this relationship awaits the conduct of more prospective and controlled longitudinal studies, as well as the further development of measurement methodologies that capture the complexity and dynamic quality of the alliance and the change process. This review has shown how such methodologies can serve as a valuable adjunct to more established data-analytic techniques. Together, these approaches hold out the promise of better aligning theory and research on the alliances of borderline patients with clinical practice—something that is, after all, the goal of both researchers and clinicians.

ACKNOWLEDGMENT

This work was supported in part by the McLean Hospital Psychosocial Research Fund and by Psychiatric Institutes of America.

REFERENCES

Adelman, S. A. (1885). Pills as transitional objects: A dynamic understanding of the use of medication in psychotherapy. *Psychiatry, 48*, 246–253.
Adler, G. (1979). The myth of the alliance with borderline patients. *American Journal of Psychiatry, 136*, 642–645.
Alexander, L. B., & Luborsky, L. (1986). The Penn Helping Alliance Scales. In L. S. Greenberg & W. M. Pinsof (Eds.), *The psychotherapeutic process: A research handbook*. New York: Guilford Press.

Allen, J. G., Deering, C. D., Buskirk, J. R., & Coyne, L. (1988). Assessment of therapeutic alliances in the psychiatric hospital milieu. *Psychiatry, 51*, 291–299.

Allen, J. G., Newsom, G. E., Gabbard, G. O., & Coyne, L. (1984). Scales to assess the therapeutic alliance from a psychoanalytic perspective. *Bulletin of the Menninger Clinic, 48*, 383–400.

Allen, J. G., Tarnoff, G., & Coyne, L. (1985). Therapeutic alliance and long-term hospital treatment outcome. *Comprehensive Psychiatry, 38*, 871–875.

Barrett-Lennard, G. T. (1962). Dimensions of therapist response as causal factors in therapeutic change. *Psychological Monographs, 76*(43, Whole No. 562).

Benjamin, L. S. (1982). Use of Structural Analysis of Social Behavior (SASB) to guide interventions in therapy. In J. Anchin & D. Kiesler (Eds.), *Handbook of interpersonal psychotherapy*. New York: Pergamon Press.

Benjamin, L. S. (1987). Use of the SASB dimensional model to develop treatment plans for personality disorders: I. Narcissism. *Journal of Personality Disorders, 1*, 43–70.

Binder, J. L., Henry, W. P., & Strupp, H. H. (1987). An appraisal of selection criteria for dynamic psychotherapies and implications for setting time limits. *Psychiatry, 50*, 154–166.

Book, H. E. (1987). Some psychodynamics of noncompliance. *Canadian Journal of Psychiatry, 32*, 115–117.

Bordin, E. S. (1979). The generalizability of the psychoanalytic concept of the working alliance. *Psychotherapy, 16*, 252–260.

Bowers, M. B., Jr., & Greenfeld, D. G. (1980). Medication and psychotherapy in outpatients vulnerable to psychosis. In J. S. Strauss, M. Bowers, T. W. Downey, S. Fleck, S. Jackson, & I. Levine (Eds.), *The psychotherapy of schizophrenia*. New York: Plenum.

Budman, S. H., Soldz, S., Demby, A., Feldstein, M., Springer, T., & Davis, M. S. (1989). Cohesion, alliance, and outcome in group psychotherapy. *Psychiatry, 52*, 339–350.

Butler, S. F., & Strupp, H. H. (1986). Specific and nonspecific factors in psychotherapy: A problematic paradigm for psychotherapy research. *Psychotherapy, 23*, 30–40.

Clarkin, J. F., Hurt, S. W., & Crilly, J. L. (1987). Therapeutic alliance and hospital treatment outcome. *Hospital and Community Psychiatry, 38*, 871–875.

Colson, D. B., & Coyne, L. (1978). Variation in staff thinking on a psychiatric unit: Implications for team functioning. *Bulletin of the Menninger Clinic, 42*, 414–422.

Docherty, J. P. (1985). The therapeutic alliance and treatment outcome. In R. E. Hales & A. J. Frances (Eds.), *Psychiatry update* (Vol. 4). Washington, DC: American Psychiatric Press.

Docherty, J. P., & Fiester, S. J. (1985). The therapeutic alliance and compliance with psychopharmacology. In R. E. Hales & A. J. Frances (Eds.), *Psychiatry update* (Vol. 4). Washington, DC: American Psychiatric Press.

Eaton, T. T., Abeles, N., & Gutfreund, M. J. (1988). Therapeutic alliance and outcome: Impact of treatment length and pretreatment symptomatology. *Psychotherapy, 25*, 536–542.

Eisenthal, S., Emery, R., Lazare, A., & Udin, H. (1979). "Adherence" and the negotiated approach to patienthood. *Archives of General Psychiatry, 36*, 393–398.

Feister, A. R., & Rudestam, K. E. (1975). A multivariate analysis of the early dropout process. *Journal of Consulting and Clinical Psychology, 43,* 528–535.

Flick, S. N. (1988). Managing attrition in clinical research. *Clinical Psychology Review, 8,* 499–515.

Foreman, S. A., & Marmar, C. R. (1985). Therapist actions that address initially poor therapeutic alliances in psychotherapy. *American Journal of Psychiatry, 142,* 922–926.

Frank, A. F. (1985, December). *The therapeutic alliance: Advances in conceptualization and measurement.* Paper presented at the annual meeting of the American Psychoanalytic Association, New York.

Frank, A. F., & Brody, S. (1987). *The Therapeutic Alliance Interview Schedule: A preliminary study of the alliance with borderline patients.* Unpublished manuscript.

Frank, A. F., & Gunderson, J. G. (1990). The role of the therapeutic alliance in the treatment of schizophrenia: Relationship to course and outcome. *Archives of General Psychiatry, 47,* 228–236.

Frieswyk, S. H., Allen, J. G., Colson, D. B., Coyne, L., Gabbard, G. O., Horwitz, L., & Newsom, G. (1986). Therapeutic alliance: Its place as a process and outcome variable in dynamic psychotherapy research. *Journal of Consulting and Clinical Psychology, 54,* 32–38.

Frieswyk, S. H., Colson, D. B., & Allen, J. G. (1984). Conceptualizing the therapeutic alliance from a psychoanalytic perspective. *Psychotherapy, 21,* 460–464.

Gabbard, G. O., Horwitz, L., Frieswyk, S., Allen, J. G., Colson, D. B., Newsom, G., & Coyne, L. (1988). The effect of therapist interventions on the therapeutic alliance with borderline patients. *Journal of the American Psychoanalytic Association, 36,* 697–727.

Gaston, L. (1990). The concept of the alliance and its role in psychotherapy: Theoretical and empirical considerations. *Psychotherapy, 27,* 143–153.

Gaston, L., Marmar, C. R., Thompson, L. W., & Gallagher, D. (1988). Relation of patient pretreatment characteristics to the therapeutic alliance in diverse psychotherapies. *Journal of Consulting and Clinical Psychology, 56,* 483–489.

Gerstley, L., McLellan, A. T., Alterman, A. I., Woody, G. E., Luborsky, L., & Prout, M. (1989). Ability to form an alliance with the therapist: A possible marker of prognosis for patients with antisocial personality disorder. *American Journal of Psychiatry, 146,* 508–512.

Gill, M. M., & Hoffman, I. Z. (1982). A method for studying the analysis of aspects of the patient's experience of the relationship in psychoanalysis and psychotherapy. *Journal of the American Psychoanalytic Association, 30,* 137–167.

Gomes-Schwartz, B. (1978). Effective ingredients in psychotherapy: Prediction of outcome from process variables. *Journal of Consulting and Clinical Psychology, 46,* 1023–1035.

Greene, L. R., Rosenkrantz, J., & Muth, D. Y. (1986). Borderline defenses and countertransference: Research findings and implications. *Psychiatry, 49,* 253–264.

Greenson, R. R. (1965). The working alliance and the transference neurosis. *Psychoanalytic Quarterly, 34,* 155–181.

Gunderson, J. G., Frank, A. F., Ronningstam, E. F., Wachter, S., Lynch, V. J., & Wolf, P. J. (1989). Early discontinuance of borderline patients from psychotherapy. *Journal of Nervous and Mental Disease, 177,* 38–42.

Gunderson, J. G., Kolb, J. E., & Austin, V. (1981). The Diagnostic Interview for Borderline Patients. *American Journal of Psychiatry, 138,* 896–903.

Gutheil, T. G. (1978). Drug therapy: Alliance and compliance. *Psychosomatics, 19,* 219–225.

Gutheil, T. G. (1982). The psychology of psychopharmacology. *Bulletin of the Menninger Clinic, 46,* 321–330.

Gutheil, T. G., & Havens, L. L. (1979). The therapeutic alliance: Contemporary meanings and confusions. *International Review of Psychoanalysis, 6,* 467–481.

Hartley, D., & Strupp, H. (1983). Therapeutic alliance: A contribution to outcome in brief psychotherapy. In J. Masling (Ed.), *Empirical studies of psychoanalytic theory.* Hillsdale, NJ: Erlbaum.

Horowitz, M., & Marmar, C. (1985). The therapeutic alliance with difficult patients. In R. E. Hales & A. J. Frances (Eds.), *Psychiatry update* (Vol. 4). Washington, DC: American Psychiatric Press.

Horowitz, M. J., Marmar, C. R., Weiss, D. S., DeWitt, K. N., & Rosenbaum, R. (1984). Brief dynamic psychotherapy of bereavement reactions: The relationship of process to outcome. *Archives of General Psychiatry, 41,* 438–448.

Horvath, A. O., & Greenberg, L. S. (1986). The development of the Working Alliance Inventory. In L. S. Greenberg & W. Pinsof (Eds.), *The psychotherapeutic process: A research handbook.* New York: Guilford Press.

Horvath, A. O., & Greenberg, L. S. (1989). The development and validation of the Working Alliance Inventory. *Journal of Counseling Psychology, 36,* 223–233.

Horvath, A. O., & Symonds, B. D. (1990). *The relationship between working alliance and outcome in psychotherapy: A synthesis.* Unpublished manuscript.

Horwitz, L. (1974). *Clinical prediction in psychotherapy.* New York: Jason Aronson.

Horwitz, L., & Frieswyk, S. H. (1980, December). *The impact of interpretation on therapeutic alliance in borderline patients.* Paper presented at the annual meeting of the American Psychoanalytic Association, New York.

Howard, K. I., Krause, M. S., & Orlinsky, D. E. (1986). The attrition dilemma: Toward a new strategy for psychotherapy research. *Journal of Consulting and Clinical Psychology, 54,* 106–110.

Howard, K. I., Rickels, K., Mock, J. E., Lipman, R. S., Covi, L., & Baum, N. C. (1970). Therapeutic style and attrition rate for psychiatric drug treatment. *Journal of Nervous and Mental Disease, 150,* 102–110.

Kernberg, O. F., Burstein, E. D., Coyne, L., Appelbaum, A., Horwitz, L., & Voth, H. (1972). Psychotherapy and psychoanalysis: Final report of the Menninger Foundation's Psychotherapy Research Project. *Bulletin of the Menninger Clinic, 36,* 1–275.

Klee, M. R., Abeles, N., & Muller, R. T. (1990). Therapeutic alliance: Early indicators, course, and outcome. *Psychotherapy, 27,* 166–174.

Kolb, D. E., Beutler, L. E., Davis, C. S., Crago, M., & Shanfield, S. B. (1985). Patient and therapy process variables relating to dropout and change in psychotherapy. *Psychotherapy, 22,* 702–710.

Luborsky, L. (1976). Helping alliances in psychotherapy. In J. L. Claghorn (Ed.), *Successful psychotherapy.* New York: Brunner/Mazel.

Luborsky, L., Crits-Christoph, P., Alexander, L., Margolis, M., & Cohen, M. (1983). Two helping alliance methods for predicting outcomes of psychotherapy: A counting signs vs. a global rating method. *Journal of Nervous and Mental Disease*, *171*, 480–492.

Luborsky, L., Crits-Christoph, P., Mintz, J., & Auerbach, A. (1988). *Who will benefit from psychotherapy: Predicting therapeutic outcomes*. New York: Basic Books.

Marmar, C. R., Gaston, L., Gallagher, D., & Thompson, L. W. (1989). Alliance and outcome in late-life depression. *Journal of Nervous and Mental Disease*, *177*, 464–472.

Marmar, C. R., Horowitz, M. J., Weiss, D. S., & Marziali, E. (1986). Development of the Therapeutic Alliance Rating System. In L. S. Greenberg & W. Pinsof (Eds.), *The psychotherapeutic process: A research handbook*. New York: Guilford Press.

Marmar, C. R., Weiss, D. S., & Gaston, L. (1989). Toward the validation of the California Therapeutic Alliance Rating System. *Psychological Assessment*, *1*, 46–52.

Marziali, E. (1984). Three viewpoints on the therapeutic alliance: Similarities, differences, and associations with psychotherapy outcome. *Journal of Nervous and Mental Disease*, *172*, 417–423.

Marziali, E., Marmar, C., & Krupnick, J. (1981). Therapeutic alliance scales: Development and relationship to psychotherapy outcome. *American Journal of Psychiatry*, *138*, 361–364.

Masterson, J. F. (1978). The borderline adult: Therapeutic alliance and transference. *American Journal of Psychiatry*, *135*, 437–441.

Moras, K., & Strupp, H. H. (1982). Pretherapy interpersonal relations, patients' alliance, and outcome of brief therapy. *Archives of General Psychiatry*, *39*, 405–409.

Morgan, R., Luborsky, L., Crits-Christoph, P., Curtis, H., & Solomon, J. (1982). Predicting the outcomes of psychotherapy by the Penn Helping Alliance Rating Method. *Archives of General Psychiatry*, *39*, 397–402.

O'Malley, S. S., Suh, C. S., & Strupp, H. H. (1983). The Vanderbilt Psychotherapy Process Scale: A report on the scale development and a process–outcome study. *Journal of Consulting and Clinical Psychology*, *51*, 581–586.

Orlinsky, D. E., & Howard, K. I. (1975). *Varieties of psychotherapeutic experience*. New York: Teachers College Press.

Rice, L. M., & Greenberg, L. S. (Eds.). (1984). *Patterns of change: Intensive analysis of psychotherapy process*. New York: Guilford Press.

Rosenbaum, R. L., & Horowitz, M. J. (1983). Motivation for psychotherapy: A factorial and conceptual analysis. *Psychotherapy*, *20*, 346–354.

Rush, A. J. (1985). The therapeutic alliance in short-term directive therapies. In R. E. Hales & A. J. Frances (Eds.), *Psychiatry update* (Vol. 4). Washington, DC: American Psychiatric Press.

Ryan, E. R., & Cicchetti, D. V. (1985). Predicting quality of alliance in the initial psychotherapy interview. *Journal of Nervous and Mental Disease*, *173*, 717–725.

Sachs, J. S. (1983). Negative factors in brief psychotherapy: An empirical assessment. *Journal of Consulting and Clinical Psychology*, *51*, 557–564.

Safran, J. D., Crocker, P., McMain, S., & Murray, P. (1990). Therapeutic alliance rupture as a therapy event for empirical investigation. *Psychotherapy*, *27*, 154–165.

Saltzman, C., Leutgert, M., Roth, C., Creaser, J., & Howard, L. (1976). Formation of a therapeutic relationship: Experiences during the initial phase of psychotherapy as predictors of treatment duration and outcome. *Journal of Consulting and Clinical Psychology, 44,* 546–555.

Saunders, S. M., Howard, K. I., & Orlinsky, D. E. (1989). The Therapeutic Bond Scales: Psychometric characteristics and relationship to treatment effectiveness. *Psychological Assessment, 1,* 323–330.

Skodol, A. E., Buckley, P., & Charles, E. (1983). Is there a characteristic pattern to the treatment history of clinical outpatients with borderline personality? *Journal of Nervous and Mental Disease, 171,* 405–410.

Smith, J. (1989). Some dimensions of transference in combined treatment. In J. M. Ellison (Ed.), *The psychotherapist's guide to pharmacotherapy.* Chicago: Year Book Medical.

Stanton, A. H., Gunderson, J. G., Knapp, P. H., Frank, A. F., Vannicelli, M., Schnitzer, R., & Rosenthal, R. (1984). Effects of psychotherapy in schizophrenia: I. Design and implementation of a controlled study. *Schizophrenia Bulletin, 10,* 520–563.

Suh, C. S., Strupp, H. H., & O'Malley, S. S. (1986). The Vanderbilt process measures: The Psychotherapy Process Scales (VPPS) and the Negative Indicators Scale (VNIS). In L. S. Greenberg & W. Pinsof (Eds.), *The psychotherapeutic process: A research handbook.* New York: Guilford Press.

Tichenor, V., & Hill, C. E. (1989). A comparison of six measures of working alliance. *Psychotherapy, 26,* 195–199.

Tracey, T. J. (1986). Interactional correlates of premature termination. *Journal of Consulting and Clinical Psychology, 54,* 784–788.

Tracey, T. J., & Kokotovic, A. M. (1989). Factor structure of the Working Alliance Inventory. *Psychological Assessment, 1,* 207–210.

Tracy, J. (1977). Impact of intake procedures upon client attrition in a community mental health center. *Journal of Consulting and Clinical Psychology, 5,* 192–195.

Waldinger, R. J., & Frank, A. F. (1989a). Transference and the vicissitudes of medication use by borderline patients. *Psychiatry, 52,* 416–427.

Waldinger, R. J., & Frank, A. F. (1989b). Clinicians' experiences in combining medication and psychotherapy in the treatment of borderline patients. *Hospital and Community Psychiatry, 40,* 712–718.

Waldinger, R. J., & Gunderson, J. G. (1984). Completed psychotherapies with borderline patients. *American Journal of Psychotherapy, 38,* 190–202.

Waldinger, R. J., & Gunderson, J. G. (1987). *Effective psychotherapy with borderline patients.* New York: Macmillan.

Wallerstein, R. S. (1986). *Forty-two lives in treatment: A study of psychoanalysis and psychotherapy.* New York: Guilford Press.

Wallerstein, R. S. (1989). The Psychotherapy Research Project of the Menninger Foundation: An overview. *Journal of Consulting and Clinical Psychology, 57,* 195–205.

Zetzel, E. R. (1956). Current concepts of transference. *International Journal of Psychoanalysis, 37,* 369–376.

Zetzel, E. R. (1971). A developmental approach to the borderline patient. *American Journal of Psychiatry, 127,* 867–871.

CHAPTER 11

Dialectical Behavior Therapy for Borderline Personality Disorder

MARSHA M. LINEHAN
HEIDI L. HEARD

Until very recently, behavioral and cognitive–behavioral therapists have generally neglected borderline personality disorder (BPD) in both theoretical writings and research investigations. This neglect is fast disappearing. For example, the cognitive approaches of Pretzer (1989) and of Young (1983) attempt to overcome the particular problems of traditional cognitive therapy with the borderline population, while preserving a focus on dysfunctional schemas and cognitions. Pretzer emphasizes difficulties such as establishing and retaining a collaborative relationship between the therapist and patient, maintaining a directed treatment, and achieving compliance with and completion of homework assignments. To solve these issues, Pretzer confronts them directly in the therapy session, using typical cognitive therapy methods to treat therapy-interfering behaviors. The therapist and patient examine the assumptions and cognitive distortions contributing to the therapy interference, and thus incorporate the interference into the therapy process itself. Young targets persistent dysfunctional cognitive schemas, which he hypothesizes were developed during early childhood. To identify and change these early maladaptive schemas, Young adds to the usual cognitive therapy techniques such diverse techniques as exploring current events, understanding dreams, homework assignments, and group therapy. Young also encourages the prescription of psychotropic medication, the modification of coping behaviors, and the use of the therapist in the therapeutic relationship to "re-parent" the patient.

Turner (1989) has developed a structured, cognitive–behavioral therapy for the borderline population. The treatment targets interpersonal and anxiety management skill deficits. Four cognitive–behavioral procedures characterize the therapy: (1) cognitive therapy stressing problem-solving skills, (2) self-control desensitization to stress-producing situations, (3) supportive psychotherapy, and (4) "states-of-mind" modification. The treatment consists of concurrent individual and psychoeducational group therapy. Turner has reported case study data on four patients, with very promising outcomes. Unfortunately, Pretzer and Young have published little about their treatment approaches, and no outcome data yet exist.

For the past several years, Linehan has been developing a comprehensive, behaviorally oriented outpatient psychotherapy called "dialectical behavior therapy" (DBT; Linehan, 1984, 1987b). DBT applies a broad array of behavior therapy strategies to the problems of BPD. The emphasis on behavioral assessment, data collection on current behaviors, precise operational definition of treatment targets, a collaborative working relationship between therapist and patient (including attention to orienting the patient to the therapy program and mutual commitment to treatment goals), and application of standard behavior therapy techniques all suggest a standard behavior therapy program. Four of the treatment procedures—exposure techniques, skill training, contingency management, and cognitive modification—have been prominent in behavior therapy for years. Each procedure has an enormous empirical and theoretical literature.

However, DBT has a number of distinctive, defining characteristics. Its overriding attribute is an emphasis on dialectical processes. The term "dialectical" is meant to describe both the coexisting multiple tensions that must be dealt with in treating the suicidal, borderline patient, and the thought processes and styles employed and targeted in the treatment strategies. DBT differs from standard cognitive therapy, however, in that cognitive influences are viewed as specific instances of behavior–behavior influence rather than a unique source of emotional and behavioral causality. The fundamental dialectical paradox in psychotherapy, and in DBT, is the necessity of balancing attempts to change patients with fundamental acceptance of the patients exactly as they are in the moment. Thus, DBT requires the simultaneous balancing of problem-solving strategies with validation strategies.

DBT is based on a dialectical world view, a biosocial (behavioral) theory of BPD, and a theoretical framework for understanding therapy-interfering behaviors. It is defined by specific treatment targets, treatment strategies, and therapist attitudes. In the remainder of this chapter, we discuss each of these issues in turn.

DIALECTICS

Although the theories and techniques of behavior therapy have become familiar to clinicians of various orientations, the theory and process of dialectics remain relatively novel concepts for exploration and discussion. The development and application of dialectics in Western culture can be traced to the early Greek philosophers, such as Zeno the Elder, Socrates, and Plato. These philosophers defined dialectics as a method of debate that involved refuting an opponent's argument by hypothetically accepting it and then leading the opponent to admit that it implies contradictory conclusions.

Modern Western philosophers have also employed the concept of dialectics to explain their theories. Kuhn's (1970) discourse on the nature of scientific paradigms, and Marx's theory of economic evolution (Tucker, 1978), emphasize the dialectical process of change through thesis, antithesis, and synthesis. A contemporary dictionary describes three aspects of dialectics: "Development through the stages of thesis, antithesis and synthesis"; "Any systematic reasoning, exposition or argument that juxtaposes opposed or contradictory ideas and usually seeks to resolve their conflict"; and "The dialectical tension or opposition between two interacting forces or elements" (G. C. Merriam Company, 1979).

Although seldom described as such, various aspects of dialectics appear in psychological theories. Conflict plays the leading role in Freud's theory of psychopathology. The ego may be characterized as the synthesizer of op-positional id and superego forces. Mahler's (1972) theory of the developing self includes the subphases of separation–individuation, during which the child, in order to avoid the pathology associated with complete "object loss" or "engulfing symbiosis," must balance holding onto and letting go of the caretaker. The child also learns to integrate disparate aspects of the self. With an emphasis on process and change, Basseches (1984) has recently explored the development of dialectical thinking in adults. In Coleman's work with borderline patients (Coleman, 1956; Coleman & Nelson, 1957; Nelson, 1962), dialectical concepts were employed within the "paradigmatic psycho-therapy."

The constructs of dialectics address many of the etiological and treatment issues of BPD. Given the central defining characteristic of BPD—the instability and/or extremity of emotions, relationships, identity, and behavior—the di-alectical emphasis on change, synthesis, and interrelatedness seems an essential concept to understand and apply. Borderline patients who employ rigid cognitive processing and who oscillate between extreme behavioral patterns in response to stressors could benefit from a paradigm that allows change as a natural and continuous part of life, and that accepts that the opposition of various ideas, emotions, and so forth results in change. They thus learn that judgments of "good versus bad" and "right versus wrong" fail to reflect the nature of life, and that instead a continuous process of balancing or integrating conflicting elements must occur. The borderline patient who reports "identity confusion" and unstable interpersonal relationships also learns that no element is completely independent of any other. Thoughts, behaviors, and emotions result from and produce other thoughts, behaviors, and emotions. Humans function as interdependent beings. The concept of dialectics permeates the theory and practice of DBT. It provides a structure for the etiology and behavioral patterns of BPD, and is employed as both a strategy and goal of therapy.

THEORY AND BEHAVIORAL PATTERNS

Biosocial (Behavioral) Theory

The model of BPD presented here proposes a biosocial (behavioral) theory that focuses on the interaction of emotion dysregulation and dysfunctional, emotion-invalidating environments in the pathogenesis of the disorder. The theory proposes that the characteristics commonly employed to describe and define BPD, including intense, labile emotions and interpersonal relationships, suicidal and other self-injurious behaviors, and disturbance of the self and identity, are sequelae of the effects of this fundamental interaction between emotion dysregulation and invalidating environment. Although similar to contemporary diathesis—stress models, the biosocial model retains a dialectical nature. The model assumes that the functioning of individuals and environmental conditions are continuously interactive, reciprocal, and interdependent, with each component adapting to and influencing the other. The individual and the environment thus constitute a system of change and effect. Since empirical research concerning BPD is still in the early stages, much of the theory presented here remains speculative. The hypotheses are generally derived from clinical experiences and from research in related areas.

According to this biosocial behavioral theory, the borderline individual has an initial emotional vulnerability that mediates her[1] behavior across all aspects of life. "Emotional vulnerability" refers to the individual's greater responsiveness to emotionally evocative stimuli, a responsiveness that includes both frequent and intense responses to even low-intensity or subtle stimuli. Two other aspects of emotional vulnerability, the inabilities to regulate emotional responses and to return easily to an emotional baseline, further frustrate the individual's ability to cope effectively. The mechanisms of borderline individuals' emotional dysregulation are not clear or necessarily consistent across individuals. A biological basis, at least at the adult level, however, is most likely. Recent temperament research (Strelau, Farley, & Gale, 1986; Thomas & Chess, 1986) indicates that high autonomic arousal and emotional reactivity often originate from constitutional sources. Biological factors could range from genetic influences to early environmental effects on the development of the central nervous system. Although one need not discover a common factor

---

[1] Since DBT was developed with female patients, the pronouns "she" and "her" are used to refer to patients. The use of these pronouns is meant to imply neither that BPD is unique to females nor that the treatment is applicable only to females.

among all borderline patients to explain the dysregulation, current research suggests that dysfunction in limbic system reactivity may be important. For example, Cowdry, Pickar, and Davies (1985) report that borderline patients may have an unusually low threshold for activation of the limbic structures.

Complicating the emotional vulnerability, the theory suggests, is an invalidating environment in which significant others negate the individual's experience of her own affect and cognitions. This environment can exist in either a "perfect" family (families that deny problems and appear to have little conflict) or a "chaotic" family (families obviously plagued by conflict, broken relationships, addictions, etc.). These families ignore and/or fail to tolerate negative emotions such as anger and sadness, and ascribe to each individual responsibility for his/her own problems and for the problems' resolutions. These families attribute failure and emotional pain to "attitude problems" or "laziness." The individual should simply endure through or prevail over life's many challenges. Such an environment radically simplifies the complexity of the individual and of the problem-solving process. Although an attitude of self-discipline and self-reliance may succeed in some situations and for some children's temperaments, an attitude that requires steadfast self-control threatens more failure and pain for the individual with an emotionally reactive temperament. The invalidating environment both fails to provide adequate training in emotion regulation skills and conditions a sense of shame and humiliation in response to intense, negative emotions. The environment described here resembles Chess and Thomas's (1986) concept of "poorness of fit" of the child with her environment. In such an environment, there are discrepancies and dissonances between environmental opportunities and demands on the one hand, and the child's characteristics and capacities on the other.

Child abuse, especially sexual abuse, has become an issue of particular importance in the etiology of BPD, both because of its reported frequency within the borderline population (Wagner, Linehan, & Wasson, 1989; Herman, Perry, & van der Kolk, 1989) and because of its possible dual role in the biosocial model. Abuse in childhood can certainly play the role of a major stressor, and it perhaps best exemplifies the invalidating environment. In the typical case scenario of sexual abuse, the victim is told that the molestation or intercourse is "OK" but that she must not tell anyone else. The abuse is seldom acknowledged by other family members, and if the child reports the abuse she risks being disbelieved or blamed (Tsai & Wagner, 1978).

Although generally viewed as the social stressor, child abuse may play a less obvious role as a cause of biological emotional vulnerability. Abuse may not only be pathogenic for individuals with vulnerable temperaments; it may "create" emotional vulnerability by affecting changes in the central nervous system. Shearer, Peters, Quaytman, and Ogden (1990) suggest that perpetual trauma may physiologically alter the limbic system. Thus, severe, chronic stress may have permanent aversive effects on arousal, emotional sensitivity, and other factors of temperament.

Behavioral Patterns

Linehan (1987a) has organized the borderline individual's behavioral patterns along three axes or poles: (1) "emotional vulnerability versus invalidation," (2) "active passivity versus apparent competence," and (3) "unrelenting crises versus inhibited grieving." The first member of each pair reflects strong physiological influences on emotion regulation, while the second member reflects the influences of environmental responses to the individual's emotional behaviors. This model of behavioral patterns reflects a dialectical paradigm, in that each member of the polar pair directly interacts with the other to generate a change in the individual. Although the axes are generally related to distress and dysfunctional behaviors, especially as they interfere with the therapy process, each behavioral pattern by itself need not result in negative experiences. In the pathogenesis of BPD, the interaction within each pair produces the dysfunctional processes and behaviors observed in the borderline individual. An important function of DBT is to affect the behavioral patterns in such a way that the borderline patient progresses toward a stable balance at the center of each axis, rather than oscillating between the extremes. Therapy can achieve this goal by altering specific processes (e.g., reducing emotional vulnerability and invalidation) or by altering the interaction between the processes (e.g., developing a behavioral pattern besides inhibited grieving to respond to constant crisis). As will be demonstrated, the six behavioral patterns labeled above offer explanations for the characteristics on which the revised third edition of the *Diagnostic and Statistical Manual of Mental Disorders* (DSM-III-R; American Psychiatric Association, 1987) bases its diagnostic criteria for BPD.

Emotional Vulnerability versus Invalidation

The "emotional vulnerability" presented above as part of the biosocial etiology of BPD also refers to a pattern of behaviors exhibited by the borderline individual. Frequent and intense responsiveness to emotional stimuli, as well as unmodulated and extended emotional responses, characterizes this behavioral pattern. Attempting to modulate her emotions, the borderline individual fluctuates unsuccessfully between avoiding or arresting additional stimuli and intensely overreacting to the current stimuli. Emotional responses operate as full systems processes that include sensory, cognitive, expressive, and phys-iological responses. The borderline patient's inabilities, therefore, should not be conceptualized simply as physiological dysregulation, but as emotional dysregulation involving a complex interaction of various emotional response processes. Intense emotional arousal may further interfere with the individual's behavior by interrupting more adaptive coping responses. High arousal is also associated with extreme, dichotomous thinking; rumination and avoidance; and/or attack behaviors. Finally, emotional dysregulation seems to produce a sense of being unable to predict or control one's self. The inability to control internal as well as external events, and the inability to modulate responses to those events, all contribute to the sense of dyscontrol.

"Invalidation" refers to a behavioral pattern that resembles the invalidating environment in which the borderline individual has lived. The pattern includes invalidating one's own emotional experiences, seeking from others an accurate perception of both external and internal "reality," and oversimplifying the complexity of solving problems. If an individual's emotions and beliefs have suffered from constant external invalidation, it follows that the individual may begin to doubt what she believes or feels and may become unable to trust herself. She may begin to invalidate her own perceptions and responses in the direction of congruence with the external environment. Establishing congruence with the environment often requires her to inhibit her own emotional experiences and expressions.

The borderline individual who learns to presume the invalidity of her internal responses may then seek from the external environment her self-image, long-term goals, and values, scanning her external environment for what to think and feel. A reliance on others for a self-image may contribute to the intense interpersonal relationships and efforts to avoid abandonment described in DSM-III-R. An acceptance of the expectations advocated by her environment frequently results in failure for the borderline patient. Such failure seems to produce a lack of self-confidence, if not feelings of self-hate. Given the invalidating pattern, which includes a lack of self-trust and self-confidence, a reliance on external determinants of emotions, and emotional inhibition, patients' reports of "identity" problems are not surprising. Finally, in a family that ignores negative emotions such as anger, the individual perhaps learns that only extreme behaviors elicit validation of her emotions from others. Such a family may even require suicidal behavior from the borderline individual before it will confirm the existence of a problem.

Active Passivity versus Apparent Competence

The remaining axes are derivatives of the emotional vulnerability versus invalidation dimension. The behavioral pattern of "active passivity" refers to the borderline individual's pattern of approaching problems passively and helplessly, doubting her ability to design and effect successful solutions, while simultaneously actively seeking help from the environment. As a result of emotion dysregulation, she is emotionally vulnerable; as a result of the invalidating environment, she distrusts her own experiences and perceptions. A pattern of learned helplessness, together with a tendency to seek help from others, thus develops. In addition, the borderline individual's environment generally fails to pay sufficient heed to her difficulties, and so never teaches the necessary problem-solving skills. The syndrome of active passivity may not be entirely due to learning experiences. There is some data, for example, to suggest that individuals with high autonomic reactivity are more likely to prefer passive self-regulation styles, including external regulation by the environment (Eliasz, 1985). This dependency on others for problem solving at times makes the possibility of abandonment even more threatening, and may partially explain what the DSM-III-R refers to as "frantic efforts to avoid . . . abandonment" (American Psychiatric Association, 1987, p. 347).

The "apparent competence" syndrome, at the opposite pole, refers to the occasional tendency of borderline patients to appear deceptively competent. The deception is in the mind of the observer. The very real competencies of the individual do not generalize across all relevant situations and across different mood states. For example, the person may be able to shake off depression or anxiety one day but not the next. Or she may be appropriately assertive in work settings, but unable to produce assertive responses in intimate relationships. Impulse control while in the therapist's office may not generalize to settings outside his/her office. The apparent competence further perpetuates the invalidating environment, since others, unable to perceive any disabilities, ignore or contradict the borderline individual's cries for help. Thus, this syndrome can support the therapist in "blaming the victim" and can blind him/her to areas where the patient needs assistance with learning new behavioral patterns.

Unrelenting Crises versus Inhibited Grieving

"Unrelenting crisis" refers to the state of constant emotional stress in which the borderline often exists. Repeated life traumas, emotional vulnerability, inadequate interpersonal skills, and insufficient social support (invalidating environment, unstable relationships) all contribute to constant crises. Low distress tolerance, high reactivity, and skill deficits augment the likelihood of encountering stressful situations and then exacerbate the various stressors encountered. The theory also supports the hypothesis that the borderline individual cannot easily recover to an emotional baseline, and thus experiences for a longer period the painful affect and cognitions elicited during the crisis.

In view of such acute, chronic states of crisis and an inability to tolerate or modulate them, the borderline's idea of escaping pain or numbness via suicide may seem like a viable option.

Crises usually involve a loss. Although the process of grieving is not well understood, major losses in life nonetheless appear to necessitate some period of mourning or grieving for adequate recovery to occur. "Inhibited grieving" refers to the borderline individual's inhibition or short-circuiting of the grief process. The borderline individual fears being overwhelmed by and unable to control her emotional responses if she confronts the pain and emptiness associated with acknowledging the loss. Instead, the theory asserts, she inhibits the grieving process when presented with the initial cues associated with loss or trauma. Thus, in a manner reminiscent of post-traumatic stress disorder, the individual may suffer obsessive and ruminative thoughts about losses and traumas, panic attacks, dissociative phenomena, insomnia, chronic anxiety, and other patterns associated with unresolved grief and trauma. The DSM-III-R proposes that parasuicidal behaviors may "counteract feelings of 'numbness'" (American Psychiatric Association, 1987, p. 346) that persist due to frequent, unresolved losses or crises. Given the borderline individual's frequent encounters with loss (e.g., incest, self-esteem, relationships, finances), this behavioral pattern pervades her life as thoroughly as does constant crises. The borderline individual oscillates between the extremely high reactivity of constant crisis and the underreaction of inhibited grieving.

DIALECTICAL BEHAVIOR THERAPY

DBT (Linehan, 1984) was designed to provide borderline patients with the problem-solving skills needed to cope effectively with emotional vulnerability and an invalidating environment, as well as those skills needed to cope with the behavioral patterns described above. The training of these skills defines the substance of group therapy, and the integration of the skills into daily life serves as a target in individual therapy.

Targets

Five behavioral targets, or goals, provide the focus and direction of individual DBT. The targets are presented to and discussed with the patient during the initial sessions. In order for the treatment to succeed, the therapist must obtain a commitment from the patient that she will work toward achieving the therapy's goals. The therapist focuses on the targets in hierarchical order, but will readdress a previous target if the associated dysfunctional behavior return. Indeed, readdressing previous targets is the norm, not the exception.

The first target, suicidal behaviors, applies directly to the DSM-III-R component of serious suicide ideation and parasuicidal behaviors (intentional self-injurious acts, including suicide attempts and self-mutilating behaviors). The primary attention to suicidal behaviors seems an obvious necessity, because of the association of these behaviors with subsequent suicide. Although self-mutilation may not appear immediately as serious, its association with suicide and the threat of accidental damage or death establish it as part of the primary target. If parasuicidal behavior has occurred, at least part of the subsequent therapy session focuses on the behavior. Realizing that parasuicidal behaviors serve various problem-solving functions, the DBT therapist endeavors to replace parasuicide with more adaptive coping behaviors. The attention to parasuicide informs the patient that the therapist regards the behavior as serious—an attitude that contrasts with the experiences of many patients from invalidating environments. Also, the therapist constructs a clear contingency for the patient: She cannot discuss other issues of interest until the threat of parasuicide has ceased.

After diminishing parasuicidal behaviors, the therapist confronts the second target: therapy-interfering behaviors on the part of both the patient and the therapist. "Therapy-interfering behaviors" are any responses on the part of either the patient or the therapist that threaten the conduct and continuance of the therapy. The basic notion is that therapy does not work with people who do not come to therapy. These behaviors include power struggles, being late for or missing sessions, refusal to work in sessions, noncompliance with homework or treatment guidelines, blaming the victim, and the like. The therapy-interfering behaviors often reflect generalized behavior patterns of both the patient and the therapist. For example, a power struggle in therapy may reflect a generalized fear of loss of control in situations where the other person has high power and control over important resources. Repeated noncompliance with self-monitoring assignments may reflect fundamental difficulties in self-management, especially in overcoming mood-dependent behavior patterns. The therapist and patient work together to generalize what has been learned about therapy-interfering behaviors to other comparable life situations of the patient. Since therapy involves two participants, DBT also addresses the therapist's therapy-interfering behaviors. Therapist behaviors such as rigid responses, invalidation, and withdrawal are attended to closely. Therapist behaviors may be worked on either within patient–therapist sessions (usually when the patient brings the problem up for discussion) or within the weekly supervision/consultation sessions each therapist attends.

The third target consists of remaining life-interfering and escape behaviors (i.e., those behaviors that threaten the patient's chances for a higher-quality life). These include, for example, excessive impulsiveness, substance abuse, eating disorders, and interpersonal difficulties coupled with lack of emotional control that lead to antisocial behavior (e.g., physical fights). The therapist teaches the patient about the destructiveness of escape behaviors and clarifies why the interfering behaviors should cease. Thus, the first strategy with these behaviors is commitment to change.

After accomplishing the first three behavioral targets, DBT addresses two issues that remain for many patients: post-traumatic stress and respect for self. Recent research has explored the prevalence of post-traumatic stress and its manifestations in the borderline population (Coons, Bowman, Pellow, & Scheider, 1989; Goodwin, Cheeves & Connell, 1990). Most of these studies have focused on child abuse or adult sexual abuse as the primary traumatic event. Post-traumatic stress follows parasuicidal, therapy-interfering, and life-interfering behaviors as a treatment target for a simple reason: The individual must be able to stay alive, stay safe, and stay in therapy if the treatment of post-traumatic symptomatology is to succeed. Through a focus on the life- and therapy-threatening behaviors, the patient acquires skills that will help her cope more effectively with the process of resolving a traumatic past.

Self-respect, the final target, encompasses the fostering of various positive "self-" aspects such as self-respect, self-trust, and self-soothing. The target focuses on the patient's ability to love herself and to trust her own "sense of self," her emotions and behaviors. Self-respect, self-esteem, and concern for one's self play a fundamental role and are influenced by validation, identity, and control. Although success with previous targets presumes at least a moderate level of self-validation and self-control, many patients remain confused about issues of identity as they discover that they need not define themselves in terms of emotional states, behaviors, or diagnostic labels. Self-trust—confidence in and assurance of one's self—interacts significantly with self-respect. The skills training and validation by the therapist enhance the patient's self-trust by providing her with the sense that she accurately perceives her environment and with the ability to respond effectively to it. Finally, Adler's concept of self-holding (Buie & Adler, 1982) is addressed as the patient learns to care for herself and to cope with emotional distress.

Basic Skills

DBT is based on a "capability" conception of behavioral functioning. This model, first proposed by Wallace (1966, 1967), suggests that behavior is a joint function of the ability to produce a particular response and the incentives in the situation to produce the behavior. The absence of a desired behavior can be due to behavioral inability (i.e., a skill deficit), to behavioral inhibition, or to lack of incentives or reinforcers in the situation. Likewise, the presence of dysfunctional behaviors can be due to the absence of competing functional behaviors or to the absence of necessary self-control behavioral repertoires. The ability to achieve the therapy targets in DBT requires a number of basic skills. These skills, taught both in individual therapy and in skill-focused therapy groups, can be divided into five groups: (1) emotion regulation skills, (2) distress tolerance skills, (3) interpersonal skills, (4) self-management skills, and (5) a group of skills called "core skills" in DBT. These core skills are behavioral capabilities drawn from the meditation and Eastern psychology practices; they include the skills of observing, describing, participating spontaneously, being nonjudgmental, being mindful, and focusing on what is effective in a given situation.

Given the emotional lability and intensity that characterize BPD, the training of emotional regulation skills plays an essential role in the treatment of the disorder. An equally important role, however, is played by distress tolerance training, which prepares the patient to accept her emotions and environment as they are in the moment. A dialectic thus operates between these two groups of skills. Distress tolerance concerns the ability to observe and acknowledge one's emotions, thoughts, and environment without attempting to change or control any variable. The training teaches the patient to accept both her emotions and her current environment in nonjudgmental ways. The therapist must clarify for the patient that distress tolerance does not equal "giving in" or "giving up," but that in many situations tolerating discomfort will actually result in preferred outcomes. The borderline patient's behavioral repertoire often includes the requisite social skills of meeting and conversing with people, and thus she appears socially competent. Skills for coping with interpersonal conflict, however, are often absent or inhibited by fear. The interpersonal skills training provides interpersonal problem-solving skills essential for the development and maintenance of stable relationships. Self-management skills are a general group of skills intended to enable the patient to gain and maintain other specific abilities. Here, the patient learns to set realistic goals and to perform behavioral analysis; she also learns contingency management and relapse prevention skills.

Strategies

The DBT therapist approaches these targets with five grand sets of strategies: (1) dialectical strategies, (2) stylistic strategies, (3) basic strategies, (4) case management strategies, and (5) integrative strategies. The grand sets all contain at least one dialectical pair of substrategies. Each of the subsets, in turn, is described by the various techniques employed to operate the strategies.

Dialectical Strategies

The dialectical strategies define DBT and permeate the therapy structure and application. The therapist must respond to the dialectical tension that occurs during therapy by balancing change strategies with acceptance strategies (e.g., persistence vs. flexibility). The therapist models dialectical thinking through various techniques, including paradox, unresolved ambiguity, and cognitive challenging. Such modeling enables the patient to discover that truth is not absolute, but that it evolves and develops. Furthermore, dialectical strategies dictate a flexible approach to therapy interactions, emphasizing fluid, continuous, and responsive movement of the therapist; a nonrigid setting of boundaries around problems encountered; a holistic view, always looking for what is missing in the current problem formulation; and attention to the oppositions occurring in each moment of the interaction.

Stylistic Strategies

The therapist employs two sets of complementary stylistic strategies in his/ her general interactions with the patient. Reciprocal vulnerability strategies, the first set, consist of the therapist's responsive and self-disclosing behaviors. To convey interest and understanding, the therapist's responses should reflect the content of the patient's communications, rather than some specific, previously written script. The therapist also discloses aspects of himself/herself that model coping with problems or that validate the patient's perception of the therapist.

Irreverent communication strategies, the second set, temporarily "unbalance" the patient by shifting her emotional response or by introducing her to a new viewpoint. Procedures include a prosaic reaction to maladaptive behaviors, taking the patient more seriously than she intended, direct confrontation of the patient's "crazy" behavior, and unorthodox responses. For example, if the patient says, "I'm thinking about killing myself," the therapist might respond, "That would make it difficult to come to therapy, wouldn't it?" The balancing of the sarcasm and indifference of the irreverent communication strategies with the sincerity, warmth, and responsiveness of the reciprocal vulnerability strategies demonstrates a dialectic that promotes the patient's cessation of thinking and behaving in the extreme.

Basic Strategies

Basic strategies include a number of problem-solving/change strategies and behavioral techniques (exposure, cognitive modification, contingency management, skill training), balanced by a number of validation/acceptance strategies. Problem-solving strategies involve a two-step process. The first step requires the patient to identify her problem. DBT teaches her to recognize dysfunctional behaviors, such as self-mutilating behavior, as indicators of an existing problem. The patient then learns to conduct a behavioral analysis on the problem:

tracing the problem's origin to the environmental and behavioral stimuli, identifying her various reactions to the problem, and hypothesizing explanations for those reactions. After problem recognition, the patient proceeds to the next step of the strategy, solutions. Having recognized particular behaviors as maladaptive responses, she must alter her behavioral chain and develop adaptive solutions. Unfortunately, the borderline patient often lacks both the internal and the external resources needed to propose and effect adaptive solutions. At this point, the therapist may employ other techniques to help the patient obtain the necessary resources. Skill training techniques are aimed to increasing coping capabilities. Cognitive modification techniques are used to modify rules, expectancies, and beliefs interfering with adaptive coping. Contingency management techniques are used to increase incentives for adaptive coping and to reduce incentives for maladaptive coping. In contrast to many behavior therapy applications, relationship contingencies are emphasized heavily in DBT. Exposure techniques are aimed at reducing fear-related and guilt/shame-related response patterns inhibiting adaptive coping. In particular, DBT stresses exposure to negative emotional responses to reduce the often automatic, conditioned inhibition and shame associated with negative emotions (especially anger) among borderline individuals.

Balancing the focus on change associated with problem-solving strategies, validation strategies require a nonjudgmental acceptance of the patient in the moment and an active search for the wisdom in the moment of the patient's response. In validation, the therapist searches for the nugget of gold in the pail of sand, so to speak. Once the nugget is found, the therapist reflects this wisdom back to the patient. (Change strategies focus on the sand.) Validation usually involves three steps: (1) observing and describing the patient's emotional, cognitive, or behavioral reactions and patterns; (2) empathizing with the patient's position, and (3) communicating whatever essential wisdom exists in the response. It is the third step that is essential and differentiates validation from ordinary (but also essential) reflection and empathic responding. This type of validation may help to clarify the borderline individual's confused sense of identity as she begins to accept and trust her own perceptions and ideas. With the "cheerleading" procedure, the therapist encourages the patient by finding, reflecting, and highlighting the patient's inner strengths and resources. The DBT therapist has faith in the patient's value and motivation to develop, grow, and change.

Whereas the validation strategies provide an excellent example of the acceptance aspect of the primary dialectic, the capability enhancement strategies demonstrate the change aspect. Through the procedures of skill acquisition, skill strengthening, and skill generalization, the therapist works with the patient to actively improve her problem-solving skills (e.g., using skills during therapy, finishing homework). Capability enhancement strategies focus on changing the borderline patient's behavioral patterns from those of a passive victim to those of an active problem solver. Each target level of DBT necessitates the enhancement of behavioral coping techniques. Capability enhancement operates as an essential strategy in the prevention of impulsive and self-mutilating behaviors.

Based on operant learning, contingency management strategies concern the therapist's arrangement of environmental contingencies in such a way that he/she reinforces only functional, adaptive behaviors and does not reinforce suicidal or other dysfunctional behaviors. Essential to the contingency strategies is the ability of the therapist to avoid appeasing the patient, even in the face of high-risk or highly aversive behaviors, while simultaneously soothing and validating the patient's difficulties, thereby avoiding punishing and blaming the patient. In practice, this balance is enormously difficult to strike. Whereas contingency management strategies directly affect behavioral patterns, cognitive modification strategies modify behavior by employing verbal procedures to change the cognitive rules that mediate and/or accompany behavior. The verbal procedures consist of contingency clarification and cognitive restructuring.

The DBT therapist employs exposure strategies when the patient's problem involves fear, anxiety, or guilt. Although these emotions may be problematic by themselves, they may also inhibit adaptive coping skills, reflect unresolved post-traumatic stress, or interfere with discussing emotional topics in therapy. The exposure techniques employed by the therapist include emitting behaviors that elicit problematic aversive emotions, using imagery, and discussing stimulus events associated with aversive emotional responses. It is essential, of course, for exposure to occur in an environment that does not further reinforce the targeted emotion. Thus, exposure is done in conjunction with an emphasis on patient coping strategies (such as relaxation, breathing, observing, and cognitive restructuring), as well as therapist soothing behaviors (such as cheerleading, validating, and praise).

Case Management Strategies

Like the stylistic strategies, the case management strategies consist of two sets of strategies that balance each other. Focusing on interpersonal skills, the consultant strategy enhances the patient's ability to request services and interact effectively with other professionals. The DBT therapist consults with the patient about how to interact with other service providers, such as physicians, case workers, and lawyers. The therapist refuses to consult directly with other professionals about the patient's treatment. This strategy thus attempts to reduce the borderline individual's problem-solving pattern of active passivity, and to enhance the patient's power directly and minimize the therapist's power. Nor does the therapist intervene for or defend the other professional to the patient.

Although the consultant strategy advocates that the patient actively solve her problems, the DBT therapist acknowledges that the patient may lack the requisite skills in some crucial situations. Environmental interventions, in situations where outcomes are important but the patient has little power, allow the therapist to intervene on the patient's behalf. Situations where this is likely include preventing involuntary hospitalization and sending mandatory progress reports to insurance or welfare agencies. The therapist also complies with laws concerning the protection of other individuals.

Integrative Strategies

There are a number of integrative strategies that combine dialectical, stylistic, basic, and case management strategies in specific ways to address common problems in treating borderline patients. Structural strategies are a group of procedures describing the structure of individual sessions and of the course of therapy. The therapist guides individual sessions according to session-beginning, targeting, and session-ending procedures. The procedures are designed to enhance the patient's comfort during a session and her well-being following a session, as well as to insure that the hierarchical targets described above are addressed in a direct fashion during each session. Relationship strategies focus on developing a strong, positive relationship between the therapist and the patient. Relationship strategies also include techniques designed to enhance and solve problems within the therapist–patient relationship. Thus the borderline individual learns how to maintain and stabilize at least one interpersonal relationship. Generalization to other interpersonal relationships, however, is not assumed, but rather is actively and directly addressed.

The crisis strategies integrate various procedures that direct the therapist's behavior when a patient's emotional crisis requires the therapist's immediate attention. The therapist also integrates several strategies and procedures when he/she operates the compliance enhancement strategies. These strategies surface when the patient exhibits therapy-interfering behavior. Finally, the therapist employs the suicidal behavior strategies in a session immediately following any parasuicide. These strategies include an in-depth focus on the parasuicidal behavior, a complete behavioral analysis of the event, and a problem-solving analysis designed to prevent future events.

THERAPIST'S ROLE

The DBT therapist plays very active roles throughout the therapy session, actively engaging the patient in a therapeutic alliance at each point. To maintain this alliance with the patient, the therapist must constantly strive to establish a dialectical balance within the therapy session between expectations of and directions for change on the one hand, and acceptance of and responsiveness to the patient's current state on the other.

Two dimensions, "unmoving centeredness versus compassionate flexibility" and "benevolent demanding versus nurturing," reflect behavioral aspects of change and acceptance (Linehan, 1989). "Unmoving centeredness" requires therapists to observe their own personal limits, maintain contingencies they have set for patients, and endure extreme attempts by the patients to elicit positive responses from the therapists for negative behaviors. A therapist must also exhibit compassionate flexibility by adapting his/her responses as specific situations recommend. This absence of rigidity in the therapist not only enhances the therapeutic alliance; it also models more effective coping behavior for the patient. Whereas "benevolent demanding" refers to the therapist's recognition of the patient's current capabilities and resources, "nurturing" refers to the therapist's acknowledgment of the patient's current inabilities. Skills training and environmental intervention are reflections of this emphasis on nurturing in DBT. The balance of this dimension is particularly essential when encountering the behavioral patterns of active passivity versus apparent competence. Without benevolent demanding, the therapist reinforces active passivity. Without nurturing, the therapist becomes invalidating by oversimplifying the difficult process of therapy. As therapy and the patient progress, the fulcrum on which these poles are balanced moves, and thus the position of the therapist on each pole is ever-changing and must be flexible.

The balancing act of a therapist becomes much more precarious with a borderline patient who often exhibits lethal, extreme responses. The therapist struggles to help the patient learn to integrate emotions and thoughts, to move toward a synthesis rather than oscillating between extremes. If the therapist fails to push hard enough, inertia results, but if he/she pushes too hard, the patient may fall. Nor can the concept of balance be made extreme: If the patient steps backward and almost falls off of the stage into the pit, the therapist cannot "balance" the situation by stepping back behind the stage curtain! DBT requires a mature therapist who remains sensitive to the patient's needs while maintaining the targets of the therapy.

TREATMENT OUTCOME

Outcome results with DBT to date are encouraging. In a randomized design (Linehan, Armstrong, Suarez, Allmon, & Heard, in press), 46 women meeting criteria for BPD with a history of at least two parasuicidal acts were assigned to DBT or to a community "treatment as usual" group. The DBT consisted of weekly individual and group therapy, conducted by experienced therapists trained in DBT. Subjects in the study were then assessed at 4-month intervals for 1 year of treatment. Half have so far been followed through a 1-year posttreatment follow-up. Data analysis suggests that DBT effectively reduces both the frequency and lethality of parasuicidal behavior. Compared to those receiving community treatment as usual, DBT patients had less frequent episodes of parasuicide, less parasuicidal behavior during each episodes, and less medically severe parasuicidal behavior. In addition, DBT patients had fewer inpatient psychiatric days during the treatment year. DBT patients also had a low dropout rate from therapy; 83% remained in treatment the entire year. These reductions in suicidal behavior and psychiatric inpatient days occurred in spite of no differential effect of treatment on ameliorating self-reports of depression or hopelessness. Follow-up analyses are now being conducted. At the 18-month point, the DBT group still had significantly fewer parasuicidal episodes. At the 1-year follow-up date, treatment gains were not lost, but the control group's gains were such that significant differences between the groups no longer held.

In a separate but related study (Linehan, Heard, & Armstrong, 1991), we examined whether giving our group therapy in conjunction with ongoing individual treatment as usual in the community would be effective. The question here was whether simply teaching skills in a group format might be effective. Our results suggested that such an approach is not effective. We found no significant improvement in the DBT group patients relative to the controls on any measure.

DBT is one of the few cognitive–behavioral psychotherapies developed specifically for BPD, and currently is the only psychosocial treatment of any sort that has been evaluated using a randomized design with a control group comparison. As noted, the treatment appears to reduce the frequency and lethality of suicidal behaviors. In addition to improving the patients' quality of life, such a reduction has important economic implications. Reductions in parasuicide mean fewer emergency room visits and fewer medical and psychiatric hospital stays, all of which are great financial costs to either the patients or the community. Additional analyses underway include the effect of DBT on variables such as the patients' interpersonal problem-solving skills, their ability to function successfully at work, and their satisfaction with life. Treatment research on DBT is only beginning, and the future research possibilities are both numerous and promising.

REFERENCES

American Psychiatric Association. (1987). *Diagnostic and statistical manual of mental disorders* (3rd ed., rev.). Washington, DC: Author.

Basseches, M. (1984). *Dialectical thinking and adult development*. Norwood, NJ: Ablex.

Buie, D. H., & Adler, G. (1982). The definitive treatment of the borderline personality. *International Journal of Psychoanalytic Psychotherapy, 9*, 51–87.

Chess, S., & Thomas, A. (1986). *Temperament in clinical practice.* New York: Guilford Press.

Coleman, M. L. (1956). Externalization of the toxic introject: A treatment technique for borderline cases. *Psychoanalytic Review, 43,* 235–242.

Coleman, M. L., & Nelson, B. (1957). Paradigmatic psychotherapy in borderline treatment. *Psychoanalysis, 5,* 28–44.

Coons, P. M., Bowman, E. S., Pellow, T. A., & Scheider, P. (1989). Post-traumatic aspects of the treatment of victims of sexual abuse and incest. *Psychiatric Clinics of North America, 12*(2), 325–335.

Cowdry, R. W., Pickar, D., & Davies, R. (1985). Symptoms and EEG findings in the borderline syndrome. *Journal of Psychiatry and Medicine, 15,* 201–211.

Eliasz, A. (1985). Mechanisms of temperament: Basic functions. In J. Strelau, F. H. Farley, & A. Gale (Eds.), *The biological bases of personality and behavior: Theories, measurement techniques, and development* (Vol. 1). Washington, DC: Hemisphere.

G. C. Merriam Company. (1979). *Webster's new collegiate dictionary.* Springfield, MA: Author.

Goodwin, J. M., Cheeves, K., & Connell, V. (1990). Borderline and other severe symptoms in adult survivors of incestuous abuse. *Psychiatric Annals, 20*(1), 22–32.

Herman, J. L., Perry, J. C., & van der Kolk, B. A. (1989). Childhood trauma in borderline personality disorder. *American Journal of Psychiatry, 146,* 490–495.

Kuhn, T. S. (1970). *The structure of scientific revolutions* (2nd ed.). Chicago: University of Chicago Press.

Linehan, M. M. (1984). *Dialectical behavior therapy for treatment of parasuicidal women: Treatment manual.* Unpublished manuscript, University of Washington.

Linehan, M. M. (1987a). Dialectical behavior therapy for borderline personality disorder: Theory and method. *Bulletin of the Menninger Clinics, 51,* 261–276.

Linehan, M. M. (1987b). Dialectical behavior therapy: A cognitive behavioral approach to parasuicide. *Journal of Personality Disorders, 1,* 328–333.

Linehan, M. M. (1989). Dialektische verhaltenstherapie bei borderline-personlichkeitstorungen [Dialectical behavior therapy: A treatment for borderline personality disorder]. *Praxis der Klinischen Verhaltensmedizin und Rehabilitation, 2,* 220–227.

Linehan, M. M., Armstrong, H. E., Suarez, A., Allmon, D., & Heard, H. L. (in press). Behavioral treatment of chronically parasuicidal borderline patients. *Archives of General Psychiatry.*

Linehan, M. M., Heard, H. L., & Armstrong, H. E. (1991). *Treatment modes of Dialectical Behavior Therapy for chronically parasuicidal borderline patients.* Unpublished manuscript, University of Washington.

Mahler, M. S. (1972). On the first three subphases of the separation–individuation process. *International Journal of Psycho-Analysis, 53,* 333–338.

Nelson, M. C. (1962). Effect of paradigmatic techniques on the psychic economy of borderline patients. *Psychiatry, 25,* 119–134.

Pretzer, J. (1989). Borderline personality disorder. In A. Freeman (Ed.), *Clinical applications of cognitive therapy.* New York: Plenum Press.

Shearer, S. L., Peters, C. P., Quaytman, M. S., & Ogden, R. L. (1990). Frequency and correlates of childhood sexual and physical abuse histories in adult female borderline inpatients. *American Journal of Psychiatry, 147*(20), 214–216.

Strelau, J., Farley, F. H., & Gale, A. (Eds.). (1986). *The biological bases of personality and behavior: Psychophysiology, performance, and applications* (Vol. 2). Washington, DC: Hemisphere.

Thomas, A., & Chess, S. (1986). The New York Longitudinal Study: From infancy to early adult life. In R. Plomin & J. Dunn (Eds.), *The study of temperament: Changes, continuities and challenges.* Hillsdale, NJ: Erlbaum.

Tsai, M., & Wagner, N. N. (1978). Therapy groups for women sexually molested as children. *Archives of Sexual Behavior, 7*(5), 417–427.

Tucker, R. C. (Ed.). (1978). *The Marx–Engels reader* (2nd ed.). New York: Norton.

Turner, R. M. (1989). Case study evaluations of a bio-cognitive behavioral approach for the treatment of borderline personality disorder. *Behavior Therapy, 20,* 477–489.

Wagner, A. W., Linehan, M. M., & Wasson, E. J. (1989, November). *Parasuicide: Characteristics and relationship to childhood sexual abuse.* Poster presented at the conference of the Association for Advancement of Behavior Therapy, Washington, DC.

Wallace, J. (1966). An abilities conception of personality: Some implications for personality measurement. *Journal of Reproductive and Infant Psychology, 21,* 132–138.

Wallace, J. (1967). What units shall we employ? Allport's question revisited. *Journal of Transpersonal Psychology, 31,* 56–64.

Young, J. (1983, August). *Borderline personality: Cognitive therapy and treatment.* Paper presented at the annual convention of the American Psychological Association, Philadelphia.

CHAPTER 12

Psychodynamic Psychotherapy of the Borderline Patient

JOHN F. CLARKIN
HAROLD KOENIGSBERG
FRANK YEOMANS
MICHAEL SELZER
PAULINA KERNBERG
OTTO F. KERNBERG

Although clinicians seeking characterological change in patients with borderline personality disorder (BPD) commonly employ forms of long-term psychoanalytically oriented psychotherapy, there have been very few studies of the process and efficacy of this treatment. BPD represents a highly prevalent type of character pathology (Kass, Spitzer, & Williams, 1983; Koenigsberg, Kaplan, Gilmore, & Cooper, 1985), and research on long-term psychotherapy of whatever orientation is dramatically underrepresented within the overall field of psychotherapy research. Thus, a major imbalance exists between a most prevalent type of psychotherapy (i.e., long-term psychotherapy for severely personality-disordered patients) and the almost exclusive focus in psychotherapy research on brief psychotherapies with significantly less ill patients.

An early empirical study on the effects of long-term psychotherapy of borderline patients was the Psychotherapy Research Project of the Menninger Foundation (Kernberg, 1973; Wallerstein, 1986). Some of the findings from this study support the hypothesis that the best treatment for nonpsychotic patients with borderline personality organization (BPO) may be the combination of an expressive approach and as much environmental structuring, external to the treatment hours, as the patient needs. This approach contrasts with a purely supportive psychotherapy, in which substantial structure is provided during the treatment hours.

BORDERLINE PERSONALITY ORGANIZATION AND BORDERLINE PERSONALITY DISORDER

BPO (Kernberg, 1975) is a theoretical conceptualization of patients who experience identity diffusion, who utilize primitive defenses (e.g., projective identification, splitting), and whose reality testing is adequate (nonpsychotic) but may be variable in intense interpersonal relations. These dynamic concepts are difficult to operationalize and measure reliably. Some of these concepts, especially the notion of identity diffusion, were used by the architects of the *Diagnostic and Statistical Manual of Mental Disorders*, third edition (DSM-III; American Psychiatric Association, 1980) and included in the criterion set for BPD on Axis II. However, theoretical constructs and clinical experience suggest that the group of patients with BPO is a more extensive group than those with five or more of the eight criteria for BPD in DSM-III Axis II (Clarkin & Kernberg, in press).

Since the concept of BPO is difficult to measure reliably and selects a more heterogeneous group of patients, we have focused our research on the BPD patient as defined by the eight criteria in DSM-III-R (American Psychiatric Association, 1987), Axis II. The BPD concept is narrower than the BPO concept, and will include patients with BPO. The other advantage in using BPD patients is that there are reliable instruments for assessing the presence of this disorder, and our results can be generalized to other studies that use these widely accepted criteria.

RATIONALE FOR PSYCHODYNAMIC TREATMENT

As with most disorders that are difficult to treat, many intervention strategies have been advocated for BPD patients. Notable among these are supportive psychotherapy (e.g., Zetzel, 1971), cognitive–behavioral treatment (Linehan, 1987), forms of expressive psychodynamic psychotherapy (Waldinger, 1987), and various pharmacotherapies (Soloff, 1989). Although all of these approaches address the behavioral dyscontrol and dysphoric affective states of BPD patients, psychodynamic treatment specifically aims to modify the hypothesized pathogenic mechanisms that impair the patient's capacity to form stable relationships with others and to maintain an integrated sense of self. It is possible that psychodynamic therapy may produce more broadly based character change and more enduring improvement for appropriate patients than the other proposed treatment methods. On the other hand, many think that dynamic treatment can only be used for a healthier subset of BPD patients.

Study of the psychodynamic psychotherapy of BPD patients could shed light upon the extent to which it meets this promise, demonstrate its overall effectiveness, elucidate the process of psychodynamic psychotherapy, and generate criteria for patient selection or patient–therapist matching. In embarking on such a program, we have begun with a project to develop research structures and methodological tools, and to examine the feasibility of such a long-term study of psychodynamic psychotherapy of BPD patients.

GOALS AND OBJECTIVES

This study was designed to develop methodologies for the investigation of psychodynamic psychotherapy of borderline patients. In order to insure that the therapy actually delivered in the study would conform to the treatment model, several of us have operationalized the treatment in a manual (Kernberg, Selzer, Koenigsberg, Carr, & Appelbaum, 1989). In addition to developing methods to insure the delivery of the specified treatment, we sought to develop measures for therapist, patient, and process variables that might be valid in the context of psychotherapy of borderline patients. We also sought to study the frequency of early dropout from treatment, to determine the extent to which this might limit the feasibility of long-term psychotherapy research with borderline patients. The specific objectives were as follows:

1. To develop a program for training therapists in the practice of an operationally defined (i.e., manualized) psychodynamic psychotherapy for borderline patients.
2. To develop a reliable method for measuring therapists' adherence to the psychodynamic treatment.
3. To develop a reliable method for assessing the skill with which therapists employ the psychotherapy.
4. To examine the frequency of early dropout, and to generate hypotheses for its occurrence.
5. To monitor the course of clinical change, and to identify patterns of change in order to test the feasibility of several standard change measures with a borderline population.
6. To determine whether standard measures of therapeutic alliance have reliability and predictive validity when applied to the treatment of BPD patients.

It should be emphasized that we did not intend to conduct an outcome study; this would have been premature, given the lack of instruments and prior research on long-term therapies. Rather, we intended to prepare the way for a process study, and at a later date to compare the effectiveness of this dynamic treatment with other (yet to be specified) standard treatments for the borderline patient.

METHODOLOGY

Patients

Female patients between the ages of 18 and 45 who received an initial clinical diagnosis of DSM-III Axis II BPD in their regular treatment contacts (in both the inpatient and outpatient systems of the New York Hospital—Westchester Division) and did not meet exclusionary criteria were approached by a member of the research team for potential participation in the study. If the patient was willing to give informed consent, she was tested with the Structured Clinical Interview for DSM-III (SCID) and the Structured Clinical Interview for DSM-III Personality Disorders (SCID-II) to ascertain whether inclusionary and exclusionary criteria were met.

Patients with any of the following Axis I or Axis II conditions were excluded: organic brain syndrome, mental retardation, schizophrenia, bipolar disorder, substance abuse disorder, and antisocial personality disorder. All patients had at least an eighth-grade education. We chose to restrict the sample to female patients to increase subject homogeneity. Since most BPD patients treated in clinical settings are female, this choice selected a clinically important group of patients.

Therapists

A total of 28 therapists treated the 31 patients in the study to date; these included faculty psychiatrists, as well as advanced psychiatry and psychology trainees. Therapists with a range of experience were selected in order to assess any possible relationship between years of experience and ability to adhere to the manualized therapy with skill. The faculty therapists ($n = 4$) had more extensive experience, and two of the four were psychoanalysts. All therapists had some prior therapeutic experience with borderline patients, on either an inpatient or an outpatient basis.

Psychotherapy

Each patient was assigned to a psychotherapist by the research coordinators. The treatment was carried out in two 45-minute sessions per week, and no limit to the treatment duration was specified (non-time-limited treatment). The treatment was studied for its first 2 years unless either patient or therapist initiated a termination or transfer prior to that time. The first 10 sessions and 10-session blocks at 6-month intervals were videotaped; all other sessions were audiotaped. The psychotherapy was conducted according to the manual for psychoanalytic psychotherapy with borderline patients written by Kernberg et al. (1989).

Medication

Although psychotropic medications of every class have been advocated for the treatment of BPD patients, there is as yet no consensus that a medication is the treatment of choice for these patients or specific subgroups of them. Antidepressant medication, however, is indicated for the treatment of severe major depression, and this disorder often coexists with BPD. We therefore chose to include the option for antidepressant medication treatment of those BPD patients in our study who also met DSM-III-R and clinical criteria for major depression. Such patients might enter the study on medication or might be placed on medication during their psychotherapy.

The decision about the indications for medication was made by a patient's treating psychotherapist in conjunction with a psychopharmacologist affiliated with the project, who saw the patient for a consultation. Patients who were receiving medication during the study were assigned a separate psychiatrist who prescribed and regulated the medication. This psychiatrist remained in open communication with each patient's psychotherapist, who in turn shared information with him when he deemed it necessary for the treatment.

The type, dosage, and duration of medication usage were recorded, along with dates of pharmacotherapy sessions. Although we realize that the use of medication complicates analysis and interpretation of process variables, we have made provision for it for ethical reasons. We plan to examine any associations between the introduction of medication and changes in therapeutic alliance, psychotherapy skill level, and adherence characteristics.

Therapist Training and Supervision

The therapists attended a 12-session seminar taught by Otto F. Kernberg and colleagues on the psychoanalytic treatment of BPD patients. It was during this time that the trainees read and studied the treatment manual (Kernberg et al., 1989). The lectures were augmented by videotapes of psychoanalytic psychotherapy with BPD patients as done by senior therapists. As the study has progressed, we have also collected illustrative videotapes of trainees to be used in the training as well. The construction of a library of training videotapes has been a major side product of the study to date.

The therapists were supervised on a weekly basis by the senior members of this research team. The supervision focused upon developing and maintaining the skillful execution of the psychotherapy as described in the manual. Supervisors sampled audiotapes and/or videotapes of the sessions, judged the skillfulness and accuracy of the therapy, and provided explicit feedback accordingly.

Rating of Therapist Adherence to the Treatment Manual

Because one major goal of this study was to assess the training of therapists in a manualized long-term dynamic psychotherapy, special attention was given to the development of instruments to assess reliably the therapists' adherence to the treatment method as defined in the manual. Assessment of adherence was carried out by rating transcripts of individual sessions. Raters identified 10 broad categories of themes present in the patients' material, and the extent to which the therapists addressed those themes following the principles of priority defined in the treatment manual. Each therapist intervention was classified into 1 of 16 defined intervention types. Adherence to the technique could be measured by the extent to which a therapist followed the principle of priorities in addressing a patient's themes, and by the extent to which the therapist made use of expressive psychotherapeutic techniques in the process.

Therapist skill was measured by means of a 22-item Likert scale applied to videotaped sessions. In the development of the scale, items were derived from existing scales, and additional items considered by our group to be especially important in work with borderline patients were added.

Measuring the Course of Change

A battery of instruments to assess patient change were administered prior to treatment, at 4-month intervals during treatment, at termination (for both treatment completers and early terminators), and at 6- and 12-month post-termination follow-ups. An attempt was also made to evaluate early terminators at 6 months to 1 year after termination. Symptomatic behavior was measured via a number of self-report instruments—the Symptom Checklist–90 (SCL-90; Derogatis, Lipman, & Covi, 1973), the Beck Depression Inventory (BDI; Beck, Ward, Mendelson, Mock, & Erbaugh, 1961), and the Buss–Durkee Hostility Inventory (Buss & Durkee, 1957)—as well as a semistructured interview, the Schedule for Affective Disorders and Schizophrenia, Change

Version (SADS-C; Spitzer & Endicott, 1978). Social adjustment, including leisure time, vocational functioning, and social functioning, was assessed with the Social Adjustment Scale—Self-Report (SAS-SR; Weissman & Bothwell, 1976).

PRELIMINARY FINDINGS

Continuation of Patients in Treatment

When compared with other diagnostic groups, borderlines prematurely terminate treatment at twice the rate of neurotics and patients with other personality disorders, and at four times the rate of schizophrenics (Skodol, Buckley, & Charles, 1983). By 6 months of treatment, only 40–77% of borderline patients continue in treatment (Gunderson et al., 1989; Waldinger & Gunderson, 1984).

It should not be surprising that borderline patients seem more likely than many other patient groups to terminate therapy prematurely, as a number of the criteria for DSM-III-R BPD suggest such behavior. For example, patients who get into intense, conflicted relationships characterized by idealization and devaluation may well be likely to terminate the relationship with a therapist. Also, patients who are angry and manifest this anger both verbally and behaviorally may be likely to bolt angrily from treatment. Patients who are impulsive with food, alcohol, relationships, and so on may act in such a way as to end treatment precipitously. And, finally, patients who are self-destructive—both in direct suicidal behavior and in more indirct ways—may self-destructively terminate their own treatment and other pathways to improvement.

A major question in this pilot project concerned the incidence of premature terminations. To date, we have evaluated and begun treatment contact with a total of 31 patients. In our form of psychodynamic therapy for a borderline patient, therapy does not begin until the patient and therapist agree upon a treatment contract that specifies the roles and obligations of both parties. This contract takes place at the beginning of the patient–therapist contact, usually within the first six sessions. As of this writing, 7 patients (23%) ended treatment contact prior to or during the contract-setting period. By 12 weeks 13 patients dropped out prematurely, yielding a cumulative 42% dropout rate by 12 weeks.

The dropout rate in our pilot work has been comparable to that reported by others in both pharmacotherapy and psychotherapy studies. Our dropout rate of 42% at the 12-week point compares favorably with the 67% rate reported by Skodol et al. (1983) in their outpatient study, and the 48% rate reported by Goldberg et al. (1986) in their outpatient medication study. By insisting on setting at treatment contract at the beginning, we may have stimulated early dropouts, but at a later point we may have obtained better compliance, in part because the issues of engagement were faced early in treatment.

Follow-Up of Remainers versus Terminators

To explore the patients' experience of the therapy as related to dropout or continuation in treatment, we contacted the first 18 patients admitted to the study some 6 months to 1 year after initation of treatment. A standardized interview format was utilized in a telephone contact of some 30 minutes' duration. Information was obtained on each patient's perceptions of the therapy and the therapist, and conscious reasons for the premature termination if that had occurred. The most striking finding in our contact with the seven patients who remained in therapy was their perception of structure of the treatment (i.e., contract settings, limit setting) as needed and as supportive of their attempts to introduce organization in their chaotic lives.

We were interested in finding out how each patient and therapist negotiated (or failed to negotiate) the treatment ending. When asked about this process, five of the 11 patients who dropped out said that they did not discuss the ending. Of the five patients who did not discuss the ending, all four of the four early dropouts did not discuss the ending, and the fifth was a late dropout. In general, then, none of the early dropouts discussed the termination, and the majority of late dropouts (six of seven) did discuss the termination.

Although previous authors such as Gunderson have found that the more pathological patients are more likely to drop out, a preliminary investigation of our data suggested that there was no difference symptomatically between the remainers and the dropouts. However, the remainers may have had more structure in their lives. Six of the seven remainers were either full-time students or working, while only four of the 11 dropouts were working. It would appear that remainers are more likely to be engaged in productive activity that insures a scheduled, routinized life.

Therapeutic Alliance

The concept of therapeutic alliance has received much attention in the psychotherapy research literature (Docherty, 1985; see also Chapter 10, this volume). In reference to borderline patients, who have such high dropout rates, the positive alliance can be seen as an important process *outcome*. At the point at which a borderline patient achieves a stable and somewhat cooperative relationship with the therapist, some of the significant borderline pathology has been altered.

By definition, borderline patients have unstable interpersonal relations involving idealization and devaluation, uncontrolled anger, and identity diffusion; hence, they will have serious difficulty forming a treatment alliance with a therapist. Therefore, we did not put much value in the existing measures of therapeutic alliance, which were developed in studies of patients without borderline pathology. We have used several measures of the alliance that rely on self-report from therapist and patient. We are currently utilizing the self-report California Psychotherapy Alliance Scales—Patient Version (CALPAS-P), and the CALPAS—Independent Rater Version (CALPAS-R) (Marmar, Horowitz, Weiss, & Marziali, 1986), on a sample of early therapy audiotapes to arrive at a judgment as to whether or not these scales reflect patient–therapist alliance and therapist behavior. The scales measure patient working capacity, both negative and positive patient contributions, patient commitment, working strategy consensus, and therapist understanding and involvement. In a subset of our BPD patients rated with the CALPAS ($n = 18$), therapeutic alliance was lower than that for a group of college counseling center clients (contrasting-group means). In preliminary analyses, the CALPAS-R measure of therapist understanding and involvement was the only scale that significantly differentiated dropouts from remainers.

Therapist Adherence to the Manual

A major goal of the present investigation was to assess our ability to teach a dynamic treatment for borderline patients. Our methods of teaching have been described earlier in this chapter. In order to assess the delivery of the treatment, two rating scales were developed for different phases of the treatment: (1) rating of the setting of the treatment contract between patient and therapist, and (2) rating of sessions after the setting of the treatment contract for verification that the dynamic approach was being followed.

Contract Setting

In our form of therapy, a contract between therapist and patient is made orally at approximately the fifth and sixth sessions. The therapist explains the tasks and roles of therapist and patient that are seen as essential for the treatment to proceed, and explores the patient's understanding and acceptance of these conditions. This contract is based upon the ways in which this particular patient's pathology will probably threaten the treatment. We devised a rating scale that enables a rater to assess (from session transcripts) the patient's contribution to the contract-setting process, the therapist's contribution and exploration in this process, and the consensus that emerges between the two participating parties.

The first question is this: How well did the trainees do in setting the terms of the contract with the BPD patients? In general, the therapists did follow the specifics of the contract setting, noting with the patients the roles of patient and therapist. However, the flexibility and skill with which this contract setting was carried out seemed to vary tremendously. From another point of view, our ability to teach the contract setting was dependent upon the native skills of those therapists to be flexible and skillful with patients, especially difficult patients.

A second question is this: What difference did a good contract setting make? For example, did the negotiation of a contract with skill lead to continuation in treatment? In preliminary analyses, there was a trend for therapist contribution to the contract and the consensus agreement on the contract setting to distinguish the terminators from the remainers. This suggests (along with the results with the CALPAS-R, mentioned earlier) that the therapists' activity was central to the BPD patients' continuation in treatment.

Adherence to Dynamic Techniques

The manual for psychodynamic treatment of the BPD patient calls for the use of the core techniques of clarification, confrontation, and interpretation, and the maintenance of a stance of therapeutic neutrality by the avoidance of supportive techniques (suggestion, giving of advice, etc.), unless such measures are essential to control acting out and the need for them is subsequently explored interpretively. Since BPD patients make extensive use of acting-out defenses, which serve to undermine the treatment process itself, the therapist must identify these defenses and address them with highest priority to protect the treatment. The treatment manual identifies several categories of such defense themes and specifies a hierarchy of priority for addressing them, based on the immediacy of their threat to the treatment.

With these considerations in mind, a rating scale was constructed that permits identification of the type of intervention employed by the therapist, as well as the presence of specific defense or transference themes in the session and the extent to which the therapist targets these themes with specific in-terventions. Thus adherence is assessed in terms of the extent to which expressive psychotherapy techniques (clarification, confrontation, interpretation) rather than supportive ones (suggestion, approval, sympathy, etc.) are employed, and the extent to which the therapist addresses defense themes according to the hierarchy of priorities (e.g., suicidal threats, threats to the treatment, dishonesty and/or withholding, breach of the treatment contract, in-session acting out, out-of-session acting out, trivialization, transference-related themes, affect-laden themes, and childhood material).

To focus the rating and to enhance reliability, a unit of patient material directly preceding each therapist intervention was defined. For each unit, the rater scored the most prominent patient theme, the therapist interventions, and the thematic area toward which the therapist addressed the intervention.

For most patient themes and their corresponding therapist interventions, the reliability coefficients (kappas) were within acceptable ranges. Kappas for patient themes ranged from 1.00 to .83 for categories such as breach of contract, transference references, affect-laden themes, and childhood material. Kappas for direction of therapist intervention were comparable. Kappas for type of therapist intervention ranged from .76 to .60 for the interventions of information, clarification, interpretation, and confrontation. Once the reliability of the scale was established, we applied the adherence instrument to 19 sessions conducted by nine therapists to determine ranges of technique utilization. In general, the majority of therapists utilized the expressive techniques (from 68% to 98% of the time) in regard to salient themes in the hierarchy noted, and they did not utilize supportive techniques. One therapist was deviant on the session rated, utilizing expressive interventions at only a 43% level. In 5 of the 19 sessions, the therapist did not address a high-priority theme.

In future work, we will apply the adherence rating in real time to ongoing treatment, and will provide the findings to therapists and supervisors to permit correction of adherence lapses. We will also monitor the extent to which this feedback is effective.

Therapist Skill Measures

The extent to which the delivered treatment is effective is expected to depend not only on technical adherence, but also on the manner in which the therapist employs the techniques. We identified 22 specific attributes of the therapist's in-session performance and attitude that should determine the skill with which the treatment is carried out. These attributes were derived from a review of skill qualities used in other studies, with the addition of several considered particularly important in work with BPD patients. An instrument was developed to permit rating these 22 items on a 7-point Likert scale. The items may be classified into four overall categories: (1) technical skill, (2) resilience in role, (3) interest and empathy, and (4) transmission of realistic hopefulness. Technical skill includes such skills as timing of interventions, pacing of sessions, clarity of language, and tactfulness. Resilience in role refers to the therapist's ability to remain in the role of therapist without artificial rigidity in the face of the patient's use of such mechanisms as omnipotent control or projective identification, while also being able to tolerate the patient's aggression and other intense affects. Interest and empathy identify appropriate concern, warmth, and empathy. Transmission of hopefulness provides a measure of the therapist's ability to convey expertise and to instill appropriate hopefulness.

The skill-rating instrument was applied to videotapes of five sessions by three judges to determine the interrater reliability of its items. Spearman–Brown reliabilities ranged from .85 to .11, with 15 of the 22 items having reliabilities of .60 or higher. Future work will explore the relationship of skill to training and experience, and to patient outcome.

Core Conflictual Relationship Themes of Patients

We were interested in the concept of "core conflictual relationship themes" (CCRTs) as articulated and measured by Luborsky (1986; Luborsky, Crits-Christoph, Mintz, & Auerbach, 1988). We hypothesized that the CCRTs of borderline patients would be more primitive than those for neurotic patients. We were also intrigued with the possibility that CCRTs might be used as a process–outcome measure for those borderline patients who continued in treatment.

Preliminary work (Schleffer, Selzer, Clarkin, Yeomans, & Luborsky, 1989) indicates that one can identify and rate CCRTs with borderlines in psychodynamic treatment. The most prevalent themes of these BPD patients were as follows:

1. The most frequent wishes were to "avoid conflict" and to "be close to others."
2. The most frequent responses from others were "rejecting" and "oppose me."
3. The most frequent responses from self were "am angry" and "am out of control."

These themes seem consistent with borderline pathology as noted in the DSM-III-R criteria. Aside from the content of their CCRT themes, most striking was the form of the productions. The CCRTs of BPD patients were characterized by confusion between self and object, negative and positive impulses, and wish and action. There were also contradictions between the same components within one relational episode and between relational episodes created later in the same session. Our impression is that borderlines' themes and level of differentiation are different from those of neurotic patients, but direct comparison of CCRTs produced by borderline and nonborderline patients in dynamic therapy is needed.

In the future, we will utilize the CCRTs as a focus of change for each individual patient. We also will utilize the CCRT as a focus of attention or lack of attention by the therapist. That is, although our treatment manual does not relate to CCRTs as such and how they are to be addressed, we will investigate with transcripts how they are employed by therapists using our manual. As noted above, the fact that the CCRTs of borderlines seem to reflect borderline pathology in content and process would make them a natural focus for intervention, especially when the relational episode is one involving the therapist himself/herself (i.e., transference).

Patients' Condition over Time

One of the difficulties in any kind of research with borderline patients is the lack of instrumentation to measure borderline pathology across time. The field of psychotherapy research is equipped to perform a clinical trial of the brief treatment of depression, in large part because there are existing measures of depression that can be used to assess this symptom complex over time. Of course, symptom measures such as the SCL-90 and the BDI have relevance to borderline patients (because they often experience depression), and can be used in a treatment study of BPD patients. It is a common observation, however, that symptoms such as depression and anxiety are quite variable in borderline patients; furthermore, borderlines tend to overreport symptoms. More important than a borderline's highly fluctuating self-report of symptoms is the change in underlying structures of the personality, including identity organization, level of defensive maneuvers, and the coherence of self that enables smooth social functioning and toleration of anxiety.

Given these difficulties, we attempted in this study to utilize existing and recognized measures of symptoms, such as the BDI, the SCL-90, and the SADS-C; in addition, we developed our own semistructured interview and rating scale for assessment of the eight borderline criteria on a dimensional scale (Kernberg & Clarkin, in press). Thus, we are able to provide some preliminary information on the measurement of these specific borderline behaviors as exhibited by our patients during their treatment. This information may enable us not only to assess patient change over time, but also to understand better the process of change in borderline patients. We do not know at present, for example, which borderline behaviors are most likely to change first. Nor do we know which behaviors are most difficult and resistant to change.

We were, of course, not blind to therapy, nor did we have control patients; however, we did attempt to rate the improvement of six patients who had received a sufficient amount (over 6 months) of the treatment, in order to provide some preliminary data. We arrived at a rating of these six patients after 6 months to 5 years of treatment on the following: (1) symptom improvement, (2) improvement in pathology specific to borderlines (as measured by an expanded SCID-II and with information from the therapist), and (3) work/social relations improvement. These three areas were assessed in different ways. Symptom improvement was based upon the patient's self-report on the SCL-90, the BDI, and the Buss–Durkee Hostility Inventory. Improvement on the eight criteria of BPD was rated on a scale of 1–6 (3 represented the criterion level in DSM-III-R); this rating was based on data from an interview (expanded SCID-II) with the patient, as well as on data from the therapist and supervisor. The third area, social adjustment (involving work, school, friends, intimacy, and leisure time), was assessed with the SAS-SR.

The first thing to note is the extent of change on the eight criteria of borderline pathology. As noted earlier, our consensus ratings of change on each of the eight criteria were not made blindly, and our own biases were free to operate. In addition, there was no control group, and any changes could have been due simply to the passage of time. However, we did pool information; moreover, some of the behaviors utilized in the criteria could be rated more or less objectively and were readily apparent (e.g., impulsive alcohol abuse, suicidal behavior).

After at least 6 months in treatment, five of the six patients no longer met critera (at least five of the eight) for the BPD diagnosis (see Table 12.1). Since each criterion was rated on a scale of 1–6, a patient could receive a total score of 15–48. The mean pretreatment score for the six patients was 28.8, and after at least 6 months in treatment the mean score was 16.5 (see Table 12.2). As Table 12.1 indicates, the order of criteria in terms of extent of change shown (from most to least) was as follows: suicidal ideation, impulsivity, affective instability, emptiness and boredom, anger, identity diffusion, fear of abandonment, and unstable interpersonal relations.

TABLE 12.1. Changes in BPD Criteria

Criterion	Mean change	Number (%) exhibiting criterion who showed change	Number still meeting criterion
Suicidal ideation	3.5	6/6 (100%)	0
Impulsivity	1.8	4/5 (80%)	1
Affective instability	1.5	3/3 (100%)	0
Emptiness and boredom	1.5	2/5 (40%)	3
Anger	1.3	3/4 (75%)	1
Identity diffusion	1.3	2/6 (33%)	4
Fear of abandonment	1.0	3/4 (75%)	1
Unstable interpersonal relations	1.0	2/5 (40%)	3

TABLE 12.2. Changes in Six Treatment Remainers

Patient	BPD criteria	Symptoms	Social adjustment
1	Total score changed from 24 to 10; all seven criteria improved	BDI, Buss–Durkee, SCL-90 all improved	Work, friends same; dating improved
2	Total score changed from 31 to 15; went from six criteria to two	No change	Work, dating improved
3	Total score changed from 32 to 17; all seven criteria improved	Buss–Durkee and SCL-90 a little worse	School and friends improved
4	Total score changed from 25 to 15; went from six criteria to two	Little change; BDI went from 25 to 18	Friends improved; dating introduced; began working full-time
5	Total score changed from 26 to 22; went from seven criteria to five	No change	No change
6	Total score changed from 28 to 19; went from eight criteria to four	No change	No change
Overall findings	Mean total score went from 28.8 to 16.5; one patient still BPD	Three no change, two worse, one improved	Four improved

Prior research (Hurt et al., 1990) has established three clusters of BPD criteria. The most robust cluster, the Impulse cluster, shows a high correlation between suicidal behavior and impulsive behavior. It is interesting to note in reference to the changes in our patients that the Impulse cluster (suicide ideation and impulsivity) changed the most and the Identity cluster (identity diffusion and fears of abandonment) changed the least. This is difficult to interpret with the present limited data set. It may be, for example, that suicidal and impulsive behaviors are overt acts that are more easily assessed than such constructs as identity diffusion and fear of abandonment. On the other hand, it may mean that if borderline patients do successfully engage in a structured treatment approach, their impulsive behavior is the first area to show change;

more complex phenomena, such as identity diffusion and fear of rejection and abandonment, may be more difficult to alter.

In the area of social adjustment, four of the six patients reported improvements in friendship patterns, heterosexual behavior, and/or work relations (see Table 12.2). Finally, mixed results were obtained for symptomatology as measured by self-report instruments. Only one patient showed considerable change for the better on these symptom inventories; three showed no change, and one patient showed some worsening.

SUMMARY AND CONCLUSIONS

It is possible at this point to evaluate the findings of this pilot study and to suggest directions for future research with the dynamic treatment of the borderline patient.

We have been able to assess BPD pathology in a number of patients, and have recruited a sample to engage in a long-term dynamic treatment. We have been able to describe a subset of these patients in terms of general symtpoms, BPD pathology along a continuum, and social/work functioning. We have also held a seminar in the dynamic treatment of BPD patients, have produced a manual to guide therapists through the course of such treatment, and have provided supervision in the manual's use.

The dropout rate from dynamic treatment is high, and special attention must be paid to keeping these patients in treatment. One possibility is that patients who are more suited for supportive therapy must be specified before treatment assignment. Another possibility is that therapists preselected for flexibility in relating to angry patients may have greater success in using dynamic techniques with this population. A third possibility that lends itself to empirical investigation is the use of adjunctive medication to control the Impulse cluster of criteria, in order to induce patients into treatment.

We have been successful in measuring therapist adherence to the treatment manual in terms of both contract setting and the use of dynamic techniques around salient patient themes. The scales for rating adherence to the treatment have shown that therapists are variable in their performance. Most adhere to the specific techniques described in the manual. However, more important and more difficult to assess are therapist skill and flexibility in general; some trainees adhere to the techniques in a very rigid and wooden fashion. We must improve our teaching techniques to overcome such lack of skill, or become more selective in the choice of therapists to be trained.

We have been able to distinguish different types of borderline patients. These types, described in terms of three clusters of criteria (Impulse, Anger, and Identity), may prove useful in selecting patients for dynamic versus supportive treatments. We have been able to chart the course of symptoms in these patients across time. The salient symptom clusters that seem most important are (1) BPD criteria; (2) other symptoms, such as depression and anxiety; (3) work or school functioning; (4) friends and intimate relations; and (5) the nature of the relationship with the therapist. In general, when change occurs the BPD criteria improve, and there is some improvement in interpersonal relations (such as contact with friends and dating).

The nature of the relationship with the therapist is both a prognostic sign and a measure of patient progress. To date we have used conventional measures of therapeutic alliance, such as the CALPAS-R, and preliminary findings support the importance of therapist skill in the early phases of the treatment alliance.

We have used the CCRT in an attempt to ascertain the nature of conflictual interpersonal material for borderline patients, and to see how our therapists address such themes. It is our impression at the moment that the CCRTs produced by borderlines are more primitive and fragmented than the CCRTs other researchers have noted in patients who are closer to the neurotic level of personality organization.

The accuracy of symptom assessment over time by a BPD patient on self-report instruments (such as the SCL-90 and the Buss–Durkee) is hard to evaluate. It may be that the reporting is accurate. Alternatively, it may be that the subjective mood of the patient on the day of testing has an influence on the reporting of symptoms for the recent past. This subjective mood of the patient may also be a manifestation of the state of the transference toward the therapist at that point in time. Chance is involved in what day the assessment is made. One method of counteracting the error variance might be to utilize a time-series analysis of self-reports from multiple points in time. In contrast, it is our impression that the assessment of actual behaviors (e.g., self-mutilation, suicide attempts) involves objective behavior that the patient can and does accurately describe.

We have conducted this research with the attitude that dynamic treatment may be a successful and in-depth treatment for an as yet unspecified subgroup of BPD patients. In this study, in fact, we have found that a subgroup of patients do adhere to and take part in this long-term treatment process. This pilot result, however, is heavily confounded in the present data by the experience and overall ability of the therapists. Of the six patients who remained in treatment for a substantial period of time, three were with faculty members (experienced therapists), two were with exceptionally talented trainee therapists, and one was with a trainee therapist of moderate skill. In contrast, of the 13 patients who dropped out of treatment by 12 weeks, only one had a faculty therapist, and another had a relatively talented trainee. The rest had moderately skilled to weak trainee therapists.

Given this caveat, what impression do we have of the patients who might benefit from dynamic treatment? History of seriousness and extent of pathology (within the borderline range without psychosis that we studied) will probably not distinguish responders from nonresponders. Rather, we think that the patients' history of treatment attempts and attitude to treatment, and their perceived need for treatment, are most important. A majority of our treatment remainers reported that they had had numerous failed treatments before, and felt that the current treatment was important and pivotal for them. During this treatment, the majority of remainers also had a regular work/school routine. It was as if they could fit the regularity and routine of the therapy into that structure. We would add that severity of symptoms/pathology is not necessarily synonymous with poor or nonexistent functioning in work or school. To summarize, the remainers (and potential responders) to dynamic treatment are those BPD patients who (1) have failed in treatment before and are currently motivated to work at treatment and change in their lives, and (2) who are currently engaged in a structure of some success in work/ school. Of course, these attributes are probably not specific to dynamic treatment, as responders to nondynamic and behavioral–supportive treatments may be so characterized. On the other hand, patients who are not functioning in work/school may respond (at least initially) better to a structured, behavioral program that calls for less internal structure from the patients themselves than does the dynamic treatment.

Another of our general impressions is that therapist skill is harder to teach (and to assess reliably) than therapist adherence to the manual per se. The contract-setting phase of treatment may serve as an illustration. This early phase of treatment requires that the therapist be simultaneously structured and flexible with a patient who often is resistant, has magical beliefs about treatment, and is angry from prior treatment attempts. After taking our training program in dynamic treatment, all of the therapists in the present study set forth the details of the treatment contract as specified by the manual. However, it was in the flexible negotiation of that contract as understood by the patients with their own idiosyncrasies that the therapists were more variable. In this regard, we are not surprised by the recent interest in and assessment of the impact of the particular therapist on the treatment outcome. In fact, we would suspect that this impact would be more pronounced with a more disturbed patient population (e.g., borderlines); with a therapy that is longer in duration; and with more dynamic aspects of therapy that involve the use of judgment and timing (as opposed to very specific behavioral strategies and techniques).

The examination of the treatment of borderline patients presents many challenges to the psychotherapy research enterprise. We believe that the serious nature of borderline pathology precludes any brief treatment as being little more than crisis intervention. On the other hand, the long-term treatments that are called for by the pathology present many research problems, including the choice of a control group, therapist adherence to a long-term manualized treatment, and the possibility of extensive patient dropout over a long-term intervention.

ACKNOWLEDGMENT

The study described in this chapter was partially funded by the Fund for Psychoanalytic Research, the American Psychoanalytic Association.

REFERENCES

American Psychiatric Association. (1980). *Diagnostic and statistical manual of mental disorders* (3rd ed.). Washington, DC: Author.

American Psychiatric Association. (1987). *Diagnostic and statistical manual of mental disorders* (3rd ed., rev.). Washington, DC: Author.

Beck, A. T., Ward, C. H., Mendelson, M., Mock, J., & Erbaugh, J. (1961). An inventory for measuring depression. *Archives of General Psychiatry, 4*, 561–571.

Buss, A. H., & Durkee, A. (1957). An inventory for assessing different kinds of hostility. *Journal of Consulting Psychology, 21*, 343–348.

Clarkin, J. F., & Kernberg, O. (in press). Diagnosis and etiology of borderline pathology. In J. Paris (Ed.), *Borderline personality disorder*. Washington, DC: American Psychiatric Press.

Derogatis, L. R., Lipman, R. S., & Covi, L. (1973). The SCL-90: An outpatient psychiatric rating scale—preliminary report. *Psychopharmacology Bulletin, 9*, 13–27.

Docherty, J. P. (Sect. Ed.). (1985). The therapeutic alliance and treatment outcome. In R. E. Hales & A. J. Frances (Eds.), *Psychiatry update: Annual review* (Vol. 4). Washington, DC: American Psychiatric Press.

Goldberg, S. C., Schulz, C., Schulz, P. M., Resnick, R. J., Hamer, R. M., & Friedel, R. O. (1986). Borderline and schizotypal personality disorders treated with low-dose thiothixene vs. placebo. *Archives of General Psychiatry, 43*, 680–686.

Gunderson, J. G., Frank, A. F., Ronningstam, E. F., Wachter, S., Lynch, V. J., & Wolf, P. J. (1989). Early discontinuance of borderline patients from psychotherapy. *Journal of Nervous and Mental Disease, 177*(1), 38–42.

Hurt, S. W., Clarkin, J. F., Widiger, T., Fyer, M., Sullivan, T., Stone, M., & Frances, A. (1990). Evaluation of DSM-III decision rules for case detection using joint conditional probability structures. *Journal of Personality Disorders, 4*, 121–130.

Kass, F., Spitzer, R. L., & Williams, J. B. W. (1983). An empirical study of the issue of sex bias in the diagnostic criteria of DSM-III Axis II personality disorders. *American Psychologist, 38*, 799–810.

Kernberg, O. F. (1973). Summary and conclusions of "Psychotherapy and psycho-analysis: Final report of the Menninger Foundation's psychotherapy research project." *International Journal of Psychiatry, 11*, 62–103.

Kernberg, O. F. (1975). *Borderline conditions and pathological narcissism*. New York: Jason Aronson.

Kernberg, O. F., & Clarkin, J. F. (in press). The development of a disorder-specific manual: The treatment of borderline personality disorder. In N. E. Miller, J. Docherty, & L. Luborsky (Eds.), *Psychodynamic treatment research*. New York: Basic Books.

Kernberg, O. F., Selzer, M. A., Koenigsberg, H. W., Carr, A. C., & Appelbaum, A. M. (1989). *Psychodynamic psychotherapy of borderline patients*. New York: Basic Books.

Koenigsberg, H. W., Kaplan, R. D., Gilmore, M. M., & Cooper, A. M. (1985). The relationship between syndrome and personality disorder in DSM-III: Experience with 2462 patients. *American Journal of Psychiatry, 142*, 207.

Linehan, M. M. (1987). Dialectical behavior therapy: A cognitive approach to parasuicide. *Journal of Personality Disorders, 1*, 328–333.

Luborsky, L. (1986). *The core conflictual relationship theme method: Guide to scoring and rationale*. Unpublished manuscript.

Luborsky, L., Crits-Christoph, P., Mintz, J., & Auerbach, A. (1988). *Who will benefit from psychotherapy: Predicting therapeutic outcomes*. New York: Basic Books.

Marmar, C., Horowitz, M., Weiss, D., & Marziali, E. (1986). The development of the therapeutic alliance rating system. In L. Greenberg & W. Pinsof (Eds.), *The psychotherapeutic process: A research handbook*. New York: Guilford Press.

Schleffer, E., Selzer, M., Clarkin, J. F., Yeomans, F., & Luborsky, L. (1989, May). *Rating CCRTs with borderline patients*. Paper presented at the annual meeting of the American Psychiatric Association, San Francisco.

Skodol, A., Buckley, P., & Charles, E. (1983). Is there a characteristic pattern to the treatment history of clinical outpatients with borderline patients? *Journal of Nervous and Mental Disease, 171*, 405–410.

Soloff, P. H. (1989). Psychopharmacologic therapies in borderline personality disorder. In A. Tasman, R. E. Hales, & A. J. Frances (Eds.), *Review of psychiatry* (Vol. 8). Washington, DC: American Psychiatric Press.

Spitzer, R. L., & Endicott, J. (1978). *Schedule for Affective Disorders and Schizophrenia—Change Version (SADS-C)* (3/1/78—3rd ed.). Washington DC: National Institute of Mental Health, Clinical Research Branch Collaborative Program on the Psychobiology of Depression.

Waldinger, R. J. (1987). Intensive psychodynamic therapy with borderline patients: An overview. *American Journal of Psychiatry, 144*, 267–274.

Waldinger, R. J., & Gunderson, J. (1984). Completed psychotherapies with borderline patients. *American Journal of Psychotherapy, 38*, 190–202.

Wallerstein, R. S. (1986). *Forty-two lives in treatment*. New York: Guilford Press.

Weissman, M. M., & Bothwell, S. (1976). The assessment of social adjustment by patient self-report. *Archives of General Psychiatry, 33*, 1111–1115.

Zetzel, E. R. (1971). A developmental approach to the borderline patient. *American Journal of Psychiatry, 127*, 43–47.

CHAPTER 13

Group Treatment of Borderline Personality Disorder

HEATHER MUNROE-BLUM

The difficulties associated with individual psychotherapy for borderline personality disorder (BPD) have been well described (Gunderson, 1984; Munroe-Blum & Marziali, 1988). Individual psychotherapy with BPD has been associated with high early dropout rates and generally poor clinical and social outcomes (Gunderson, 1984; Munroe-Blum & Marziali, 1988; Waldinger & Gunderson, 1984). Some believe that individual psychotherapy may do more harm than good (Dawson, 1988; Friedman, 1975; Frances, Clarkin, & Perry, 1984). The studies that have been conducted to assess the effectiveness of individual psychotherapy for BPD are limited in number and generally suffer from methodological weaknesses, such as limited sample size, lack of a control group, retrospective assessments, and measurement problems (Gunderson, 1982, 1984; Munroe-Blum & Marziali, 1988). Nonetheless, there is considerable indication that individual psychotherapy may not be the primary treatment of choice for BPD. Certainly no evidence exists to the contrary. What, then, are the alternatives?

Although group treatment has long been conducted for mixed diagnostic groups of patients, including borderlines, group psychotherapy has historically been viewed as inappropriate for BPD. The disruptive behaviors and demands for exclusive attention typically associated with BPD have been viewed as counterproductive to the development of group cohesiveness and group growth (Munroe-Blum & Marziali, 1988). It might also be argued that therapists have been unwilling to engage in the treatment of a group of patients with BPD. This more or less pervasive attitude about the inappropriateness of group treatment for BPD, and the continued reliance on individual psychotherapy in the absence of its demonstrated effectiveness, are reflective of the fallacy of letting theory guide practice in the absence of empirical validation of treatment approaches. Somewhat surprisingly, in spite of the practice dominance of individual psychotherapy in the treatment of BPD, a number of therapists have utilized group approaches. Although the data are just beginning to accrue, it appears that patients with BPD are capable of achieving improved outcomes through participation in group treatment.

In this chapter, aspects of the conceptual justification for testing group approaches to the treatment of BPD are explored; the existing literature on group studies is reviewed; and contributions of the literature to the future treatment and study of BPD are discussed.

CONCEPTUAL JUSTIFICATION FOR GROUP TREATMENT

BPD can best be described in terms of seven identifying features: impulsivity, low social role achievement, manipulative suicidal behaviors, heightened affect, mild psychotic disturbances, intolerance of being alone, and disturbed close relationships (Gunderson, Kolb, & Austin, 1981). It makes sense that a particular intervention strategy should be promoted for BPD only to the extent that it might feasibly, or demonstrably, correct the problems inherent in this disorder (Munroe-Blum & Marziali, 1988). Group treatment for BPD can be viewed as addressing a majority of the problems associated with the disorder.

We (Munroe-Blum & Marziali, 1988) and Aronson (1989) draw on the work of a range of authors (particularly Stone & Gustafson, 1982; Horwitz, 1977, 1980, 1987; Wong, 1980; and Schreter, 1981) to propose useful ways in which group treatment may achieve positive outcomes related to BPD characteristics:

1. Group therapy can be helpful in diluting the transference relationship, by providing multiple targets of emotional investment and a more controlled therapeutic regression than in individual psychotherapy; this provides the opportunity for identification with other patients as well as the therapist(s).
2. With multiple social role models, a range of feedback, and multiple interpersonal interactions, certain maladaptive social patterns are highlighted, and the opportunities for learning are enhanced.
3. It is likely that patients can more readily accept advice and instruction from peers or in collaboration with peers than from a therapist alone.
4. Group members may serve as an interpersonal buffer for patients anxious about being too close to the therapist.
5. The more schizoid patients may benefit from the stimulation and interaction in a group.
6. Peer pressure can help set limits for members with poor control over impulsive behaviors.

7. Group treatment can provide a benign holding environment that promotes positive personal exploration and enhances individual capacity to deal with affect-laden issues.

Although this overview may describe the potential advantages of group treatment for BPD, it does not answer important related questions such as the following: What specific model and structure should be used for group treatment? Should group treatment be offered in conjunction with other treatments? What are the necessary related characteristics of the therapist? Is using cotherapists advisable? Marziali and I have noted elsewhere (Munroe-Blum & Marziali, 1988) that in treatment of BPD therapeutic errors may be the rule rather than the exception. This is as likely to be true of group as of individual treatment. Traditional group approaches may not be useful with BPD; rather, population-specific therapeutic strategies may best be utilized in promoting therapeutic success in group treatment. Although the empirical testing of group approaches to the treatment of BPD is in its early stages, some group studies exist. Their findings can contribute to useful formulations of group strategies for treatment of BPD and can provide a backdrop for future treatment studies.

REVIEW OF EXISTING LITERATURE ON GROUP TREATMENT

The literature describing aspects of group treatment for BPD is overwhelmingly based on the clinical impressions and case illustrations of seasoned therapists. Although the most effective test of treatment effects would come from a well-conducted experimental or quasi-experimental study design, only two randomized, controlled trials have been initiated on this topic (one of these is currently in progress). Experimental approaches allow for control of a number of potential sources of bias, which might contaminate one's ability to look at the pure effects of the treatment under study; however, other methodological strategies can be employed to add precision to the measurement of effects, even in the absence of experimental design. Inclusion of standard and psychometrically sound diagnostic procedures, selection of representative patients samples, standardization of the therapeutic maneuver, measurement of cointervention(s), predetermination and adequate assessment of outcomes, and complete patient follow-up are some of these approaches.

The literature addressing group treatment of BPD spans nearly 40 years (see Table 13.1 for summary). The literature identified in this chapter was drawn from the references of key books and review articles, as well as the results of a computerized Medline search that spanned roughly the past 15 years. Approximately 19 articles and one book were identified that had relevance for group treatment of BPD. Of these, only the reports of three studies (Macaskill, 1982; Munroe-Blum & Marziali, 1988; Linehan, 1987a, 1987b) specify clearly the diagnostic criteria used in selection of patients, the therapeutic approach of the group treatment, and the particular outcomes of interest and how these were measured. Only two studies could be found that utilized control groups and random allocation of patients to treatment (Munroe-Blum & Marziali, 1991, and Linehan, 1987a, 1987b).

Two key conceptual debates dominate the three decades of literature. The first debate concerns whether treatment groups should be homogeneous groups comprised only of patients with BPD, or heterogeneous groups of patients with mixed diagnoses. The second debate concerns whether group should be adjunctive to other treatment (primarily individual psychotherapy) or should be the primary treatment approach.

The early articles (Knight, 1953; Spotnitz, 1957; Feldberg, 1958; Hulse, 1958) referred primarily to patients with "borderline psychosis," "incipient schizophrenia," or "borderline schizophrenia"; these were essay-style articles with some case illustrations, theoretically driven by psychoanalytic interpretations and formulations. Of these four articles, only that by Knight made reference to group treatment as adjunctive to individual psychotherapy. The other authors proposed group treatment as the primary approach and appeared to be recommending analytic groups of mixed patients, though this was not always clearly specified. At this early stage in the literature, the authors attempted to specify patient features (Hulse, 1958) and features of the therapy (Spotnitz, 1957) that would promote positive outcomes. Worthy of note is the fact that Spotnitz (1957) cautioned therapists against an overly interpretive intervention style, and encouraged therapists to be supportive and to provide structure without being overly intrusive or controlling.

Tabachnick (1965), in keeping with a reliance on case illustration and an essay-style approach, proposed that group combined with individual treatment would provide complementarity of treatment for patients with schizoid and borderline features, particularly those experiencing problems related to isolation. He suggested that the combined treatment would allow for a splitting of the transference: The negative features of the transference would be enacted within the group, allowing for a more productive use of the individual psychotherapy.

Horwitz (1977, 1980, 1987) proposed the use of combined sequential treatments and viewed the group as preparing the patients to make productive use of individual psychotherapy. Horwitz's articles showed a disciplined clinical attention to case material, and his proposals stemmed from the careful study of eight cases. Horwitz did not present the specific diagnostic characteristics of these cases, but defined the patient population as patients with borderline and narcissistic features, which were related to ego capacity versus characterological traits. He identified four patient indicators for group treatment:

TABLE 13.1. Overview of Literature on Group Treatment

Study or studies	Population(s)	Study method	Treatment	Outcome
Knight (1953), Spotnitz (1957), Feldberg (1958), Hulse (1958), Tabachnick (1965), Horwitz (1977, 1980, 1987), Wong (1980), Roth (1980, 1982), Kibel (1980), Stone & Gustafson (1982), Slavinska-Holy (1983)	"Borderline psychosis," "borderline schizophrenia," "incipient schizophrenia," "borderline and narcissistic states" (diagnostic criteria generally vague). Sample size: 1 to 10.	Clinical experience, case illustrations, group illustrations.	Sequential group–individual; concurrent group–individual; homogeneous patient groups; heterogeneous patient groups.	Combined treatment provided reciprocity, complementarity of treatment; group allowed for dilution of transference, controlled therapeutic regression, control of behavior, social learning, dilution of countertransference.
Schreter (1981)	Somaticizing borderline patients (vague diagnostic criteria). Sample size: 12.	Before–after.	Insight-oriented, diagnostically heterogeneous group.	Group contributed to decreased use of medical services, decreased emergency contacts with therapists, improved emotional coping, and improved interpersonal relations.
Macaskill (1982)	Borderline female patients (specific criteria). Sample size: 9.	Before–after or retrospective study.	Focal, interpretive homogeneous group treatment.	Improved self-understanding; gains from altruistic behaviors.

Munroe-Blum & Marziali (1988)	Borderline patients (specific diagnostic criteria). Sample size: 8.	Before–after.	Sequential individual–group, time-limited.	Benefits to cotherapists for group; sequence was unfavorable, perhaps due to switching therapists between treatments; those who stayed in group made clinical gains for the most part.
Linehan (1987a, 1987b)	Parasuicidal borderline women (specific diagnostic criteria). Sample size: 22.	Randomized, controlled trial.	Combined individual–group dialectical behavior therapy versus community treatment as usual.	Decreases in parasuicidal episodes, severe behaviors, symptoms, and treatment dropouts, and improved work status, for those receiving experimental treatment.
Munroe-Blum & Marziali (1991)	Borderline patients (specific diagnostic criteria). Sample size: 60+.	Randomized, controlled trial.	Time-limited relationship management group versus individual treatment as usual.	Forthcoming.
Salvendy (1989)	Severe borderlines (specific diagnostic criteria). Sample size: unknown.	Before–after.	Time-limited group—individual induction.	Group as adjunct only; small gains, if any.

demandingness, egocentrism, social isolation and withdrawal, and social deviance. He viewed group treatment as providing the patients with the opportunity to dilute the transference, to explore affects, to attain emotional gratification, and to express hostility productively. Horwitz was one of the first authors to describe the positive (as opposed to negative) effects of group treatment for the therapist, stating that it may also allow for a dilution of the countertransference.

Wong (1980) proposed simultaneous individual and group treatment for patients with unspecified borderline and narcissistic features. Using his clinical experiences and illustrations from groups of identity-impaired patients, he described the therapist's subjective responses to group treatment. Roth (1980, 1982) proposed that a six-type, group-related diagnostic schema, derived from the individual psychoanalytic work of Rosenfeld (1978), would add clarity to analytic group psychotherapy of borderline and narcissistic patients. He suggested that groups of these patients move through at least four stages of development, and that this developmental group process (and the related provision of multiple "objects") is beneficial to the individual patients. Although Roth's proposals are interesting and may be testable, they have not yet been empirically substantiated.

Kibel (1980), also relying on clinical experience and case illustrations, promoted combined individual and group psychotherapy for borderline and narcissistic patients; he reaffirmed the reciprocity of the two treatments, as identified earlier by Tabachnick (1965). Kibel acknowledged the spectrum of psychopathology represented in this patient population, and incorporated group theory into treatment formulations for these patients. He recommended that each group be composed whenever possible with reference to such patient characteristics as ego structure, motivation, and psychological-mindedness.

Schreter (1981), in the first formal investigation of group treatment for patients including borderlines, conducted a before–after study of 12 somaticizing patients. The group was conceptualized as an insight-oriented experience; however, confrontation was limited, especially in the early stages of the group. Although standardized diagnostic criteria do not appear to have been applied, the patients clearly had many borderline features. At outcome patients appeared to have decreased their use of medical services, increased their capacity for dealing effectively with affect-laden material, and improved their interpersonal relationships. Of note is the observation that in this therapy patients were encouraged to phone their group therapist in cases of emergency, but rarely did so.

Stone and Gustafson (1982) proposed specific techniques in group psychotherapy of narcissistic and borderline patients. Using clinical experience and case illustrations, they suggested a developmental approach to the individual patient and to assessing the fit between individual and group development. They viewed the working alliance as a goal, rather than as an intermediate step in group treatment. They noted that not enough is known about the use of interpretation and the management of noninterpretive relationships in a group. They identified a role for an active and supportive, but nonintrusive and noninterpretive, therapeutic stance.

Macaskill (1982) conducted the first study of a homogeneous group of borderlines. Patients were diagnosed systematically, using the critera of Gunderson and Singer (1975), and were treated with focal, interpretive group therapy. Nine female patients reported their individual progress according to Yalom's 12 therapeutic factors (Yalom, 1975). Overall, the patients rated themselves as having made positive gains as a result of the group. In particular, they reported that their self-understanding or insight had increased, and that they had been helped through the opportunity to help others (altruism). Macaskill's findings provide some support for the unique merits of group treatment, as altruistic behaviors cannot be readily expressed in individual treatment.

Slavinska-Holy (1983) proposed combined individual treatment and diagnostically homogeneous group treatment. Drawing on her clinical experience and using case vignettes, she asserted the reciprocity of the two treatments for managing the transference and for promoting learning. Slavinska-Holy proposed specific therapeutic techniques, including the active use of role play.

In 1988, Marziali and I (Munroe-Blum & Marziali, 1988) first proposed time-limited group psychotherapy for BPD. We cited the lack of empirical support for the individual treatment of BPD, the adances in classification of the disorder, and the nature of the disorder as indications for the usefulness of testing time-limited group approaches. We also drew on findings of a pilot study in which sequential treatment (10 individual sessions followed by 16 sessions in a homogeneous group) was explored in a before–after fashion. Fourteen subjects qualified for the pilot treatment study on standardized diagnostic criteria. Of these, eight were eligible for the study. Although the study suffered from treatment dropouts at the rate generally reported (50%), several conclusions followed from the investigation. First, the individual induction to the group was unsuccessful: All patients reported difficulty in making the transition from the individual to the group phase of treatment, as well as difficulty in switching therapists. Second, all but one of those who participated in the group manifested improvements on standardized outcome assessments. These improvements included less depression and/or anxiety, more satisfying interpersonal contacts, and enhancement of self-appraisal skills. Third, a cotherapy group model had advantages for patients and therapists. Based on this early experience, we have launched a randomized, controlled trial (Munroe-Blum & Marziali, 1991).

In this trial (still in progress), a relationship management therapy model (Dawson, 1988) applied to short-term (cotherapist-led) group treatment of a diagnostically homogeneous group of patients with BPD is being compared to individual "treatment as usual" of borderline patients with the same characteristics. Patients are diagnosed by means of the Diagnostic Interview for Borderlines (DIB; Gunderson et al., 1981). Patients from the McMaster University Department of Psychiatry Clinics are assessed on a number of reliable and valid measures of clinical, social, and behavioral outcomes at several follow-up intervals. The experimental intervention is manual-guided. Therapists for both treatments have similar levels of experience and represent a range of professional disciplines. Patients are followed in the study, regardless of their compliance with the assigned treatment. Over 60 patients have been randomly assigned to the treatments to date. Many patients have found the group treatment to be acceptable, and treatment outcome comparisons are to be reported shortly. It is anticipated that this study will produce considerable information on the usefulness of a particular time-limited group approach in the treatment of BPD.

The only other randomized trial study of treatment for BPD has been conducted by Marsha Linehan and colleagues at the University of Washington. Linehan investigated the use of combined individual and group dialectical behavior therapy (Linehan, 1987a, 1987b) for 22 parasuicidal BPD women, diagnosed by means of the DIB and other standardized assessments. In this study, the experimental treatment was manual-guided, and subjects were assessed over several follow-up intervals. At outcome the experimental group had less parasuicidal episodes, less severe dysfunctional behaviors, a decrease in symptoms, a decrease in treatment dropout, and improved work status, in comparison with control subjects who received community treatment as usual (Linehan, 1987a, 1987b).

In 1989, Salvendy published a paper describing a study of a time-limited group approach in which individual induction by nongroup therapists took place over two sessions and an insight-oriented, cognitive–behavioral model of group treatment was then utilized. Group treatment lasted 16 sessions, and cotherapists were employed. Salvendy concluded from his study that this time-limited group treatment posed difficulties for therapists and patients. Among other things, patients rated the group as lasting too short a time. Salvendy proposes that time-limited group treatment might best be used as an adjunct to individual treatment. Although this paper presents a nice description of the group process and techniques, the lack of detail regarding the diagnostic criteria applied in selecting patients, the number of patients enrolled in and completing the study, and the number of follow-up assessments raises some question about the author's conclusions.

To summarize the overall contributions of this broad literature, it is worthy of note that with a few exceptions, it is driven by psychoanalytic formulations. Furthermore, only two or three studies have been conducted that meet any of the scientific or methodological criteria necessary to begin to demonstrate the effectiveness of group treatment for BPD. Moreover, the papers that have been written do little to delineate the merits of one group approach versus another, or of group treatment alone versus group treatment as an adjunct to individual treatment. On the other hand, numerous senior and respected clinicians convincingly describe the acceptability of a range of group approaches for both therapists and patients, and provide strong theoretical and clinical justification for group approaches. One well-conducted study (that by Linehan) provides convincing evidence in support of one particular combined individual–group approach. Data will shortly be forthcoming from another randomized trial describing the effects of a time-limited group approach (Munroe-Blum & Marziali, 1991) to BPD treatment. Group treatment can provide a forum within which to incorporate approaches that directly promote self-sufficiency and improved social role performance for those with BPD.

IMPLICATIONS FOR FUTURE RESEARCH AND TREATMENT

It appears from the literature that group treatment of BPD is acceptable to patients and can contribute to positive clinical and behavioral outcomes. Although specific group approaches and treatment effects remain to be tested, a number of guidelines might be adopted for group treatment of BPD. Cotherapy models can provide support to both therapists and patients. There may be reciprocal benefits to using group therapy as an adjunct to individual therapy. When combined treatment models are employed, it may be useful to use the same therapists for both treatments. It is worth exploring the use of group treatment in preparing patients for individual treatment, but probably not the reverse. Both time-limited and longer-term group approaches may contribute positively to clinical and social outcomes.

From a research perspective, we have barely begun to rigorously investigate the potential effects of any psychotherapy or psychosocial therapy for BPD. The field is greatly in need of experimental and quasi-experimental study designs to assess the relative merits of group treatment versus other treatments, of one group approach versus another, and of combined treatment approaches. Although the findings of such studies may only confirm the judgments of experienced clinicians, they will contribute much to the effective training of new clinicians and to the planning of treatment services for this often ill-managed group of patients. Group approaches are particularly worthy of investigation, because they constitute acceptable, rational, and efficient treatment with strong potential to improve the clinical and behavioral functioning of patients with BPD.

REFERENCES

Aronson, T. A. (1989). A critical review of psychotherapeutic treatments of the borderline personality. *Journal of Nervous and Mental Disease, 177*(9), 511–528.

Dawson, D. (1988). Treatment of the borderline patient: Relationship management. *Canadian Journal of Psychiatry, 33*(5), 370–374.

Feldberg, T. M. (1958). Treatment of "borderline" psychotics in groups of neurotic patients. *International Journal of Group Psychotherapy, 8,* 76–84.

Frances, A., Clarkin, J., & Perry, S. (1984). *Differential therapeutics in psychiatry: The art and science of treatment selection.* New York: Brunner/Mazel.

Friedman, H. J. (1975). Psychotherapy of borderline patients: The influence of theory on technique. *American Journal of Psychiatry, 132,* 1048–1052.

Gunderson, J. G. (1982). Empirical studies of the borderline diagnosis. In L. Grinspoon (Ed.), *Review of psychiatry* (Vol. 2). Washington, DC: American Psychiatric Press.

Gunderson, J. G. (1984). *Borderline personality disorder.* Washington, DC: American Psychiatric Press.

Gunderson, J. G., Kolb, J. E., & Austin, F. (1981). The Diagnostic Interview for Borderline Patients. *American Journal of Psychiatry, 138,* 896–903.

Gunderson, J. G., & Singer, M. T. (1975). Defining borderline patients: An overview. *American Journal of Psychiatry, 132,* 1–9.

Horwitz, L. (1977). Group psychotherapy of the borderline patient. In P. Hartocollis (Ed.), *Borderline personality disorders.* New York: International Universities Press.

Horwitz, L. (1980). Group psychotherapy for borderline and narcissistic patients. *Bulletin of the Menninger Clinic, 44,* 181–200.

Horwitz, L. (1987). Indication for group psychotherapy with borderline and narcissistic patients. *Bulletin of the Menninger Clinic, 51,* 248–260.

Hulse, W. C. (1958). Psychotherapy with ambulatory schizophrenic patients in mixed analytic groups. *Archives of Neurology and Psychiatry, 79,* 681–687.

Kibel, H. (1980). The importance of a comprehensive clinical diagnosis for group psychotherapy of borderline and narcissistic patients. *International Journal of Group Psychotherapy, 30,* 427–440.

Knight, R. P. (1953). Borderline states. *Bulletin of the Menninger Clinic, 17,* 1–12.

Linehan, M. M. (1987a). Dialectical behavior therapy: A cognitive behavioral approach to parasuicide. *Journal of Personality Disorders, 1,* 328–333.

Linehan, M. M (1987b). Dialectical behavior therapy for borderline personality disorder: Theory and method. *Bulletin of the Menninger Clinic, 51,* 261–276.

Macaskill, N. D. (1982). Therapeutic factors in group therapy with borderline patients. *International Journal of Group Psychotherapy, 32*(1), 61–73.

Munroe-Blum, H., & Marziali, E. (1988). Time-limited, group psychotherapy for borderline patients. *Canadian Journal of Psychiatry, 33,* 364–369.

Munroe-Blum, H., & Marziali, E. (1991). [Time-limited group treatment of borderline personality disorder]. Study in progress.

Rosenfeld, H. (1978). Notes on the psychopathology and psychoanalytic treatment of some borderline patients. *International Journal of Psycho-Analysis, 59,* 215–222.

Roth, B. E. (1980). Understanding the development of a homogeneous identity-impaired group through countertransference phenomena. *International Journal of Group Psychotherapy, 30,* 405–426.

Roth, B. E. (1982). Six types of borderline and narcissistic patients: An initial typology. *International Journal of Group Psychotherapy, 32,* 9–27.

Salvendy, J. T. (1989). Short-term group psychotherapy with severe borderlines. *Group Analysis, 22,* 309–316.

Schreter, R. K. (1981). Treating the untreatables: Group experience with somaticizing borderline patients. *International Journal of Psychiatry, 10*(3), 205–215.

Slavinska-Holy, N.M. (1983). Combining individual and homogeneous psychotherapies for borderline conditions. *International Journal of Group Psychotherapy, 33,* 297–312.

Spotnitz, H. (1957). The borderline schizophrenic in group psychotherapy: The importance of individualization. *International Journal of Group Psychotherapy, 7,* 155–174.

Stone, W. N., & Gustafson, J. P. (1982). Technique in group psychotherapy of narcissistic and borderline patients. *International Journal of Group Psychotherapy, 32*(1), 29–47.

Tabachnick, N. (1965). Isolation, transference-splitting, and combined therapy. *Comprehensive Psychiatry, 6,* 336–346.

Waldinger, R., & Gunderson, J. (1984). Completed psychotherapies with borderline patients. *Archives of General Psychiatry, 38,* 190–202.

Wong, N. (1980). Combined group and individual treatment of borderline and narcissistic patients: Heterogeneous versus homogeneous groups. *International Journal of Group Psychotherapy, 30,* 389–404.

Yalom, I. D. (1975). *The theory and practice of group psychotherapy* (2nd ed.). New York: Basic Books.

CHAPTER 14

Multimodal Treatment of Borderline Personality Disorder

ROBERT J. WALDINGER

Borderline personality disorder (BPD) is notoriously difficult to treat, and mental health professionals routinely utilize more than one treatment modality in their efforts to address the multiple and varied problems associated with this diagnosis. The majority of borderline patients—both inpatient and outpatient—receive some form of psychotherapy and a trial of at least one medication during the course of treatment (Soloff, 1981; Skodol, Buckley, & Charles, 1983). In addition to pharmacotherapy and individual psychodynamic therapy of the expressive or supportive variety, borderline patients may also receive cognitive and behavioral therapies, group therapy, family therapy, marital therapy, hospital milieu treatment, day hospitalization, or community residential treatment. Often these treatments run concurrently, and together they comprise our armamentarium in the struggle to alleviate the dramatic and often life-threatening symptoms of this disorder.

Despite the frequency with which clinicians use multiple treatment modalities with borderline patients, there is a striking absence of research in this area. Medline and Mental Health Abstracts computer searches of the literature from 1966 through 1989 revealed only 11 articles dealing specifically with combinations of treatment modalities for patients with BPD (Kretsch, Goren, & Wasserman, 1987; Linehan, 1987; Roth & Stiglitz, 1971; Shapiro, Shapiro, Zinner, & Berkowitz, 1977; Slavinska-Holy, 1983; Stein, 1981; Stone, Stone, & Hurt, 1987; Tucker, Bauer, Wagner, Harlam, & Sher, 1987; Waldinger & Frank, 1989a; Wong, 1980a; Zinner, 1978). Of these studies, only five used empirical approaches that moved beyond the level of the individual case report (Kretsch et al., 1987; Linehan, 1987; Stone et al., 1987; Tucker et al., 1987; Waldinger & Frank, 1989a).

How might we account for this paucity of research? Certainly, the problems facing investigators in other areas are applicable to the study of multimodal treatment:

1. Before the publication of the *Diagnostic and Statistical Manual of Mental Disorders*, third edition (DSM-III), there was no consensus about the diagnosis of BPD. Even now, controversy surrounds the diagnosis, and empirical efforts to demarcate the boundaries of the disorder with increasing precision continue.

2. Few of the treatment modalities used with borderline patients have been standardized, making it difficult for investigators to insure that the treatments under study are specified adequately and are delivered with a reasonable degree of uniformity. Moreover, many clinicians argue that manualized treatments inhibit the therapist and thereby limit the efficacy of the therapeutic endeavor.

3. Long-term psychosocial treatments, the mainstay of most approaches to BPD, are labor-intensive and therefore expensive. Funding for the study of these modalities has been limited.

4. Outcome measures specific to the treatment of BPD are not well developed, and there is disagreement about which variables are the most important indicators of improvement.

In addition to these constraints, which affect all treatment research with borderline patients, the study of multimodal treatment has its own special complications:

1. How the investigator chooses to define a multimodal treatment condition may vary considerably. The component treatments may be administered concurrently or consecutively or intermittently; moreover, they may be weighted equally, or one may be an adjunct to another or considered of secondary importance.

2. Multiple modalities require multiple comparison groups. Thus, larger numbers of subjects are needed than is the case in single-modality studies (e.g., placebo-controlled medication trials).

3. Control over the delivery of treatment is more complicated and requires increased monitoring as additional modalities are added to a study design.

4. Outcome research has not established definitively which individual treatments are most effective with borderline patients. As a result, there are no clear guidelines for researchers to use when deciding on which combinations of treatments warrant the most intensive investigation. For example, it is not yet clear whether expressive or supportive techniques (or some mixture of these) are most effective with borderline patients. Thus, it would be difficult to decide which type of individual psychodynamic psychotherapy to include as a treatment condition in a multimodal treatment outcome study.

Research on BPD may well follow the course of treatment research in schizophrenia. In the latter case, initial empirical studies were aimed at improved definition of the syndrome, while treatment studies were largely confined to case reports of intensive individual psychotherapies. This was followed by a period of more systematic and large-scale controlled clinical trials that pitted one modality (intensive individual psychotherapy) against another (pharmacotherapy). As clinicians and researchers became increasingly aware of the limitations of this unimodal approach to the treatment of schizophrenia, investigators began to pay more attention to other treatment modalities (e.g., family psychoeducational treatment) and to combinations of modalities. A similar shift away from an emphasis on intensive psychodynamic therapy alone may be occurring in the treatment of BPD (Aronson, 1989). To date, however, the existing work on multimodal treatment of BPD remains rudimentary and preliminary; thus, any discussion of this work must of necessity yield more questions than answers. Since there are so many possible combinations of treatments that might be used with borderline patients, it would be impossible to cover all of them. The following discussion is therefore limited to those combinations of treatments that are most often cited in the literature, and that have been the subjects of the few existing empirical studies. These are (1) hospital treatment and individual psychotherapy, (2) group psychotherapy and individual psychotherapy, (3) pharmacotherapy and individual psychotherapy, and (4) family therapy and individual psychotherapy. Discussion focuses on the rationale for each combination, the empirical work done to date, and the implications of this preliminary work for future research.

HOSPITAL TREATMENT AND INDIVIDUAL PSYCHOTHERAPY

Rationale

The combination of individual psychodynamic therapy and hospital treatment has long been advocated for the treatment of BPD (see, e.g., Masterson, 1972; Kernberg, 1975; Gunderson, 1984). Many rationales for this combination have been put forward in the literature, and the following are among the most common:

1. *Engagement.* Borderline patients are difficult to engage in psychotherapy, and a sizeable proportion leave treatment precipitously in the early phases (Gunderson et al., 1989). Hospitalization can afford many patients a supportive environment in which they can begin to negotiate a relationship with a psychotherapist; in effect, it enables some patients to form an early treatment alliance (Eppel, 1988).

2. *Containment of acting out.* Individual psychotherapy often activates negative transference feelings early in the treatment of borderline patients, and these feelings may prompt patients to act in ways that are destructive to themselves, to others, and to the treatment. Prolonged and serious acting out of transference feelings for the psychotherapist may make meaningful psychotherapeutic work impossible. To the extent that hospitalization curtails acting out, it may be essential to the progress of psychotherapy with some borderline patients (Gunderson, 1984).

3. *Access to data.* Borderline patients commonly manifest disparate modes of functioning in different settings and in different relationships. The hospital milieu becomes a field in which borderline patients can display a wide range of pathogenic internalized object relations in their interactions with staff members and other patients (Kernberg, 1984). Information about these intrapsychic constellations may be less available to an individual psychotherapist working in isolation on an outpatient basis, and therefore the constellations may be less amenable to psychotherapeutic intervention than they would be while the patient is hospitalized.

4. *Provision of a holding environment.* Individual psychotherapy may stir up feelings of such intensity that borderline patients sometimes find the psychotherapeutic work unbearable without added support. The hospital provides a holding environment that helps patients weather the storms of a psychotherapeutic relationship during difficult phases of treatment (Adler, 1985). Hospitalization may facilitate certain kinds of work (e.g., the exploration of childhood trauma) that require an atmosphere of physical and emotional safety in order to proceed.

Empirical Work

Two studies bearing on the combination of individual psychodynamic psychotherapy and hospital treatment are worth noting. Neither of these studies focused expressly on combined therapy. Individual psychotherapy was simply one modality used during and after hospital treatment, and each study made some effort to look at the interaction of the hospital stay and individual psychotherapy.

The first study, by Stone et al. (1987) at the New York State Psychiatric Institute, examined a group of 500 patients, 224 of whom were diagnosed retrospectively as having BPD. (The remainder consisted predominantly of patients with other personality disorders, schizoaffective disorder, and schizophrenia.) Patients were selected on the basis of their amenability to psychoanalytically oriented psychotherapy; and they were admitted to the hospital specifically for this treatment. During hospitalization, the psychotherapy was conducted three times per week by psychiatry residents under supervision. After discharge, the frequency and duration of psychotherapy varied considerably.

The hospital treatment included group treatment, family therapy, rehabilitation, and pharmacotherapy, all used in varying combinations with different patients. The average length of hospital stay was 12.5 months, and the range was from 3 to 42 months. Hospital staff members were described as psychoanalytically oriented.

The psychotherapy condition was even less standardized than the hospital treatment. There were no guidelines for the conduct of the therapies, and no standard framework to which all treatments adhered. Treatment varied with the particular resident and supervisor involved in each case, and therapies were not monitored as they progressed.

Investigators made retrospective DSM-III diagnoses of BPD, based on re-examination of charts. Follow-up interviews were conducted with each patient by telephone. The time at follow-up ranged from 10 to 23 years after discharge from the hospital. Data also were collected in interviews with the patients' psychotherapists at the time of follow-up. The study compared patients with borderline, schizophrenic, and schizoaffective disorders with respect to rates of suicide and rehospitalization, work and marriage histories, fertility rates, and scores on the Global Assessment Scale (GAS).

The authors noted that some borderline patients who originally were deemed amenable to psychoanalytically oriented psychotherapy dropped out of treatment after 3 to 4 months, and yet functioned at a very high level at follow-up. They could not therefore conclude that psychoanalytically oriented psychotherapy was essential to these patients' recovery. Those patients who were rated by their therapists as having benefitted most from individual psychotherapy were rated as having high motivation, high psychological aptitude, high suicidality, and low impulsivity at the outset of treatment. They were also rated as high on likeability.

As noted above, this study was not truly multimodal, insofar as its main objective was to examine the effects of long-term hospitalization on the course and outcome of BPD. Neither the hospital treatment nor the individual psychotherapy was studied in a prospective, systematic way. Neither condition was standardized, and no attempt was made to monitor these treatments for consistency as they proceeded. From this study, it is difficult to isolate the specific effects that either hospital treatment or individual psychotherapy had on the course of the borderline disorder. It is not possible to draw conclusions from this study about the differential effects of psychotherapy alone, hospital treatment alone, and the two in combination.

The second study was done by Tucker et al. (1987) at the New York Hospital–Cornell Medical Center, Westchester Division. It was a prospective, 2-year study of 40 patients diagnosed as having borderline personality organization (Kernberg, 1977) and treated on a long-term inpatient unit that specialized in borderline disorders. All patients received individual psychotherapy as part of a treatment program that included group psychotherapy, task groups, patient government, and other therapeutic activities. Among the explicit goals of hospital treatment were improvement in patients' interpersonal relationships, facilitation of a lasting discharge from the hospital, and facilitation of patients' ability to use individual psychotherapy on an outpatient basis.

To evaluate outcome, structured interviews were carried out on admission and at 1 and 2 years after discharge from the hospital. Interview material was scored by independent raters, and patients were assessed with respect to current symptoms, treatment, employment, education, and social life. Ratings on the GAS were also made.

Only 25 of the 40 study patients remained in the hospital longer than 6 months, thereby fulfilling the criterion of being in intermediate or long-term treatment. At both the 1-year and 2-year follow-ups, the majority of these patients were in outpatient psychotherapy. They were more likely to remain in continuous psychotherapy during the 2 years after discharge than they had been in the 2 years prior to hospital admission; there was also a trend toward their remaining with the same therapist throughout the post-discharge years. Patients had significantly fewer hospitalizations in the 2 years after discharge than in the 2 years before admission. These data suggest that hospital treatment facilitates continuance in subsequent outpatient psycho-therapy, but they do not provide information about the relationship between hospital treatment and the outcome of individual psychotherapy.

The authors also found that longer hospital stays were correlated with increased continuance in psychotherapy, a greater likelihood of remaining in treatment with the same therapist, and fewer rehospitalizations after 1 year. However, this correlation did not hold at the 2-year follow-up. The authors concluded that outcome beyond the first year after discharge may not be related to length of hospitalization. They tempered this conclusion with the observations that the number of patients in the study was small; that patients with longer lengths of hospital stay may have been more impaired on admission; that a 2-year follow-up may have been inadequate to assess change; and that the assessment measures used in this study were not specifically geared to borderline psychopathology.

The conclusions that can be drawn from this study about the interaction between hospital treatment and individual psychotherapy are limited in other ways. Not only was the study sample small, but it included a relatively het-erogeneous group of patients. All patients were diagnosed as having borderline personality organization, but not all met the more narrow DSM-III criteria for BPD. Neither the hospital treatment nor the individual psychotherapy was standardized in terms of duration or content.

Nevertheless, the hospital treatment was more uniform than in other studies, in that all patients were treated in homogeneous groups and on one unit specifically designed for borderline disorders. It also was carried out prospectively, using multiple pre- and posthospitalization assessments of both social functioning and psychiatric symptoms.

Further Investigation

The combination of individual psychodynamic therapy and hospital treatment is widely used in working with borderline patients and warrants further systematic investigation. Ideally, research should be carried out using standardized treatments, comparing groups given each treatment alone and in combination. A great deal of preliminary work must be done before such research can be carried out. Manuals for psychotherapy and milieu treatment need to be developed, and protocols for implementing these treatments need to be devised.

Investigators need to distinguish between engagement and continuance in treatment on the one hand, and outcome on the other. The first goal of any treatment is engagement, and a great majority of borderline patients terminate psychotherapy prematurely (Waldinger & Gunderson, 1984). Hospital treatment may facilitate engagement in individual psychotherapy, and may promote continuance in psychotherapy after discharge; yet it may have little effect on the long-term course and outcome of BPD, as was suggested in the study by Tucker et al. (1987).

Investigators must also determine the respective roles of hospital treatment and individual psychotherapy in any given study design. Is hospitalization meant to be an adjunct to and facilitator of individual psychotherapy, and therefore used on an as-needed basis for purposes of alliance building and crisis management? Or is the goal of hospital treatment to provide a setting in which borderline patients can display a fuller range of maladaptive behaviors than can be elicited in a psychotherapists's office, and to offer a therapeutic milieu in which patients can understand and alter these behaviors? The study by Tucker et al. was based on the latter model, whereas the conceptualization of the role of the hospital in the study by Stone and his group was less clear.

The interaction of different types of individual psychotherapy and hospital treatment must also be investigated. The studies discussed above employed intensive psychotherapy and lengthy hospital stays, but other combinations are certainly possible. Intensive exploratory psychotherapy commonly stirs up intense affects and fosters regression that patients and treaters feel safer managing in the hospital. In this way, intensive psychotherapy may foster longer hospital stays. Conversely, supportive psychotherapies, which focus on the management of current problems and on the bolstering of adaptive defenses, may emphasize a rapid return to higher levels of social and occupational functioning and thereby may foster shorter hospital stays. The synergism between the two modalities studied must be given careful attention in any study design.

GROUP PSYCHOTHERAPY AND
INDIVIDUAL PSYCHOTHERAPY

Rationale

For decades, the combination of psychoanalytically oriented group therapy and individual therapy has been advocated as useful for borderline patients.

Initially, group treatment was mentioned in the literature only as a possibly useful adjunct to individual therapy (Kernberg, 1975; Knight, 1953). More recently, clinicians have described the distinct advantages that combined treatment affords over either modality alone. Horwitz (1980, 1987) and Wong (1980a, 1980b) cite several ways in which group treatment can enhance individual therapy:

1. Group psychotherapy dilutes the intense transference that many borderline patients experience in individual treatment; it thus minimizes the likelihood of uncontrolled therapeutic regression.

2. Group treatment highlights certain maladaptive character traits, especially demandingness, egocentrism, greed, and envy. The group provides patients with the opportunity to recognize, reduce, and control maladaptive behaviors, while individual therapy can support the recognition and alteration of these behaviors.

3. Group therapy facilitates the internalization of new self-representations and object representations by providing opportunities for multiple identifications.

4. Group treatment decreases the isolation of more socially withdrawn borderline patients, and provides these patients with numerous models for taking social risks.

5. The group therapy situation asks that the egocentric patient find a balance between working on his/her own problems and investing in helping others with their problems.

6. Via peer pressure, groups can exert a controlling functioning for patients who have poor impulse control.

There is disagreement in the literature about the most desirable structure for combining individual and group treatment for borderline patients. This disagreement centers on two issues: (1) whether group and individual therapy should be conducted by one treater or two, and (2) whether groups should be homogeneous with respect to diagnosis (i.e., composed entirely of borderline patients) or heterogeneous (including patients with different diagnoses).

Stein (1981) distinguishes between "combined" and "conjoint" therapies. Combined therapy involves the simultaneous use of individual and group treatments conducted by the same psychotherapist, whereas conjoint therapy involves the use of different cooperating treaters in the two modalities. Stein advocates a multimodal approach, but he does not specifically state whether combined or conjoint treatment is preferable. In one of the early descriptions of combining group and individual psychotherapy, Roth and Stiglitz (1971) used a conjoint approach with 23 borderline and psychotic outpatients. They reported that the intrapsychic splitting facilitated by the use of two therapists was manageable in most cases and could be therapeutically useful. Wong's (1980a, 1980b) clinical experience leads him to the opposite conclusion: He recommends a combined approach for all borderline patients, in order to avoid facilitating intrapsychic splitting.

With respect to the composition of the group, Slavinska-Holy (1983) advocates homogeneity for several reasons: (1) Homogeneous groups allow for the use of therapeutic techniques designed to address the stage-specific developmental arrests of the borderline patient; (2) homogeneity resolves the group therapist's long-standing dilemma regarding whether to treat the group as a whole or individuals within the group; and (3) homogeneous groups afford patients the opportunity to teach one another about insights particular to borderline psychopathology, thereby reinforcing these insights for themselves. By contrast, Wong (1980a) advocates heterogeneity for groups in which borderline patients are treated. He argues that a preponderance of borderline patients in a group creates an atmosphere of intense oral demands, rage, envy, and devaluation of the therapist. This in turn leads group members to become discouraged and demoralized, and places therapists at risk for unmanageable countertransference reactions.

Linehan (1987; see also Chapter 11, this volume) has developed an alternative to psychodynamically oriented therapy for parasuicidal borderline women, called "dialectical behavior therapy"; it is an offshoot of cognitive—behavioral therapies. She has designed a year-long program of treatment that includes weekly individual therapy and twice-weekly group therapy. The approach is highly structured and directive, with a focus on teaching patients general problem-solving skills, interpersonal skills, and strategies for regulating emotions and tolerating distress. Linehan is currently conducting a study that compares this multimodal dialectical behavior therapy to treatment as usual in the community (Chapter 11 reports preliminary results). It will be interesting to see how this multimodal treatment compares with combined group and individual psychodynamic treatments and with single modalities.

Empirical Work

Only one study has specifically addressed the combination of individual and group treatments. Kretsch et al. (1987) studied patterns of change of borderline patients treated in psychodynamically oriented individual and group psychotherapy. They followed 25 patients who met DSM-III criteria for BPD, and compared this group with 18 patients diagnosed as "neurotic." Patients were treated in weekly group psychotherapy and weekly individual psychotherapy over a number of years. Treatment was designed on an individualized basis, such that some patients began in individual psychotherapy, others in group and individual therapy, and others in group therapy alone. Changes in the mode of treatment used were made as each patient's clinical situation warranted, so that patients received different therapeutic combinations at different times.

Patients were assessed independently by group and individual psycho-therapists after 3 years of treatment, and again after 4 years of treatment, using Bellak's Ego Functions Assessment Scale (Bellak, Hurvich, & Gediman, 1973). This scale measures 11 ego functions: reality testing, judgment, reality sense, control of drives, object relations, thinking processes, regression in the service of the ego, defense mechanisms, stimulus barrier, autonomous functioning, and synthetic functions.

The investigators reported results of these assessments for patients in group therapy, individual therapy, and conjoint therapy. They found that the borderline and neurotic patients in individual psychotherapy (with or without conjoint group therapy) showed significant improvement in ego functioning between the third and fourth years of treatment, relative to baseline. However, the profiles of change for patients as rated by their group psychotherapists were complex: Borderline patients in group treatment showed improvement on all subfunctions of Bellak's scale. By contrast, neurotic patients in group treatment showed improvement in some ego functions, whereas other ego functions (most notably reality testing, reality sense, and object relations) were rated as more disturbed over time.

The authors concluded that at similar temporal stages in therapy, group treatment strengthens ego functioning for borderline patients, whereas it lowers ego defenses for neurotic patients. They further conclude that group treatment is "either a stronger stimulant to or a more appropriate setting for eliciting pronounced changes in ego functioning" than individual therapy (p. 110).

This study has significant limitations. Diagnosis was made by independent raters on the basis of clinical interviews, but the criteria used to diagnose neurotic patients were not specified. Ratings of ego functioning were made by the therapists. Although they were kept unaware of the purpose of the study, they were by no means independent observers. The treatments were not manualized or otherwise standardized, so that patients received varying combinations of group and individual therapy at various times. In analyzing their results, the authors did not separate out those patients in one modality from those in conjoint treatment when analyzing the effects of single modalities. Thus, for example, patterns of change for patients in individual therapy were reported without distinguishing those patients in individual therapy alone from those in conjoint treatment.

Issues for Investigation

Despite its limitations, the Kretsch et al. (1987) study makes an interesting suggestion: that group treatment not only fosters changes that are different from those seen in individual treatment, but also affects different diagnostic groups in different ways. Patterns of change reported by group therapists were different from those reported by individual therapists. These differences might have been due to observer bias or to the particular settings in which the observations took place. Further studies of multimodal treatment might attempt to sort out the differential effects of group and individual treatment, to look at how patients appear to function in different therapeutic settings, and to distinguish the effects of multimodal treatment on borderline patients from those in other diagnostic categories.

The technical and theoretical approaches to individual and group therapy that are most effective with borderline patients have yet to be elucidated, and this leaves the area of multimodal treatment without guidelines for which treatments to include in research protocols. Ideally, comparative studies of psychodynamic approaches and cognitive–behavioral approaches (such as Linehan's) will lay the groundwork for future investigation of the efficacy of combined modalities.

The question of whether combined or conjoint therapy is more effective with borderline patients remains a matter of opinion based on anecdotal information. The question is of central importance to clinicians who are called upon to design treatment plans for borderline patients, and it warrants further research.

PHARMACOTHERAPY AND INDIVIDUAL PSYCHOTHERAPY

Rationale

In the past decade, pharmacotherapy has been used with increasing frequency in the treatment of BPD. As noted at the outset of this chapter, a majority of borderline patients receive a trial of at least one psychotropic agent during the course of their treatment (Soloff, 1981; Skodol et al., 1983). Although medication is commonly used for concurrent Axis I disorders (e.g., major depressive episode), recent studies have shown certain psychotropics to be of modest efficacy in alleviating some of the symptoms of the borderline syndrome itself (Soloff et al., 1986; Goldberg et al., 1986; Gardner & Cowdry, 1986; Cowdry & Gardner, 1988).

There is reason to believe that the combination of psychotherapy and pharmacotherapy may be advantageous in the treatment of BPD. Many borderline patients are incapacitated by depressive symptoms, impulsivity, and mild cognitive distortions, all of which can sometimes be ameliorated by medication. This, in turn, may facilitate the work of psychotherapy (Waldinger & Frank, 1989b).

Empirical Work

To date, there has been virtually no empirical work on the combination of pharmacotherapy and psychotherapy (individual or otherwise) in the treatment of BPD. Among the recent studies of pharmacotherapy, the double-blind placebo-controlled study of amitriptyline and haloperidol conducted by Soloff et al. (1986) used medication "in addition to the usual group, milieu, or individual therapies available on the inpatient units" (p. 692). Outpatients in that study were seen in weekly psychotherapy, in addition to their visits to the psychopharmacologist. However, Soloff et al. made no attempt either to control for or to study the interpersonal therapies delivered to their study patients.

In an effort to identify psychosocial factors that influence psychotherapists' decisions about whether or not to use medication with borderline patients, a colleague and I (Waldinger & Frank, 1989a) surveyed 40 psychiatrists in private practice about their prescribing practices with borderlines whom they treated in individual psychodynamic psychotherapy. This survey corroborated the clinical impression that therapists' decisions about whether and when to use medication with borderline patients are strongly influenced by psychosocial factors. Therapists were most likely to prescribe medications when they felt pessimistic about patients' capacity to benefit from psychotherapy, and they were rarely willing to prescribe for patients who had a history of substance abuse or suicide attempts. Most therapists in this survey believed that medication use often strengthened the therapeutic alliance with their borderline patients and rarely weakened it. Although most of the 40 psychiatrists surveyed did the prescribing for the borderline patients whom they treated in psychotherapy, some stated a preference for having another physician serve as pharmacotherapist while they themselves continued to do the psychotherapy.

This survey was not a study of the effects of multimodal treatment on the course and outcome of BPD. Rather, it was an attempt to look at how clinicians currently make decisions about introducing pharmacotherapy during ongoing individual psychotherapy with borderline patients, as well as some of the consequences of the decision to do so.

Issues for Investigation

Despite its limitations, our survey (Waldinger & Frank, 1989a) raises some interesting questions for further research. Given the current paucity of guidelines for clinicians who consider combining pharmacotherapy and psychotherapy for borderline patients, the factors that influence their decisions warrant further study. Treatment compliance is also an important area for future research, as medication abuse appears to be quite common among borderline patients. Therapists in this study reported that on average, 47% of the medicated patients in each therapist's practice abused medication at some point in treatment. Because it often elicits intense negative transference reactions, psychodynamic therapy may exacerbate medication misuse. However, insofar as it provides a holding environment for borderline patients, psychotherapy may facilitate compliance. It would thus be useful to study medication compliance in the presence or absence of an ongoing psychotherapy.

The question of combined versus conjoint therapy (i.e., one or two treaters) is of particular relevance to the combination of pharmacotherapy and psychotherapy. Combined treatment has the potential advantage of affording one clinician an overview of the entire treatment, which may be invaluable in attempting to distinguish medication effects and side effects from reactions to the therapist and to other important people in the patient's life. Conjoint treatment, on the other hand, may decrease the likelihood of medication abuse by separating the act of prescribing from the intense, transference-laden environment of the psychotherapy. These two treatment frames need further systematic study.

In designing future research on the combination of pharmacotherapy and psychotherapy, investigators must develop a standard treatment manual for pharmacotherapy. Obviously, there is great variation in the types of interactions that occur between prescriber and borderline patient, and many pharmacotherapists deliver supportive and sometimes even exploratory treatment in the course of brief medication interviews. The pharmacotherapy condition must be standardized and monitored just as carefully as the psychotherapy condition in any study of multimodal treatment.

FAMILY THERAPY AND INDIVIDUAL PSYCHOTHERAPY

No empirical work has been done on the combination of family therapy and individual psychotherapy, and there are few case reports in the literature. Many individual psychotherapists, such as Gunderson (1984), have mentioned the usefulness of family therapy as an adjunctive technique. However, the writers discussed below have specifically advocated the combination of family and individual therapy as more effective than either modality alone, particularly for borderline adolescents. Shapiro et al. (1977) studied borderline adolescents and observed that the working alliance between patient and individual psychotherapist was consistently facilitated by the active participation of the individual therapist in concurrent conjoint family therapy. Zinner (1978) summarized the advantages of a combined treatment approach over the exclusive use of each component. He noted that a borderline adolescent usually seeks treatment in a crisis situation (e.g., a suicide attempt) in which the family is intensely involved, and a multimodal approach considers the family as both a locus of the problem and a resource for its solution. The adolescent's arrested development is seen as tied to the family's unconscious motivations and fears. To the extent that these are uncovered in family therapy, they provide important material for the patient's individual psychotherapy as well as the family work. New perspectives gained by the adolescent in individual psychotherapy can be introduced into the family treatment, and family reactions to the adolescent's age-appropriate behaviors can be observed and modified. Without combined treatment, the gains made by the adolescent in individual therapy are often met with intense resistance in the family and cannot be sustained. Concurrent family therapy can prevent this process and mobilize the family's resources for positive change. Concurrent couples treatment is also seen as helpful in this model.

Because no systematic studies of this multimodal approach have been carried out, it is impossible to evaluate its utility beyond the evidence of anecdotal reports. Moreover, it is not clear that psychodynamically oriented family therapy is the modality of choice in a multimodal treatment frame. In recent years, the approaches of the structural and strategic schools of family therapy have appeared promising in the treatment of difficult patients (see, e.g., Minuchin, 1974; Haley & Hoffman, 1967; Hoffman, 1981). These approaches have been outside the mainstream of psychiatry, largely because they redefine problems as systemic and view individual diagnoses and psychodynamics as largely irrelevant (Aronson, 1989). They offer potentially valuable techniques that should be examined in studies of combined family and individual psychotherapy.

SUMMARY AND DISCUSSION

This chapter brings into bold relief the paucity of information about combined treatment approaches for BPD currently available. Multimodal treatment is now standard care for borderline patients, which makes this gap in our knowledge particularly important and glaring. This review has attempted to highlight issues relevant to the empirical study of combined treatment. These issues are summarized below.

1. *The nature of multimodal treatment.* What constitutes a multimodal treatment varies considerably from one clinical setting to another. In much of the clinical literature on combined treatment, one modality is central, and others are adjunctive. One modality may be used to prepare the patient for treatment in another (e.g., hospitalization as a means of engaging a patient in individual psychotherapy), or as a means of eliciting clinical data that can then be worked with in another. Investigators must be clear about the relative roles of different treatments in a combined framework, as well as the rationale for assignment of these roles.

2. *Time frame.* Combined treatment often connotes the use of two or more modalities simultaneously. However, the provision of multiple therapies on an ongoing basis (e.g., medication and group psychotherapy) is by no means the only arrangement that falls into the category of multimodal treatment. Therapies may be sequential rather than concurrent, or one therapy may be ongoing while others are added intermittently. Different treatments may be appropriate for different phases of the disorder (e.g., hospitalization and

large-group work during an initial crisis, followed by day treatment and small-group work, followed by individual outpatient psychotherapy).

3. *One or more treaters*. The issue of combined versus conjoint treatments is most clearly discussed in the literature on group and individual psychotherapy. It is also particularly relevant in combining pharmacotherapy and various forms of psychotherapy. Although we have outlined elsewhere the potential advantages and disadvantages of "splitting the treatment" (Waldinger & Frank, 1989b), there is to date no empirical evidence for the greater utility of a one- or two-treater strategy in working with borderline patients.

4. *Manualizing treatments for empirical investigation*. Treatments must be standardized if meaningful comparisons of their efficacy are to be made. This is true not only for the individual, group, and family psychotherapies, but also for pharmacotherapy and hospital treatment. Hospital treatment is itself multidimensional, and researchers must attempt to identify and operationalize the active ingredients in hospitalization for borderlines in order to study it in combination with other modalities. Comparison of combined treatment approaches with single treatments and with other combinations of treatments will be more feasible once manuals for each modality have been written and tested.

5. *Monitoring the treatment process*. None of the studies reviewed here attempted to monitor the delivery of treatment while it occurred. Such monitoring would be essential to insure that treatments were delivered with some degree of uniformity.

6. *Measuring the outcome of treatment*. Outcome measures specific to the resolution of borderline psychopathology have not been well developed. There is debate about whether such specially tailored instruments are needed, or whether more general assessments (e.g., the GAS) are satisfactory measures of change in borderline patients. Several issues pertaining to outcome are unique to the study of multimodal treatments:

a. *Synergism*. Investigators must consider the ways in which various combinations of treatments may enhance or detract from one another.

b. *Compliance*. Combined treatments may facilitate or impede patients' ability to comply with treatment. Dropout rates are high among patients with BPD (Gunderson et al., 1989), and it would be useful to analyze the effect of multimodal treatments on continuance and compliance.

c. *Multiple fields of observation*. The study by Kretsch et al. (1987), in which group and individual therapists performed independent ratings of the same patient over a 1-year time span, illustrates the complexities of assessing patients in different settings. Changes that appear in one modality may not appear in another, and these differences may yield important information about how particular therapies work.

As empirical research on single treatment modalities continues, it will lay the groundwork for more systematic study of combined approaches. Such work is sorely needed, as clinicians remain eager for guidelines that will enable them to plan more rational treatments for their borderline patients.

REFERENCES

Adler, G. (1985). *Borderline psychopathology and its treatment.* Northvale, NJ: Jason Aronson.

Aronson, T. A. (1989). A critical review of psychotherapeutic treatments of the borderline personality: Historical trends and future directions. *Journal of Nervous and Mental Disease, 177,* 511–528.

Bellak, L., Hurvich, M., & Gediman, H. (1973). *Ego functions in schizophrenics, neurotics and normals.* New York: Wiley.

Cowdry, R. W., & Gardner, D. L. (1988). Pharmacotherapy of borderline personality disorder: Alprazolam, carbamazepine, trifluoperazine, and tranylcypromine. *Archives of General Psychiatry, 45,* 111–119.

Eppel, A. B. (1988). Inpatient and day hospital treatment of the borderline: An integrated approach. *Canadian Journal of Psychiatry, 33,* 360–363.

Gardner, D. L., & Cowdry, R. W. (1986). Positive effects of carbamazepine on behavioral dyscontrol in borderline personality disorder. *American Journal of Psychiatry, 143,* 519–522.

Goldberg, S. C., Schulz, C., Schulz, P. M., Resnick, R. J., Hamer, R. M., & Friedel, R. O. (1986). Borderline and schizotypal personality disorders treated with low-dose thiothixene vs. placebo. *Archives of General Psychiatry, 43,* 680–686.

Gunderson, J. G. (1984). *Borderline personality disorder.* Washington, DC: American Psychiatric Press.

Gunderson, J. G., Frank, A. F., Ronningstam, E. F., Wachter, S., Lynch, V. J., & Wolf, P. J. (1989). Early discontinuance of borderline patients from psychotherapy. *Journal of Nervous and Mental Disease, 177,* 38–42.

Haley, J., & Hoffman, L. (1967). *Techniques of family therapy.* New York: Basic Books.

Hoffman, L. (1981). *Foundations of family therapy: A conceptual framework for systems change.* New York: Basic Books.

Horwitz, L. (1980). Group psychotherapy for borderline and narcissistic patients. *Bulletin of the Menninger Clinic, 44,* 181–200.

Horwitz, L. (1987). Indication for group psychotherapy with borderline and narcissistic patients. *Bulletin of the Menninger Clinic, 51,* 248–260.

Kernberg, O. F. (1975). *Borderline conditions and pathological narcissism.* New York: Jason Aronson.

Kernberg, O. F. (1977). The structural diagnosis of borderline personality organization. In P. Hartocollis (Ed.), *Borderline personality disorders: The concept, the syndrome, the patient.* New York: International Universities Press.

Kernberg, O. F. (1984). *Severe personality disorders.* New Haven, CT: Yale University Press.

Knight, R. P. (1953). Borderline states. *Bulletin of the Menninger Clinic, 17,* 1–12.

Kretsch, R., Goren, Y., & Wasserman, A. (1987). Change patterns of borderline patients in individual and group therapy. *International Journal of Group Psychotherapy, 37,* 95–112.

Linehan, M. M. (1987). Dialectical behavior therapy for borderline personality disorder. *Bulletin of the Menninger Clinic, 51,* 261–276.

Masterson, J. F. (1972). *Treatment of the borderline adolescent: A developmental approach.* New York: Wiley.

Minuchin, S. (1974). *Families and family therapy.* Cambridge, MA: Harvard University Press.

Roth, S., & Stiglitz, M. (1971). The shared patient: Separate therapists for group and individual psychotherapy. *International Journal of Group Psychotherapy, 21,* 44–52.

Shapiro, E. R., Shapiro, R. L., Zinner, J., & Berkowitz, D. A. (1977). The borderline ego and the working alliance: Indications for family and individual treatment in adolescence. *International Journal of Psycho-Analysis, 58,* 77–87.

Skodol, A., Buckley, P., & Charles, E. (1983). Is there a characteristic pattern to the treatment history of clinical outpatients with borderline personality? *Journal of Nervous and Mental Disease, 171,* 405–410.

Slavinska-Holy, N. (1983). Combining individual and homogeneous group psychotherapies for borderline conditions. *International Journal of Group Psychotherapy, 33,* 297–312.

Soloff, P. H. (1981). Pharmacotherapy of borderline disorders. *Comprehensive Psychiatry, 22,* 535–543.

Soloff, P. H., George, A., Nathan, R. S., Schulz, P. M., Ulrich, R. F., & Perel, J. M. (1986). Progress in the pharmacotherapy of borderline disorders. *Archives of General Psychiatry, 43,* 691–697.

Stein, A. (1981). Indications for concurrent (combined and conjoint) individual and group psychotherapy. In L. R. Wolberg & M. L. Arons (Eds.), *Group and family therapy 1981.* New York: Brunner/Mazel.

Stone, M. H., Stone, D. K., & Hurt, S. W. (1987). Natural history of borderline patients treated by intensive hospitalization. *Psychiatric Clinics of North America, 10,* 185–206.

Tucker, L., Bauer, S. F., Wagner, S., Harlam, D., & Sher, I. (1987). Long-term hospital treatment of borderline patients: A descriptive outcome study. *American Journal of Psychiatry, 144,* 1443–1448.

Waldinger, R. J., & Frank, A. F. (1989a). Clinicians' experiences in combining medication and psychotherapy in the treatment of borderline patients. *Hospital and Community Psychiatry, 40,* 712–718.

Waldinger, R. J., & Frank, A. F. (1989b). Transference and the vicissitudes of medication use by borderline patients. *Psychiatry, 52,* 416–427.

Waldinger, R. J., & Gunderson, J. G. (1984). Completed psychotherapies with borderline patients. *American Journal of Psychotherapy, 38,* 190–202.

Wong, N. (1980a). Combined group and individual treatment of borderline and narcissistic patients: Heterogeneous versus homogeneous groups. *International Journal of Group Psychotherapy, 30,* 389–404.

Wong, N. (1980b). Focal issues in group psychotherapy of borderline and narcissistic patients. In L. R. Wolberg & M. L. Arons (Eds.), *Group and family therapy 1980.* New York: Brunner/Mazel.

Zinner, J. (1978). Combined individual and family therapy of borderline adolescents: Rationale and management of the early phase. *Adolescent Psychiatry, 6,* 420–427.

PART FIVE

CONCLUSIONS

CHAPTER 15

Borderline Personality Disorder: Research Implications

M. TRACIE SHEA

The preceding chapters describe the wealth of knowledge that has been accumulated on various aspects of borderline personality disorder (BPD), as well as some of the obstacles that have impeded interpretations of research findings and conclusive answers to the many compelling questions that remain. Research on various aspects of BPD is covered, including questions of etiology, diagnosis, and treatment. The purpose of this chapter is to highlight some of the predominant methodological issues relevant to research in this area, and to discuss possible strategies for dealing with them. The chapter begins by discussing issues and strategies associated with definition and diagnosis of BPD, followed by a similar discussion of issues associated with assessment. Methodological considerations more specific to studies of treatment and of etiology are then addressed.

DEFINITION AND DIAGNOSIS

One of the major unresolved issues in research on BPD concerns its defining features and boundaries. The *Diagnostic and Statistical Manual of Mental Disorders*, third edition (DSM-III) provided an important advance, with the introduction of standardized criteria for diagnosis of all the personality disorders. Nonetheless, substantial heterogeneity within samples of patients diagnosed with BPD clearly remains. As noted by Clarkin, Widiger, Frances, Hurt, and Gilmore (1983), there are numerous possible combinations of the eight BPD criteria, and thus multiple ways of meeting the criteria. There is also considerable heterogeneity introduced by the concurrent presence of other Axis II disorders, as most patients meeting criteria for BPD also meet criteria for various other Axis II disorders. Another source of heterogeneity is the presence of concurrent Axis I disorders. Again, most patients with BPD have a history (either current or past) of at least one, and often multiple, Axis I disorders. As a result, even careful diagnostic procedures using state-of-the-art interviews do not insure comparability within or across samples of patients diagnosed with BPD.

A number of strategies have been proposed to deal with the heterogeneity issue. The optimal approach for any study, of course, will depend on the research question. For certain types of validation or classification studies, for example, heterogeneity is desirable, and one would not want to restrict the sample. Studies of etiology or treatment, on the other hand, may be handicapped by the variance introduced by excessive heterogeneity. For these latter types of studies, a number of strategies may be considered.

Attempts have been made to deal with heterogeneity in regard to the constellation of criteria met for the BPD diagnosis by using empirical data to establish more homogeneous subtypes of patients meeting the criteria. Hurt, Clarkin, Munroe-Blum, and Marziali (Chapter 9), for example, have identified three subsets of criteria from the eight DSM-III criteria: an Identity cluster, an Affect cluster, and an Impulse cluster. Various combinations of these clusters, or core problems, yield potentially more homogeneous subgroups of patients. Although Hurt et al.'s chapter focuses on the relevance of the core problems and subtypes for treatment studies, this approach is also relevant to etiological studies.

A similar but slightly different approach may be particularly relevant to psychosocial treatment intervention studies. A number of psychosocial treatment approaches have been developed or described specifically for the treatment of BPD, including dialectical behavior therapy (see Linehan & Heard, Chapter 11) and psychodynamic treatment (see Clarkin et al., Chapter 12). Modifications of cognitive therapy have also been described for treatment of BPD (e.g., Beck, Freeman, & Associates, 1990; Young & Swift, 1988). Each of these treatment approaches has provided conceptualizations of the core pathology of the disorder, derived from the theoretical perspective of the treatment, with the therapeutic rationale, strategies, and interventions following from the definition of the core pathology. For treatment efficacy studies, assessment should insure that all patients have this core pathology, which should be required in addition to meeting criteria for the diagnosis. For example, the core pathology of BPD that is outlined by Benjamin in Chapter 8 involves the presence of a morbid fear of abandonment, and the wish for protective nurturance. The perception of abandonment or of deprivation will result in rage—or, in interpersonal terms, in a change from friendly dependency on a nurturer to hostile control. It would be critical in a treatment study of psychotherapy using the Structural Analysis of Social Behavior (SASB) interpersonal model to assess and require this specific aspect of borderline pathology. This insures a critical element of sample homogeneity that is intrinsically relevant to the research question.

The core pathology approach can also be helpful in reducing the overlap with other personality disorders, by its use in differential diagnosis. Benjamin (in press), for example, defines the core pathology of each of the Axis II disorders in terms of her system, the SASB. By elaborating the core (interpersonal) criteria for each disorder, she emphasizes the importance of context and motivation for some criteria; these factors help to elucidate the differences among disorders in behaviors that may appear similar. For example, anger or rage for the borderline is typically precipitated by abandonment. In contrast, the anger displayed by an individual with narcissistic personality disorder is more likely to be precipitated by failure or criticism. Use of this approach should in principle reduce the number of misdiagnosed borderlines, or false-positive cases. It should also reduce the number of artifactual diagnoses of "comorbid" Axis II disorders, which may make a sample appear to be more heterogeneous than it really is.

Another approach that may be helpful in increasing homogeneity is the identification of dimensions of behavior or traits that may cut across different personality disorders, and may or may not be present within a specific disorder. Focusing on such dimensions may result in detection of relationships that may be missed by focusing on samples of patients defined by diagnostic classes. In Chapter 5, Widiger, Miele, and Tilly discuss the advantages of using dimensional measurement (i.e., avoiding the use of artificial distinctions and the loss of information necessitated by categorical diagnosis) and improving interrater reliability of assessment. A demonstration of the benefits of using cross-cutting dimensions of behavior is provided by Links in Chapter 3, in his citation of a finding by Silverman et al. (1987) regarding familial patterns of psychopathology. Chronic affective instability and chronic impulsivity were found to be significantly more common in relatives of borderline patients than in the relatives of patients with other personality disorders and the relatives of schizophrenic patients; by contrast, the morbid risk of major affective disorders, schizophrenic disorders, alcoholism, drug abuse, or antisocial personality disorder did not differ among the relative groups. As Silverman et al. (1987) suggest, the traits may be a more fruitful avenue for discovering inherited psychobiological substrates of the genetic aspects of BPD (as well as other personality disorders) than the diagnosis.

The work of Siever and Coccaro (Siever, Klar, & Coccaro, 1985; Siever et al., 1987; Coccaro et al., 1989) provides another compelling example of the importance of investigating traits or dimensions rather than diagnoses, with their finding of a relationship between central serotonin function and impulsive suicidal and aggressive behaviors. Coccaro (in press), from a review of the clinical psychobiological literature, also suggests that dimensions of behavior may be a more valid and clinically relevant means of viewing personality disorder.

With regard to heterogeneity introduced by the concurrent presence of Axis I disorders, again optimal strategies depend on the research question. If the focus of the research is on diagnostic classification or the relationship between BPD and Axis I disorders, clearly heterogeneity in terms of Axis I disorders is desirable. This is likely not to be the case for treatment intervention studies, where the presence of Axis I disorders may influence treatment response. One strategy for treatment studies is to exclude patients with at least some current Axis I disorders, such as a current episode of major depression. Another is to stratify patient assignment to treatment on the basis of common and relevant Axis I disorders, or at least to include these disorders as covariates in statistical analyses.

ASSESSMENT

Diagnostic Assessment

There has been considerable progress in the diagnostic assessment of BPD, with the development of several structured and semistructured interviews, as well as self-report measures. Chapter 6, by Reich, provides a thorough review of the available measures. Despite these advances, however, limitations in the current state of assessment are apparent in the poor agreement across measures, as also described by Reich. Given the absence of knowledge concerning the relative validity of the various assessment measures and approaches, at this point it seems advisable to include measures from multiple perpectives—for example, clinical interview plus self-report, therapist diagnosis, and/or informant interview. A conservative approach would require a positive diagnosis from multiple perspectives. Given that test–retest reliability for assessment at the diagnostic level also tends to be low, a repeated diagnostic assessment to confirm the initial diagnosis should be used if possible. Also, as noted, since there is a loss of information and lower interrater reliability associated with categorical assessment, some form of continuous measurement is important. Examples of relevant variables for continuous assessment include the number of criteria met, the degree of severity of each of the criteria present, and the degree of impairment associated with the criteria or disorder.

Assessment of Change

For some studies (e.g., longitudinal or treatment studies), the assessment of change in BPD is a focus. Such assessment raises a number of issues, many of which are intrinsically tied to the quality of the initial diagnostic assessment (see Endicott & Shea, 1990, for a more extensive discussion of issues associated with assessment of change in personality disorders). The severity of the disorder, the pervasiveness and persistence of the dysfunctional behavior across situations and over time, and the degree of impairment associated with it are important aspects to capture in any investigation of change. A reduction in impairment or severity may represent a meaningful change, even if many of the criteria for the diagnosis are still present. To provide a fuller context for understanding the course of change, whether in longitudinal or treatment studies, it is also useful to assess life situations or circumstances that may affect the functioning of the patient. Certain kinds of life stresses are likely to aggravate the pathological behavior patterns, whereas other circumstances may provide enough stability to improve functioning.

Other issues important to consider are associated with the time period covered for assessment of change. With regard to measurement of functioning, assessment of the previous week or month (frequently used in outcome studies of Axis I disorders) may be misleading in studies of BPD, because there may be temporary fluctuations in the level of functioning. When one is considering change in diagnosis or number of criteria met as an outcome, an important consideration is the expected base rate of occurrence for the criteria. Behaviors associated with some of the criteria may be expected to occur less frequently (e.g., suicide attempts). If the time period covered for initial diagnostic assessment is lifetime or even 5 years, the absence of such behaviors over a 6-month interval cannot be assumed to reflect meaningful or permanent change. The interpretation of change in terms of meeting diagnostic criteria at the follow-up (based on behavior evidenced during a relatively short follow-up interval) as true change in the personality disorder may thus be misleading.

Another issue associated with assessment of personality disorders in general is the degree of inference required for judging the presence of some of the criteria. Some are more overt and fairly concrete (e.g., suicide gestures), whereas others require much more inference (e.g., identity disturbance, emptiness and boredom). These more inferential and complex criteria require more careful evaluation, and more extensive rater training and reliability checks, particularly in attempts to assess change.

The influence of the presence of a current Axis I disorder (particularly an affective disorder) on the assessment of personality traits and disorders when self-report measures are used has been noted by many (Coppen & Metcalf, 1965; Hirschfeld et al., 1983; Liebowitz, Stallone, Dunner, & Fieve, 1979; Joffe & Regan, 1988). The extent to which Axis I disorders influence assessment when structured interviews are used is unclear. However, when change in functioning is being assessed, it is particularly important not to confuse change that may be associated with the recovery from an episode of major depression (or another Axis I disorder) with change in the personality disorder. At the initial assessment, the patient's long-term and typical functioning must be assessed—either by waiting until the patient is no longer in a current episode, or by obtaining independent reports.

TREATMENT INTERVENTION STUDIES

A number of issues are more specifically associated with treatment studies of BPD. A frequently cited issue is attrition (e.g., Gunderson et al., 1989), as borderline patients are well known for noncompliance and dissatisfaction/ disappointment with the therapist or treatment approach. Those who remain in a treatment study may thus be a selectively higher-functioning subsample of borderline patients. If strategies are built into the treatment to prevent dropout, this may reduce the attrition problem. The low attrition rates reported by Linehan and Heard (Chapter 11) in a sample of severely dysfunctional borderline patients in a year-long treatment is encouraging in this regard, and suggests that if compliance with treatment is made an explicit treatment priority, attrition rates may be reduced.

A related issue associated with treatment studies of borderline patients is the level of skill and flexibility required on the part of the therapist. Requiring a minimum level of experience of therapists, and engaging in continued supervision and/or monitoring of competence, are particularly important in treatment studies with these patients. The need for flexibility on the part of the therapist must be balanced with the requirement of standardization of treatments and assessment of therapists' adherence to the treatment strategies outlined. Ideally, flexibility will be built into the standardization of treatments. Linehan (see Chapter 11) has attempted this in her dialectical behavior therapy by explicitly shifting the priorities of the interventions, depending upon the status of the patient (e.g., suicidal or not).

A difficult issue in establishing the efficacy of psychosocial treatments for any disorder concerns appropriate control groups. There has been extensive discussion of this issue in the psychotherapy research literature (e.g., Parloff, 1986), and a full discussion of this issue is beyond the scope of this chapter. Clearly, however, successful treatments of BPD are likely to be long-term, and the difficulties of designing a control condition in short-term treatment studies are magnified in studies of long-term treatments. Waiting-list, no-treatment, or attention controls are not ethical or feasible for extended periods of time. Control groups that provide part of the therapy (e.g., supportive interventions such as encouragement, feedback, and clarification), but not the specific interventions of the treatment being investigated (e.g., interpretations, identification of cognitive distortions, etc.), may be more feasible. Comparisons with such control groups would provide stringent tests of the efficacy of the specific interventions rather than of the treatment as a whole.

STUDIES OF ETIOLOGY

A consistent finding emerging from studies of etiological factors associated with BPD, and identified by Marziali (Chapter 2), Links (Chapter 3), and Stone (Chapter 4), is the presence of a history of parental hostility and abuse—particularly sexual and physical abuse—in patients with borderline pathology. As noted by Marziali, the validation of this type of trauma as specifically causal to BPD requires studies that address two limitations characteristic of most studies to date: (1) use of a prospective, rather than a retrospective, design; and (2) inclusion of control groups. Retrospective studies, although valuable in generating hypotheses, are limited by the possibility of distortions in recall. Memories and perceptions of the quality of parental relationships, in particular, may be confounded by the current pathology. Sample selection in such studies is also inherently biased against finding subjects who experience the same trauma but do not develop borderline pathology. As discussed by Marziali, prospective, longitudinal studies of high-risk subjects are needed to confirm these factors as causal, and also as *specifically* causal to borderline pathology. Retrospective studies of borderline patients without control groups do not address the possibility of diverse outcomes, including other forms of pathology, resulting from the same traumatic factors. Prospective studies of high-risk samples address this issue; they also allow investigation of the mechanisms by which early trauma results in borderline pathology, as well as of the protective factors that may reduce the risk of developing the disorder. Stone emphasizes the importance of studying positive factors or strengths (e.g., intelligence, talent, humor, etc.) as prognostic in the course of BPD. Such factors are also likely to be important in terms of the risk of developing the disorder.

Familial transmission studies are also a valuable strategy for generating hypotheses regarding the role of genetically transmitted factors, but of course are limited in terms of conclusions regarding the mechanism of transmission. This may be particularly true in the case of borderline pathology, where the features of the disorder (e.g., impulsivity and instability of affect and behavior) are conducive to the creation of a chaotic familial environment. Adoption and twin studies are needed to clarify the role of genetic factors. As noted earlier, investigations of dimensions of behavior, such as impulsivity and aggression, are likely to be more fruitful than studies of diagnostic classes in identifying genetically transmitted biological substrates.

Finally, as addressed in all of the chapters dealing with etiology, it is clear that more complex models involving the interactions of genetic and environmental factors are necessary if we are to arrive at a more comprehensive understanding of the etiology of BPD.

CONCLUDING COMMENTS

The field of research on BPD has advanced tremendously in the past 10 years. Despite the continuing need for further refinement in nosology, the standardized criteria of DSM-III have at least provided a common language and starting point for research. The development of the "first generation" of structured interviews, despite their possible limitations, has provided a methodology that improves reliability of assessment, allowing the next question—that of validity—to be addressed. Research using dimensional approaches has begun to identify important dimensions of behavior that will probably contribute to the quality of the nosological system, as well as to the quality of research on etiology and treatment. A number of psychosocial treatment approaches that have been developed or modified specifically for BPD have been "standardized"; that is, they have manuals describing the theoretical rationales, as well as specific therapeutic strategies and techniques. These include psychodynamic (Kernberg, Selzer, Koenigsberg, Carr, & Appelbaum, 1989), cognitive (Beck et al., 1990), and behavioral (Linehan, 1984) approaches. Adherence measures have been developed for some of these approaches (e.g., Koenigsberg et al., 1985). These treatments might be considered "research-ready." Although there have been few controlled studies of any psychosocial treatment, Linehan's study of dialectical behavior therapy (see Chapter 11) is an exception. This study has demonstrated the feasibility of conducting a controlled treatment study for up to a full year.

Such methodological advances, and the accumulating body of research, have moved the field closer to a position from which to address many important and compelling questions. Several directions would be valuable to pursue. Work needs to continue on the validity of the current nosology, including continued work on the identification of basic dimensions of behavior underlying various aspects of borderline pathology. Longitudinal studies, using frequent assessments, would be valuable in identifying the stability of individual criteria over time—including those that may be more stable, perhaps representing "core" criteria. Longitudinal studies would also be useful in clarifying the nature of the relationship between BPD and the Axis I disorders. For example, they would allow investigation of the degree and persistence of concurrent Axis I disorders, as well as the influence of Axis I disorders on symptoms and level of functioning of borderline patients.

Another potential benefit of longitudinal studies is the use of longitudinal data as validators of various measures and methods of initial diagnostic assessment. For example, does information from patient self-report, from clinician judgment, or from informants provide the most accurate assessment, as confirmed by longitudinal stability? Work on classification and construct validity will need to proceed interactively and in conjunction with work on assessment validity.

Although some aspects of methodology for longitudinal assessment of personality disorders need to be developed, a useful model for longitudinal study of psychopathology exists: the National Institute of Mental Health Psychobiology of Depression study, which has successfully assessed the longitudinal course of subjects with affective disorders for over 10 years (Katz, Secunda, Hirschfeld, & Koslow, 1979). A similar approach to the investigation of course in the personality disorders would be valuable.

Retrospective studies investigating developmental factors associated with BPD have consistently identified variables such as early physical and sexual abuse, which should now be investigated in prospective, longitudinal studies of high-risk subjects. Inclusion of control groups—for example, samples of subjects who have experienced different types of trauma from those associated with BPD—will allow investigation of the specificity of the relationship between the types of trauma postulated and borderline pathology. It would also be useful for such studies to include measures of temperament and other types of traits, in order to allow investigations of possible interactions between such traits (which might be conceptualized as vulnerability and protective factors) and specific environmental influences in the development of borderline pathology. Family studies of transmission patterns, focusing particularly on dimensions of behavior such as those described earlier, will provide a useful mechanism for identifying variables to be studied in subsequent twin and adoption studies, and eventually in studies of genetic transmission.

Finally, research is needed to determine the effectiveness of both psychosocial and pharmacological treatments for BPD. Ideally, such research would include studies of long-term treatments (i.e., treatments lasting more than 1 year), although methodological and feasibility issues associated with studies of such treatments remain to be resolved. Intermediate outcomes that can be assessed in studies of shorter duration would also be valuable. Examples might include investigation of therapeutic techniques that reduce attrition, or that contribute to the development of a positive therapeutic alliance.

In summary, research in the area of BPD has benefited substantially from increased attention in recent years by a range of investigators with diverse theoretical and research perspectives. Much progress has been made in dealing with difficult conceptual and methodological issues. Although future research will need to continue to address the challenging issues of methodology that remain, such research should be balanced with pursuit of the many compelling substantive questions.

REFERENCES

Beck, A. T., Freeman, A., & Associates. (1990). *Cognitive therapy of personality disorders*. New York: Guilford Press.

Benjamin, L. S. (in press). *Diagnosis and treatment of personality disorders: A structural approach*. New York: Guilford Press.

Clarkin, J. F., Widiger, T. A., Frances, A., Hurt, S. W., & Gilmore, M. (1983). Prototypic typology and the borderline personality disorder. *Archives of General Psychiatry, 45*, 348–352.

Coccaro, E. F. (in press). Psychopharmacological studies in patients with personality disorder: Review and perspective. *Journal of Personality Disorders*.

Coccaro, E. F., Siever, L. J., Klar, H., Maurer, G., Cochrane, K., Cooper, T. B., Mohs, R. C.,'& Davis, K. L. (1989). Serotinergic studies in patients with affective and personality disorders: Correlates with suicidal and impulsive aggressive behavior. *Archives of General Psychiatry, 46,* 587–599.

Coppen, A., & Metcalf, M. (1965). Effects of a depressive illness on MPI scores. *British Journal of Psychiatry, 11,* 236–239.

Endicott, J., & Shea, M. T. (1990). Measurement of change in personality disorders. *Psychopharmacology Bulletin, 25*(4), 572–577.

Gunderson, J. G., Frank, A. F., Ronningstam, E. F., Wachter, S., Lynch, V. J., & Wolf, P. J. (1989). Early discontinuance of borderline patients from psychotherapy. *Journal of Nervous and Mental Disease, 177,* 38–42.

Hirschfeld, R. M. A., Klerman, G. L., Clayton, P. J., Keller, M. B., McDonald-Scott, P., & Larkins, B. H. (1983). Assessing personality: effects of the depressive state on trait measurement. *American Journal of Psychiatry, 140,* 695–699.

Joffe, R. T., & Regan, J. J. (1988). Personality and depression. *Journal of Psychiatric Research, 22,* 279–286.

Katz, M. M., Secunda, S. K., Hirschfeld, R. M. A., & Koslow, S. H. (1979). NIMH Clinical Research Branch Collaborative Program on the Psychobiology of Depression. *Archives of General Psychiatry, 36,* 765–777.

Kernberg, O. F., Selzer, M., Koenigsberg, H., Carr, A., & Appelbaum, A. (1989). *Psychodynamic psychotherapy of borderline patients.* New York: Basic Books.

Koenigsberg, H. W., Kernberg, O. F., Haas, G., Lotterman, A., Rockland, L., & Selzer, M. (1985). Development of a scale for measuring techniques in the psychotherapy of borderline patients. *Journal of Nervous and Mental Disease, 173*(7), 424–431.

Liebowitz, M. R., Stallone, F., Dunner, D. L., & Fieve, R. F. (1979). Personality features of patients with primary affective disorder. *Acta Psychiatrica Scandinavica, 60,* 214–224.

Linehan, M. M. (1984). *Dialectical behavior therapy for treatment of parasuicidal women: Treatment manual.* Unpublished manuscript, University of Washington.

Parloff, M. B. (1986). Placebo controls in psychotherapy research: A sine qua non or a placebo for research problems? *Journal of Consulting and Clinical Psychology, 54*(1), 79–87.

Siever, L. J., Coccaro, E. F., Zemisklany, Z., Silverman, J., Klar, H., Loscenzy, M. F., Davidson, M., Friedman, R., Mohs, R. C., & Davis, K. L. (1987). Psychobiology of personality disorders: Pharmacologic implications. *Psychopharmacology Bulletin, 23,* 333–336.

Siever, L. J., Klar, H., & Coccaro, E. F. (1985). Psychobiologic substrates of personality. In H. Klar & L. J. Siever (Eds.), *Biologic response styles: Clinical implications.* Washington, DC: American Psychiatric Press.

Silverman, J. M., Siever, L. J., Coccaro, E. F., Klar, H., Greenwald, S., Rubenstein, K., Mohs, R. C., & Davidson, M. (1987, December). *Risk of affective disorder and personality disorder in the relatives of personality disorder patients.* Paper presented at the meeting of the American College of Neuropsychopharmacology, San Juan, Puerto Rico.

Young, J., & Swift, W. (1988). Schema-focused cognitive therapy for personality disorders: Part I. *International Cognitive Therapy Newsletter, 4*(5), 13–14.

CHAPTER 16

To Know Borderline
Personality Disorder

JOHN P. DOCHERTY

In this book, Clarkin, Marziali, and Munroe-Blum have undertaken a formidable, daunting task and have succeeded admirably. The foregoing chapters provide a clear, concise overview of the advances and limits in our empirically based knowledge of borderline personality disorder (BPD). To put this in a larger perspective, it is helpful to recall that in internal medicine it used to be said, "To know syphilis is to know internal medicine." This was later replaced by the aphorism, "To know lupus is to know internal medicine." Both of these expressions refer to illnesses called "the great masqueraders." Each can present with many, many manifestations—multiple and fluctuating syndrome states. In a similar manner, we might say, "To know BPD is to know psychiatry."

DIAGNOSIS

BPD is a disorder that can present manifold faces to the clinician. For a while now, we have been searching for the method in the madness of this mutative and elusive disorder. The documentation of this search is an exciting yet humbling record of the progress and limits of contemporary mental health science. Tackling the problem of BPD forces us to face fundamental flaws in our epistemic foundation. Most basically, it faces us with our lack of a common metric for the description of psychological phenomena. The orderly progress of physical science has been rooted in the appreciation of distance and its progressively refined measurement—"the long and short of it." Such an essential dimension, and the universal unit for its measurement, are not yet available in the psychological domain. As a result, BPD remains a confounding and confounded diagnosis.

In our efforts toward a better understanding of this complex, complicated, and confusing category of psychiatric diagnosis, it is useful to take a step back and consider the reason for its existence. Why do we have such a diagnosis? The purpose for its development was to help describe a group of patients who are troubling, both conceptually and practically. Conceptually, they present symptomatology that does not fit standard, syndrome-based diagnostic categories in a stable and easily identifiable fashion. Indeed, even with the excellent, hard work that has led to more refined instruments for diagnosis, we are left with a troublesome overlap with schizotypal disorder, the full range of affective disorders, some psychotic disorders, and particularly the other expressive personality disorders. Yet this should not surprise us. It was specifically to identify such a chameleon-like group of patients that this diagnostic category came into being.

The second purpose of this diagnosis is not less important and should not be forgotten. This diagnostic category was formed perhaps principally as a heuristic device. Clinicians needed guidance and consensual support in understanding and validating their experiences in the treatment of such patients. The diagnosis was developed to describe a difficult, trying, frustrating, and anxiety-inducing group of patients. In many ways, Kernberg's (1975) greatest contribution to psychiatry may be the solace that he has provided for thousands of us clinicians, who were left in painful isolation before he so clearly articulated the nature of the therapist's experience and a reasonable and conceptually coherent method of approach for helping these patients.

In essence, in our increasingly refined methodologies and instrumentation for defining and ascertaining this diagnosis, we should not lose sight of the genesis of this category. We forget, at our peril, Melissa Schmideberg's (1959) initial and essential characterization of these patients as suffering from a disorder of "stable instability." The heart of this disorder is an understanding that these patients suffer from unstable relationships, vengeful feelings, fleeting states of consolation, and a variety of more or less dangerous impulses that are more or less adequately controlled. In addition, they demonstrate an unusual degree of lability in levels of psychological compensation; hence the variety of syndromes and mixed syndrome forms they manifest over the course of time, and the perplexity they generate in the conscientious psychopharmacologist.

Much of our confusion in approaching the diagnosis of this manifestly complex group stems from a lack of appreciation in contemporary psychiatry of an essential diagnostic model of medicine. The medical model of diagnosis is an Aristotelian structural model consisting of three categories: "etiology," or first cause; "pathology" (vulnerability), or second cause; and "syndrome," or third cause. Thus, for a patient who presents with congestive heart failure, a complete diagnosis would consist of the diagnosis of the congestive heart failure itself (the syndrome diagnosis), the underlying pathology (e.g., a myocardiopathy), and the etiology (e.g., alcohol-induced).

Such a model, interestingly, is present in many contemporary systems of psychotherapy. For example, interpersonal psychotherapy of depression uses a partial structural model. First, it makes the diagnosis of depressive syndrome; then it makes a pathology diagnosis of, for example, interpersonal dispute. The pathology diagnosis then guides the direction of treatment and the selection of treatment techniques. In cognitive–behavioral therapy of depression, again the depressive syndrome is diagnosed; then an underlying pathology diagnosis involving a particular constellation of dysfunctional attitudes and negative thoughts is made, and specific treatment is directed toward this constellation. Similarly, in behavioral therapies of depression based on social learning theory, first the syndrome-level diagnosis of depression is made; then a pathology diagnosis based upon a functional analysis of a system of self-monitoring, self-evaluation, and self-reward is made. These models indicate an important direction for our field—toward a more complete diagnostic system and, with that, toward less confusion. We too often lose sight of this model, to our detriment.

It would be particularly useful to keep it in mind as we consider the category of patients that we are trying to capture with the label of BPD. As we currently use this term, we seem to be referring to a pathology level of diagnosis—that is, a structure demonstrating certain critical deficiencies. We further presume that this structure gives rise to various other symptoms, expressed as variable syndrome states. With such a model, it would not surprise us to find a great deal of comorbidity in borderline patients (e.g., affective disorders, brief psychoses, and various anxiety states). In such a model, BPD is presumed to be a more stable organization underlying these more transient syndrome manifestations. Yet, in our most common diagnostic practice, we do not adhere consistently to this conceptualization. As reflected in the revised third edition of the *Diagnostic and Statistical Manual of Mental Disorders* (DSM-III-R; American Psychiatric Association, 1987), we have developed essentially a syndrome approach to the diagnosis of this disorder; that is, we are attempting to detect this disorder through listing a compendium of "surface" phenomena. This has led to a very long list. Furthermore, this current phenomenological approach to diagnosis poses several problems. First, there is considerable overlap of these surface symptoms with symptoms we use to characterize other diagnostic entities. Second, to the extent that we do try to select items reflecting an underlying abnormal personality structure, there is difficulty in discriminating the signifiers of the personality organization from the syndrome symptoms. Third, we do not yet systematically recognize that although the personality organization may be stable in a theoretical sense, the expression of its various deficiencies may wax and wane as the system is subjected to different challenges.

All this, of course, is made even more difficult by the fact that we do not have a consensually accepted system for understanding personality organization. The "organs of personality" and their pathways of connection are not well understood. It is thus reasonable to assume that until this basic work has been accomplished, we must accept a certain amount of confusion.

As Reich's chapter (see Chapter 6) so competently summarizes, there has been considerable productive activity in the development of methods for the diagnosis and assessment of BPD. We are sharpening and, perhaps, resolving the broader conceptual differences in the use of this term and identifying a core configuration of disordered psychological function. However, significant problems remain:

1. The place, function, or value of psychotic symptoms in the definition of BPD remains problematic.

2. The various methods of diagnosis have demonstrated only very mediocre intersystem reliability. Why is this? One issue is confusion regarding the conceptual level of different symptoms; a second relates to the problem of heterogeneity, which is discussed below. A third reason, perhaps, lies in the fact that we have not quantified the core phenomena of instability. Our system still leaves too much room for independent interpretation. Take, for example, the term "lability of affect." How do we define this? How much lability of affect is needed and what are its manifestations? In regard to "impulsivity," we have the same problem: How much impulsivity? Over how long a period of time? Under what conditions? Similarly, "emptiness and boredom," "unstable and intense relationships," and, of course, "identity disturbance" require further specification of both content and context. Ultimately, of course, the problem lies not in the increasing specification of these particular manifestations; it lies in the enduring problem of the absence of a common metric for the description of psychological experience.

3. Heterogeneity of presentations of BPD is a major problem. Interestingly, Reich's review of the systems for the measurement of BPD (see Chapter 6) seems to reveal that a difficulty in any two of eight different domains will qualify a person for the diagnosis of BPD. These domains are impulsivity, unstable and intense relationships, intense and uncontrolled anger, identity disturbance, affective instability, intolerance of being alone, physically self-damaging acts, and feelings of chronic emptiness and boredom. Four of these criteria are in the affective domain, two are action criteria, one is a relationship criteron, and one is a cognitive self-appraisal criterion. The identification of these criteria and the finding that any two in general will qualify someone for a diagnosis of BPD underscores the great heterogeneity of the disorder. A patient with self-injurious impulsivity and affective instability is different from one with identity disturbance and intolerance of being alone. The conceptual necessity for permitting such heterogeneity must be questioned.

4. It is interesting to note that our current approach to this disorder lacks criteria describing typical patterns of disturbance in the thought processes of BPD patients. This is unfortunate, because disturbances of logical thought often seem to be critical processes mediating the evolution of affective instability, impulsivity, and unstable interpersonal relationships in BPD.

5. Finally, most current approaches are symptom-based. A structural approach to diagnosis is not reflected in most of this work. Yet, interestingly,

for BPD (as for depressions), psychotherapy-derived or psychotherapy-linked systems appear to be breaking new ground. Marsha Linehan's work in dialectical behavior therapy (see Linehan & Heard, Chapter 11) requires that a more fundamental diagnosis of core defects underlying the manifest symptomatology must be made in order to direct treatment; the Kernberg–Clarkin psychodynamic approach (see Clarkin et al., Chapter 12) has a similar requirement. Also very promising is the work of Benjamin using the interpersonal circumplex model (see Chapter 8). Benjamin has developed the Structural Analysis of Social Behavior to describe basic patterns or structures of interpersonal relatedness that tend to characterize certain more or less definable groups of individuals. This work reveals the increasing clarity that can be achieved by identifying structures at a deeper level than the level of manifest symptomatology (e.g., anger, impulsiveness, feelings of bordeom), where a great deal of overlap occurs. Some of this overlap can be disentangled, and the meaning of symptoms can be more accurately assessed, through a comprehension of the deeper structure of personality that generates those symptoms. Since, ultimately, personality is interpersonal, systematically identifying the disturbed interpersonal process characteristic of the personality disorder holds the prospect for much greater homogeneity of diagnosis and for a more useful connection between therapeutic strategy and etiological variables.

ETIOLOGY

It is not surprising, given the fact that we are still laboring to achieve a more clear-cut definition of BPD, that our inquiries into etiology have been limited. The methodological rigors of etiological research pull for a study of clear and stable diagnostic entities. Nonetheless, some very interesting correlational work has been accomplished with borderline patients, and this work suggests important practical considerations for current clinical care.

One observation is the correlation between early abuse (especially intrafamilial abuse, particularly sexual abuse) in females and the presence of BPD. Cross-sectional studies, as Marziali points out in her elegant review of contemporary knowledge regarding etiology in BPD (see Chapter 2), support this association. In addition, the family studies reviewed by Links (see Chapter 3) supports this association. Links notes several interesting findings. First is that BPD seems to be clearly familial: There is much greater morbid risk for BPD among first-degree relatives of patients with BPD. Alcoholism and substance abuse are also frequent among relatives of BPD patients, perhaps stemming from a similar etiological source. Most relevant, however, is the suggestion from family environment studies that a high degree of hostile control on the part of one or both parents (so-called "biparental failure and neglect") is related to the development of this disorder. As Links notes, this is very similar to the concept of "negative expressed emotion," which has been shown to exert a negative impact upon the course of schizophrenia.

Another finding supporting the importance of early abuse is Michael Stone's discovery in his work on the course of illness in borderline patients (see Chapter 4) that those patients who, for reasons stemming from early life experience, seemed to drift toward the selection of relationships with negative hostile and destructive individuals had a much poorer outcome, as might be expected. This may be a critical process that mediates early abuse and allows it to exert its pathological effect. Finally, Benjamin (Chapter 8) notes that the familial predecessors of BPD suggested by the circumplex model fit closely with this same etiological variable—namely, abandonment, incest, and abuse.

A second important etiological variable appears to be neuropsychological dysfunction. Marziali (Chapter 2) notes the high prevalence of "organic features," particularly frontal lobe signs, in patients with BPD.

At the very least, these findings suggest that, in contemporary practice, a complete diagnostic evaluation of a patient with a diagnosis of BPD should include a careful history of early abuse (particularly sexual abuse) and an adequate neuropsychological examination. The theoretical etiological force of these variables aside, their presence in a patient with BPD has direct implications for treatment planning, and the data we now have on the relatively high prevalence of these problems in patients with BPD necessitate this assessment.

Still missing, however, in the study of etiology is the elaboration of more specific and complete etiological hypotheses. How, for example, does neuropsychological dysfunction generate BPD symptomatology? What specific cognitive functions are linked to specific symptomatic defects? Are there both neurodevelopmental and neurodegenerative processes that may account for the linkages? How are these processes differentiated? Similar questions may be asked about incest: What is the psychic lesion caused by incest? What cognitive–affective processes does it affect? How are these effects measured? In brief, the more fully and precisely these etiological hypotheses can be stated, the more informative and worthwhile will be the necessary prospective studies.

THE COURSE OF ILLNESS

The long-term course of illness for BPD patients remains largely unknown. Important contributions have been made by such investigators as Michael Stone (1980) and Thomas McGlashan (1984). The interesting findings emerging from this body of work emphasize the importance of understanding course in BPD. Yet the life trajectory of these patients remains largely uncharted.

We have little idea about the systematic alterations in symptom manifestation that may occur over time. We do not yet know whether there are characteristic courses of illness that may help differentiate one form of BPD from another. Such work has a long and successful tradition in medicine, but has not yet found application in the study of the heterogeneity of BPD. Furthermore, the work that has been accomplished to date has principally been retrospective, and has been based on skewed samples derived, in general, from populations of hospitalized patients. We lack a single study of the life course of an adequately sized community sample of BPD patients.

There are, however, some key findings from current research that the clinician may usefully keep in mind. First, outcome is very variable in a population of BPD patients. Although many will have a very poor outcome, some of these patients will do extremely well. As Stone (Chapter 4) notes, among the variables that seem to relate to poor outcome are heavy familial concentration of bipolar disorder and early, chronic parental abuse. Second, no clear findings have emerged yet regarding the usefulness of particular treatments with different subgroups of BPD patients; several different therapeutic interventions seem useful in producing positive outcome. Finally, we know from the life course studies that this is a very serious and severe illness. It is, as most clinicians are aware, a lethal illness. The suicide rate is extremely high. Stone found the suicide rate of his BPD sample to be 55 times higher than that of Caucasians in the U.S. general population.

TREATMENT

Although a great deal has been learned from clinical experience about useful treatment strategies for BPD patients, acceptable treatment research is still in the very earliest stages of development. Several chapters of this book reveal the major reasons why it has been difficult to proceed smoothly with treatment research.

First, there is the problem of "retention." Successful treatment research can be most readily accomplished when it is possible to begin with matched cohorts of patients in an experimental treatment and a control treatment and to follow both groups through to completion. It is an unfortunate but highly significant fact of treatment with BPD patients that there is an extremely high attrition rate. Many if not most patients are early dropouts from treatment. Clarkin and colleagues report in their discussion of psychodynamic approaches to the borderline patient (Chapter 12) that by week 12, 42% of their patients had dropped out of treatment. This finding tends to be the rule, not the exception. As a result, contemporary investigators have come to regard retention in treatment as an initial and basic outcome variable itself in the assessment of a treatment's efficacy with borderline patients.

Frank's very interesting chapter (Chapter 10) reveals why such retention in treatment is not a trivial accomplishment. BPD patients reveal the complexity of apparently simple clinical interventions. For example, various contradictions in the BPD patient's development of a therapeutic alliance reveal a much greater complexity in this phenomenon than had been appreciated in work with neurotic patients. Some important, clinically relevant findings that have emerged in regard to the alliance are as follows:

1. The therapeutic alliances of borderline patients develop slowly; we cannot expect the same rapid formation of alliances that is seen in work with relatively healthy neurotic patients.
2. Some borderline patients come to treatment with a predisposition to form or not to form an alliance, and this does not change much over time.
3. In borderline patients, an initially strong negative affective bond may in fact lead to very positive changes later.
4. Conversely, an initially positive-seeming, compliant relationship—especially one devoid of a strong affective bond—may warn of significant later danger.

This work is at an early stage. Fortunately, several useful instruments have been developed that will contribute to a greater understanding of the vicissitudes of the development of therapeutic alliance in borderline patients. In the meantime, the problem of retention is not solved and continues to pose a significant problem for the conduct of clinical trials.

The treatment of BPD patients is not short-term; rather, clinical experience indicates that a long period of treatment, on the order of years rather than weeks, is necessary to achieve stable gains. Methodological problems associated with conducting relatively intensive long-term treatment have not yet been solved. Such problems include therapists' maintaining fidelity to and competence in a particular therapeutic approach over a long period of time, as well as the development of a methodology for establishing the competence of a therapist prior to embarking on a long-term treatment. It is simply not feasible, for example, to conduct a 2-year competency exercise prior to beginning a 2-year clinical trial.

BPD patients often require multiple therapeutic interventions—not only different kinds of social interventions, but also different pharmacological interventions necessitated by the emergence of different syndrome states. Moreover, the recurring crises that characterize these patients and the methods necessary to treat those crises would constitute deviations from most therapy protocols. The complexity of treatment necessitated by the changing, extreme, and often unpredictable clinical condition of these patients creates major methodological problems. It does not allow a smooth application of single, carefully controlled therapies. Moreover, the problems with ways in which an investigator might seek to combine treatment are very nicely illustrated by Munroe-Blum (Chapter 13), who reviews the application of group psychotherapy to borderline patients, and by Waldinger (Chapter 14), who suggests an approach to organizing multimodal treatment. With regard, for example, to group therapy, when and how should a group be introduced? Should group therapy occur prior to individual therapy? Should it be used concomitantly? Are cotherapists needed? In addition, the basic structure and content of these additional therapies need elaboration and validation.

Finally, it is important to note that although the issue has not been addressed in this volume, it is critical to consider the possibility that the combination of some treatments will interact in a negative fashion to retard or undermine the progress of the borderline patient. Such negative effects seem not too unusual in borderline patients and must be carefully considered in combined treatment prescriptions for these patients.

In the face of these problems, it is heartening to see the impressive progress that has been made in Marsha Linehan's work on the application of dialectical behavior therapy to BPD patients (see Chapter 11), and in the tenacious and creative efforts of Kernberg, Clarkin, and their colleagues to develop a systematic, verifiable psychodynamic approach to the treatment of BPD patients (see Chapter 12). These investigators have pioneered the extremely difficult application of state-of-the-art psychotherapy clinical trials methodology to the study of BPD patients. Although this work is still preliminary, some interesting findings have begun to emerge:

1. It seems difficult to treat BPD patients in group therapy alone; there does seem to be a need for an ongoing individual relationship, to manage crises and provide the motivational fuel and emotional stability to allow other treatment to proceed (see Chapters 13 and 14).
2. At least in psychodynamic therapy, therapist competence in a specific treatment approach does appear, on a preliminary basis, to be related to better outcome (see Chapter 12).
3. When compared to "treatment as usual," an active, structured treatment does appear to be more successful at containing some of the more severe manifestations of the illness (such as suicidality), at least over a period of a year (see Chapter 11).
4. External organization in the patient's life seems to be related to a greater tendency to continue in therapy (see Chapter 12).

Thus, we may begin to see the development in this next decade of several well-defined and data-supported treatments for BPD patients. With foresight, Hurt, Clarkin, Munroe-Blum, and Marziali (Chapter 9) have begun to address the next problem that will emerge. This is the problem of indications and contraindications: Which patient should get which treatment? This is a problem of great clinical importance, and already one of practical significance in other areas of psychotherapy research. Hurt et al. (Chapter 9) suggest a very interesting strategy for conducting such comparative treatment research. According to this strategy, patients would be categorized so that they might be assigned on a matched basis to a compatible or an incompatible treatment—that is, a treatment expected to help their particular problem or one expected not to. This approach to psychotherapy studies seems to me a very useful and long-overdue one. Until we establish the boundaries of a treatment's efficacy by demonstrating for whom it will *not* work, its credibility will remain in question.

In conclusion, I would simply note that one important chapter seems to be missing from this helpful and quite successful volume—namely, a chapter on coping with the borderline patient. This is not a tangential issue or one of peculiar personal concern for therapists; this is a problem for family members and coworkers, as well as for clinicians. It is a relevant and critical area for study in its own right. The lives of these patients and those around them tend to be much happier when friends, therapists, and family members learn or are taught how to cope effectively with the interpersonal and personal distress experienced and wrought by the BPD patients. In fact, it is quite remarkable how much stress can be attenuated and alleviated when such expertise is developed. This psychoeducational process requires a systematic discussion.

REFERENCES

American Psychiatric Association. (1987). *Diagnostic and statistical manual of mental disorders* (3rd ed., rev.). Washington, DC: Author.

Kernberg, O. (1975). *Borderline conditions and pathological narcissism*. New York: Jason Aronson.

McGlashan, T. H. (1984). The Chestnut Lodge follow-up study. II: Long-term outcome of borderline personalities. *Archives of General Psychiatry, 41*, 586–601.

Schmideberg, M. (1959). The borderline patient. In S. Arieti et al. (Eds.), *American handbook of psychiatry*. New York: Basic Books.

Stone, M. (1980). *The borderline syndrome: Constitution, personality and adaptation*. New York: McGraw-Hill.

Index